John D. Bisognano
G. Ronald Beck • Ryan W. Connell
(Editors)

Manual of Outpatient Cardiology

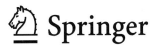 Springer

Editors

Dr. John D. Bisognano, M.D., Ph.D
Department of Internal Medicine
Division of Cardiology
University of Rochester
Medical Center
Rochester, New York
USA

Ryan W. Connell, M.D
Department of Internal Medicine
Division of Cardiology
University of Rochester
Medical Center
Rochester, New York
USA

G. Ronald Beck, M.S
Department of Internal Medicine
Division of Cardiology
University of Rochester
Medical Center
Rochester, New York
USA

ISBN 978-0-85729-943-7   e-ISBN 978-0-85729-944-4
DOI 10.1007/978-0-85729-944-4
Springer London Dordrecht Heidelberg New York

British Library Cataloguing in Publication Data
A catalogue record for this book is available from the British Library

Library of Congress Control Number: 2011941507

Foreword

All health care providers need to know how to diagnose and treat common cardiovascular diseases for one simple reason: cardiovascular diseases are common and deadly. The prevalence of cardiovascular diseases is enormous: 8% of adult Americans have diabetes, 23% of men and 19% of women smoke, 33% have hypertension, and 33% are obese [1]. In the United States, cardiovascular diseases cause over 780,000 heart attacks and 400,000 deaths each year [1]. Cardiovascular diseases are the biggest cause of death and disability across the globe [2].

However, it is challenging to keep up with the latest advancements in cardiovascular diagnostics and therapies. The pace of medical research is accelerating, with the spread of genetic testing, the explosion of clinical trials, and the proliferation of treatment guidelines.

The *Manual of Outpatient Cardiology* provides a concise and authoritative guide for a variety of health care providers who do not necessarily specialize in cardiology: primary care physicians, physician assistants, nurse practitioners, residents, and students. We have divided the book into three parts: cardiovascular diagnostics, cardiac diseases, and cardiac symptoms. We have included the most recent guidelines of both the American College of Cardiology and the American Heart Association to make this manual the most authoritative and reliable outpatient guide available.

The section on Cardiac Diagnostics is a guide to health care providers who are confronted with patients with common cardiovascular diseases, and who must choose the best and most cost-efficient set of tests. This section discusses when to use specific tests, such as stress tests and cardiac ultrasound, while weighing the risks and benefits. The chapters on Common Cardiac Diseases emphasize conditions seen every day in the clinics of general medical doctors and specialists, including common diseases such as hypertension and dyslipidemia. The final section, Approach to the Patient, summarizes the most up to date strategy to evaluate and treat common symptoms, including chest pain, dizziness, and palpitations.

We hope this *Manual of Outpatient Cardiology* will be useful to a wide range of readers who want to learn more about cardiovascular diseases encountered every day in the clinic. We thank our contributors and members of the Cardiology Division of University of Rochester Medical Center for their knowledge and expertise in preparing this book.

Rochester, NY, USA   Charles J. Lowenstein

References

1. Roger VL et al. Heart disease and stroke statistics 2011 update: a report from the American Heart Association. Circulation. 2011;123:e18–209.
2. World Health Organization: Global health observatory data repository, causes of death summary tables 2008: http://apps.who.int/ghodata/?vid=10012. June 16, 2011.

Contents

List of Contributors

Mehmet K. Aktas, M.D. Division of Cardiology –
Electrophysiology, University of Rochester
Medical Center, Rochester, NY, USA

Jeffrey D. Alexis, M.D. Division of Cardiology,
Department of Internal Medicine,
University of Rochester Medical Center,
Rochester, NY, USA

G. Ronald Beck, M.S. Department of Internal Medicine
Division of Cardiology, University of Rochester Medical
Center, Rochester, NY, USA

John D. Bisognano, M.D., Ph.D. Division of Cardiology,
Department of Internal Medicine, University of Rochester
Medical Center, Rochester, NY, USA

Robert C. Block, M.D., MPH Department of
Community and Preventive Medicine, The University
of Rochester School of Medicine and Dentistry,
Rochester, NY, USA

Andrew J. Brenyo, M.D. Division of Cardiology,
University of Rochester Medical Center,
Rochester, NY, USA

Imran N. Chaudhary, MB, BS Division of Cardiology,
University of Rochester Medical Center,
Rochester, NY, USA

Ryan W. Connell, M.D. Division of Cardiology,
Department of Internal Medicine,
University of Rochester Medical Center,
Rochester, NY, USA

M. James Doling, M.D. Division of Cardiology,
University of Rochester Medical Center,
Rochester, NY, USA

James Eichelberger, M.D. Division of Cardiology,
Department of Medicine, University of Rochester,
Rochester, NY, USA

Michael W. Fong, M.D. Division of Cardiology,
University of Southern California, Los Angeles,
CA, USA

James Gallagher, M.D. Division of Cardiology,
Department of Medicine, University of Rochester
Medical Center, Rochester, NY, USA

Blake Gardner, M.D. Division of Cardiology,
Department of Medicine, University of Rochester
Medical Center, Rochester, NY, USA

John P. Gassler, M.D. Division of Cardiology,
Department of Medicine, University of Rochester
Medical Center, Rochester, NY, USA

Norman Gray Jr, M.D. Division of Cardiology,
University of Rochester Medical Center,
Rochester, NY, USA

Melissa Gunasekera, M.D. Department of Medicine,
University of Rochester Medical Center,
Rochester, NY, USA

Burr Hall, M.D. Division of Cardiology - Electrophysiology, Department of Internal Medicine, University of Rochester Medical Center, Rochester, NY, USA

Bryan Henry, M.D. Division of Cardiology, Finger Lakes Cardiology Associates, University of Rochester, NY, USA

Theodore I. Hirokawa, M.D., Ph.D. Department of Surgery, Highland Hospital, Rochester, NY, USA

Ryan J. Hoefen, M.D., Ph.D. Division of Cardiology, Department of Medicine, University of Rochester Medical Center, Rochester, NY, USA

David T. Huang, M.D. Division of Cardiology, University of Rochester Medical Center, Rochester, NY, USA

Matthew Jonovich, M.D. Division of Cardiology, Department of Medicine, University of Rochester Medical Center, Rochester, NY, USA

Michael Katz, M.D. Division of Cardiology, Department of Medicine, University of Rochester Medical Center, Rochester, NY, USA

Peter A. Knight, M.D. Division of Cardiac Surgery, Department of Surgery, University of Rochester Medical Center, Rochester, NY, USA

Christopher D. Lang, M.D. Internal Medicine, University of Rochester Medical Center, Rochester, NY, USA

Susan F. Lien, M.D. Division of Cardiology, University of Rochester Medical Center, Rochester, NY, USA

Charles J. Lowenstein M.D. Chief, Division of Cardiology, Department of Internal Medicine, University of Rochester Medical Center, Rochester, NY, USA

Benjamin R. McClintic, M.D. Division of Cardiology, Department of Medicine, University of Rochester Medical Center, Rochester, NY, USA

Harry E. McCrea III, M.D. Division of Cardiology, University of Rochester Medical Center, Rochester, NY, USA

Craig R. Narins, M.D. Division of Cardiology and Vascular Surgery, University of Rochester School of Medicine, Rochester, NY, USA

Jason D. Pacos, M.D. Division of Cardiology, University of Rochester Medical Center, Rochester, NY, USA

Nicholas A. Paivanas, M.D. Internal Medicine, University of Rochester Medical Center, Rochester, NY, USA

Angelo J. Pedulla, M.D. Division of Cardiology, University of Rochester Medical Center, Rochester, NY, USA

Benjamin G. Plank, M.D. Division of Cardiology, Department of Medicine, University of Rochester Medical Center, Rochester, NY, USA

Mohan Rao, M.D. Division of Cardiology, Department of Medicine, University of Rochester Medical Center, Rochester, NY, USA

John E. Reuter, M.D. Division of Cardiology, University of Rochester Medical Center, Rochester, NY, USA

J. Franklin Richeson, M.D. Division of Cardiology,
University of Rochester Medical Center,
Rochester, NY, USA

Robert L. Rosenblatt, M.D., DO, FAAC Division of
Cardiology, University of Rochester Medical Center,
Rochester,
NY, USA

Eugene Storozynsky, M.D. Division of Cardiology, Highland
Hospital, University of Rochester Medical Center,
Rochester, NY, USA

John C. Teeters, M.D. Division of Cardiology,
Highland Hospital, University of Rochester Medical Center,
Rochester, NY, USA

Christine Tompkins, M.D., M.S. Division of Cardiology –
Electrophysiology, University of Rochester
Medical Center, Rochester, NY, USA

Menachem Wakslak, M.D. Department of Cardiology,
Maimonides Medical Center, Brooklyn, NY, USA

Kevin J. Woolf, M.D. Division of Cardiology,
University of Rochester Medical Center,
Rochester, NY, USA

Duncan D. Wormer, M.D. Division of Cardiology,
University of Rochester Medical Center,
Rochester, NY, USA

Part I
Cardiac Diagnostics

Chapter 1
History and Physical

Norman Gray and J. Franklin Richeson

Approaching the patient with cardiovascular disease begins with a comprehensive cardiac history and careful physical examination. During medical training, great emphasis is placed on thorough, extensive, and complete histories and physical exams. With careful focus and direction, examining the cardiac patient should lead the practitioner to a diagnosis prior to any lab or imaging tests. The goal of this chapter will be to help the reader refresh his or her bed side skills.

The Chief Complaint and History of Present Illness

The history can provide the practitioner with 90% of the information necessary to make a diagnosis. Whenever possible, the interviewer should use open-ended questioning of the patient, as answers suggested to the patient by the interviewer's questions are less apt to be true than are those volunteered without suggestion. Start with the chief complaint to better focus attention on the patient's primary problem. Examples may include chest pain, syncope, palpitations, or dyspnea.

N. Gray (✉) • J.F. Richeson
Division of Cardiology, University of Rochester
Medical Center, Rochester, NY, USA
e-mail: ngray@alumni.nd.edu

J.D. Bisognano et al. (eds.), *Manual of Outpatient Cardiology*,
DOI 10.1007/978-0-85729-944-4_1,
© Springer-Verlag London Limited 2012

Moving on from the Chief Complaint, eliciting the History of Present Illness (HPI) will occupy the lion's share of the interview. The HPI tells the story, and the practitioner's role is to re-create the scene by pulling out the necessary details to put that scene in motion. Every story has a beginning, and for the patient, defining the "beginning" may often be difficult. The patient may believe that the precipitating symptom that prompted today's visit is the "beginning," but further prompting maybe necessary to reveal the cascade of events began long ago. The beginning of events may be related to medication changes, dietary changes, or stressful events; just to name a few to consider as the HPI develops. Asking where the patient was, what they were doing, and who else was around at the beginning of events may provide additional useful clues as you hear the story.

The details of the HPI are obtained by having the patient describe all aspects of each symptom. For example, if the symptom is "discomfort," the patient needs to describe its quality (burning, stabbing, squeezing, etc.), its location, its intensity, its radiation, its duration, other accompanying symptoms, and provoking and/or alleviating factors. Every story lasts for a period of time and length of symptoms once they begin can provide additional information to the HPI. Similar experiences prior to the most recent presentation can provide helpful insight.

Using the example of Chest Pain as the Chief Complaint, consider what an appropriate HPI might consist of below. While the quality of cardiac discomfort may be variably described, most patients with ischemic Chest Pain insist that it is not a "pain," but an oppressive sensation likened to squeezing or pressure. It may occur anywhere between the nose and navel, but the central chest is the most often cited location. Ischemic Chest Pain is almost always diffuse; patients who localize the discomfort to a spot the size of a quarter do not have ischemic pain. Radiation patterns of cardiac pain also vary. Many patients may not experience symptoms outside the chest, or do so only when it becomes particularly severe. Radiation, when it does occur, is idiosyncratic: some patients feel it along the medial aspect of the arm; others experience it extending to the neck or jaw. Noting the intensity of the discomfort as a marker of damage is of little utility, except to judge whether interventions are having a salutary effect. The presence of associated symptoms may be of some diagnostic value: the presence of diaphoresis, dyspnea, nausea, and/or lightheadedness adds to the likelihood that the discomfort is of cardiac origin. For Chest Pain, the most important quality of the discomfort is its apparent provocation and alleviation. If the symptom in question is a one-time occurrence, its interpretation is problematic, as it is difficult to judge what provoked or alleviated it. If, however, the same symptom has happened repeatedly, finding the commonalities between the events may be diagnostic. Symptoms reliably occurring with exertion, versus recumbent postural changes, versus meals or periods of anxiety, greatly influence the differential diagnosis. In the same way, identifying factor that relief the discomfort, be it rest, by belching, by changing position, or by certain drugs will also strongly affect the differential diagnosis. If a common pattern can be identified, the diagnosis is made much simpler. For recurring cardiac ischemic pain, it is almost always provoked by physical or emotional stress. It is rarely pleuritic or positional, and it is rarely associated with focal tenderness.

In the upcoming chapters, a particular diagnosis underlies the discussion and will explore in more depth specific features and questions to explore in the HPI for a given Chief Complaint.

Remember that the cardiovascular system extends beyond the heart. Peripheral vascular disease, for example, especially in patients with underlying coronary disease, should be screened for and assessed when appropriate. Pulmonary symptoms may often times be mistaken for a primary pulmonary complaint when in fact other risk factors and hints in the HPI may lead to underlying cardiovascular disease.

In addition to a thorough HPI, obtaining a complete past medical history and social history play a critical role in evaluating cardiac patients. Chronic medical problems, such as valvular disease, history of arrhythmias, hypertension, and diabetes, are important risk factors that can help better contribute to a pre-test probability for diagnosis based on your history and physical examination. Inquiring about social habits such as the geographic origins of the patient, his/her educational background, occupational background, living circumstances, habits, and family structure not only helps the practitioner build a relationship with the patient but may also impact the current illness. For cardiac patients, it is particularly important to know the patient's exposure to tobacco, alcohol, and illicit drugs. One should gain an idea of the patient's daily physical exercise.

In the patient with established cardiac disease, it will be especially important to gather a complete cardiac profile of the history and prior studies and interventions. For coronary disease, gathering information such as prior heart attacks, prior interventions with or without stents, determining what type of stents are in place (coated or uncoated), coronary bypass history and grafts, what disease burden remains in the arteries and the last time they were examined, and left ventricular function, can help the practitioner gain a critical insight in what may be going on and what treatment strategies may best suit the patient. For example, many cardiac patients can recall how their initial presentations felt with their first heart attacks and asking how the current presentation compares to prior events can be a great help.

Documenting the medication history of the patient, noting dosage fluctuations, intolerances, allergies, and the patient's adherence to these often proves to be of crucial importance. Obtaining a dietary history can be a challenge and may be improved upon if another family member is present to attest to the patient's accurate portrayal. It is often helpful to have the patient recount all of the foods he/she has eaten over the past 24 h (or over a typical day), to ascertain the typical sodium and saturated fat of the diet. Medication compliance in any patient, but especially the cardiac patient, should always be addressed as non-compliance is a leading cause for changes in cardiac clinical status; the leading cause for admission to the hospital in patients with moderate to severe chronic heart failure is medication non-compliance.

Since many cardiac illnesses are familial, one should construct a pedigree of family members, noting illnesses, ages of onset, and ages at death, whenever possible. Special note should be taken if members of the family have died suddenly and unexpectedly, and if family members have been diagnosed with coronary artery disease before the age of 55.

Cardiac Physical Examination

After obtaining the History, a thorough cardiac exam is the next step in evaluating the patient. With the advancing improvements and availability of modern imaging, the skill of practitioners performing the cardiac physical exam has atrophied in our culture, but remains a necessary and valuable source of information.

The cardiac physical exam begins with accurate vital signs. Proper blood pressure measurements, most accurately obtain manually as opposed to the automated methods, with the patient resting calmly ideally for 5 min should be 120/80 in the normal patient. One should measure it at least once in both arms to assure the absence of coarctation. In patients suspected of having pericardial tamponade, one should ascertain respirophasic variation of blood pressure (known as "Pulsus Paradoxus"). To check for a Pulsus Paradoxus, inflate the cuff to supra-systolic levels, and slowly deflate it. Korotkoff sounds will first be heard at the end of expiration, and one should note the pressure at which these become audible. As the cuff is further deflated, Korotkoff sounds become audible throughout the respiratory cycle, and this pressure should be noted. The difference of these two values, the respirophasic variation, should be less than 10 torr. If it is greater than that, Pulsus Paradoxus is said to exist. This is commonly seen in obstructive airway disease and is always seen in cardiac tamponade. Of course, since systolic pressure varies widely, independent of respiration, in atrial fibrillation, measuring respirophasic variation in AF is pointless.

Heart rate is usually easy to obtain by palpating a peripheral pulse, but this method may under-count heart rate if premature beats or atrial fibrillation is present, in which case auscultation is to be preferred. A normal heart rate ranges from 60 to 100 beats per minute.

The cardiac exam extends beyond the heart. The peripheral circulation should not be forgotten. Palpate all pulses (radial, brachial, carotid, femoral, popliteal, posterior tibial, and dorsalis pedis) for amplitude and symmetry. Additionally, the carotids, femorals, and abdominal aorta should be auscultated for bruits. The characteristics and contour of pulses should be noted as they can suggest underlying pathology (the slow-rising carotid waveform of critical aortic stenosis, the waterhammer pulse of aortic regurgitation, and the spike-and-dome carotid pulse of obstructive cardiomyopathy).

Moving to the patient's right side, begin focusing on the heart portion of the cardiac examination with inspection. Start by exposing the chest and looking at the chest wall for any evidence of a right or left ventricular (RV and LV) heave or prominent apical impulse. On a normal examination, an RV impulse should not be visible; if a second impulse is noted at the left lower sternal border is noted, it is most likely due to an abnormal RV. Look for any skeletal deformities or scars to suggest prior bypass or devices underneath the skin that may represent pacemakers or ICDs. Inspect along the border of the apex of the heart to define the point of maximum impulse (PMI). A normal PMI, which may be visualized in up to 50% of patients, is a gentle outward motion located in the mid clavicular line between the fourth and fifth intercostal space. Abnormalities of the impulse include its displacement (laterally, for pressure-overload conditions, caudally and laterally for volume-overload conditions), and changes in contour of the impulse. Dysfunctional or aneurysmal left ventricles have a broader, more diffuse impulse. Pressure overload of the LV causes the impulse to be more sustained (moving outward for more than ½ of systole), while volume overload of the LV cause the excursion of the impulse to be hyperdynamic. Look for any additional impulse accompanying the PMI that could represent an S3 or S4 gallop.

Palpation of the precordium is generally performed next. Usually this can best be done with the examiner standing on the patient's right side, with the fingers of the palpating hand resting in the left interspaces. If the palpating hand is laid there passively, and pressure is exerted on top of it by the other hand, one is more sensitive to cardiac events. In palpation, one seeks the same sort of information yielded by inspection: the site and character of the apical impulse, the presence of an RV heave, and the presence of (palpable) gallops. Additionally, one may sometimes palpate pulmonic valve closure in the second left interspace, or the impulse of an ascending aortic aneurysm, and the vibration of Grade IV, or louder, cardiac murmurs.

After inspection and palpation, the next step is auscultation. Most of the auscultation is done with the diaphragm, but low-pitched sounds (gallops, and the rumble of mitral stenosis) should be sought using the bell. Since ambient noise from the examiner's hand offers interference, the hand should be relaxed on, or better yet, removed from, the stethoscope.

It is important to understand the normal heart sounds on exam, S1 and S2. The S1 component represents mitral and tricuspid valve closure and marks the beginning of systole. The S2 component marks the closing of the aortic and pulmonary valves and the beginning of diastole. Usually S2 is louder than S1 when determining the cadence of S1 and S2 in the cardiac cycle. At physiologic heart rates, diastole is longer than systole, so it is easier to discriminate S1 and S2. When the heart rate is rapid, however, it may be difficult to discern systole from diastole. This can be achieved by simultaneously palpating the carotid pulse (which is preceded by S1 and followed by S2) or viewing a simultaneous ECG tracing or arterial pressure tracing. When listening to the heart, assess if the rhythm is regular or irregular and if any pattern exists. The presence of tachycardia or bradycardia may be a clue to underlying pathology. An irregular rhythm may prove to be an underlying arrhythmia.

Once one clearly recognizes which sound is S1, one should focus on that sound. Usually it is a single sound. When there are two, rather than one, discrete sounds in the vicinity of S1, the differential includes (1) a split S1 (mitral and tricuspid closures heard separately), (2) an S4-S1 sequence, or (3) an S1-ejection click sequence. A split S1 is best heard at the apex and left lower sternal border, both sounds are high-pitched, and there may be a respirophasic widening and narrowing. An S4-S1 sequence is usually confined to the apex, and the S4 component becomes much fainter or disappears when listening with the diaphragm. An S1-ejection click sequence is heard best at the base of the heart, both sounds being high-pitched.

The second heart sound is rich in diagnostic information. The second heart sound represent the closure first of the aortic valve (A2) followed shortly thereafter by closure of the pulmonary valve (P2). Normally, aortic and pulmonary valve closure may be heard as a single sound during the latter portion of expiration, but becomes a pair of distinct sounds during the latter portion of inspiration. This of course is normal, or physiologic, splitting of S2 and stems from the delayed closure of P2 as the right side of the heart is distended by the inspiratory influx of blood. Normally, aortic valve closure is louder than pulmonic valve. When the converse pattern is heard (splitting with expiration, and closure with inspiration), that signifies paradoxical splitting of S2. Since pulmonic closure is still delayed by inspiration, paradoxic splitting of S2 must mean that aortic closure is always delayed (as in left bundle branch block, dysfunctional LV contraction) or pulmonic closure is always advanced in time (as in insertion of a bypass tract in the RV). Sometimes, S2 has a physiologic behavior (tends to close with expiration) but does not fully close, as occurs in right bundle branch block. Rarely, S2 is widely split with no changes during respiration (fixed split). In such cases, the additional influx to the RV comes from the peripheral venous system during inspiration (as is normal) but comes from the left atrium during expiration, most commonly in the presence of an atrial septal defect. A fixed split of S2 is diagnostic of ASD. When pulmonary hypertension is present, P2, as auscultated over the second left interspace is often louder than A2. In severe aortic stenosis, the A2 component becomes inaudible.

Additional heart sounds can be appreciated on auscultation outside of the normal S1 and S2 components. The S1 and S2 are high pitched sounds best appreciated with the diaphragm of the stethoscope. When listening for lower pitched sounds, such as an S3 or an S4 to be reviewed below, it is important to listen with the bell of the stethoscope.

An extra heart sound after S2, called an S3, can be normal or abnormal depending on the clinical scenario. The sound of an S3 comes from blood flow in to the left ventricle during diastole. In the young patient, an S3 can be a normal finding due to vigorous relaxation of the heart during diastole causing a negative pressure within the ventricle that draws blood in at a faster rate. This accelerated filling of the left ventricle creates an S3 sound as blood hits the wall of the ventricle early in diastole. In contrast, within the elderly patient or patient with an abnormal heart, as the relaxation of the heart muscle worsens and as the ventricular walls become stiffer and less compliant, an S3 represents abnormal filling and relaxation of the ventricle suggesting underlying cardiac pathology and diastolic dysfunction.

A fourth heart sound, referred to as an S4, can be heard before the beginning of systole and S1. An S4 is never normal. The S4 comes in the setting of atrial contraction; when the heart is under increased volumes due to underlying cardiac disease, atrial contraction, which occurs just before systole, tries to fill the left ventricle which is already under stress and volume overload. The contraction and force of blood trying to flow from the left atrium to the ventricle causes the S4 sound you hear. The S4 often times becomes more audible as patient's with underlying cardiomyopathy develop heart failure and conversely can decrease in intensity or resolve completely in patients who are in compensated heart failure and adequately volume managed.

After establishing S1 and S2 and listening for an S3 or S4, one should pay attention for any additional heart sounds. Murmurs (to be discussed in a separate chapter) can be heard in both systole and diastole and may change in character and volume based on various maneuvers during the exam. In patients with a clinical suspicion for pericardial disease, listening for a rub in different positions, especially the left lateral decubitus position, will be important in guiding the differential diagnosis.

Clinical assessment of the volume status of a cardiac patient is critical to reaching the right diagnosis and treatment plan. Inspection of the neck veins for jugular venous pressure (JVP) allow for a clinical assessment of RV preload and right sided pressures as a measurement of overall volume status. The patient should lie at an angle that allows visualization of the meniscus of the JVP to be between the clavicle and the ear. For some patients, this will be the supine position, and for others, the meniscus will be above the ear even when bolt upright. The patient's head should be turned slightly away from the side being examined. The examiner should stand on the side opposite of that being examined. This allows the examiner to view the sternomastoid tangentially (excursions coursing left-right across one's visual field are easier to appreciate than those bouncing in-line with the line of vision). One should look for lifting and falling of the sternomastoid and note the vertical height of the peak of the excursion relative to the sternal angle. If excursions are seen, but one is uncertain whether they are of arterial or venous origin, gently compress the base of the neck with a tongue blade. Gentle pressure should abolish venous, but not arterial, waveforms.

A normal venous pressure wave consists of a biphasic pulsation for each cardiac cycle representing atrial contraction (called the *a* wave) and atrial filling (called the *v* wave). Normally, the mean level of JVP should be 4–7 cm vertically above the right atrium. Since the sternal angle is 5 cm vertically above the right atrium, adding the vertical elevation of the JVP above the sternal notch provides the absolute clinical RV filling pressure. Abnormalities in the pulsation characteristics of the "a" and "v" wave can also provide useful insight. The absence of an 'a' wave (making the JV waveform monophasic) indicates atrial fibrillation. The presence of a giant 'v' wave (a common finding), along with finding a pulsatile liver, is diagnostic of tricuspid regurgitation. Cannon 'a' waves are sometimes seen (connoting A-V dissociation) when the right atrium contracts against a closed tricuspid valve.

The basics of the cardiac exam have been reviewed here. Throughout the different chapters, key physical exam findings and maneuvers will be further discussed and reviewed as they are relevant to a particular diagnosis.

Initial Diagnostic Work Up

An adequate differential after the history and physical examinations can help the practitioner determine the appropriate initial testing. Further details for a given diagnosis have been organized in the next several chapters.

The tool box of diagnostic testing for cardiac patients after the physical exam starts with the ECG. The ECG is an important diagnostic test to help rule in or out various diagnoses on the differential. Accurate interpretation of the ECG as part of the diagnostic work up is critical and will be discussed further in the next chapter. The ECG can be used to evaluate for a broad range of differential diagnoses including arrhythmias, ischemia, cardiac injury, hypertrophy, pulmonary disease, and electrolyte abnormalities, just to name a few. If available, it may be useful to compare prior ECG tracings to look for any changes suggesting a more acute diagnosis, especially in the patient with known cardiac disease and chronic changes to the ECG at baseline.

The evolution of cardiac biomarkers over the past two decades has greatly improved the ability to objectively test for cardiac myocyte damage. Today's standard cardiac biomarkers include troponin I, troponin T, CKMB, and CK. Troponin I and troponin T are proteins within cardiac muscle tissue that are part of the tropomyosin complexes responsible for cardiac myocyte contraction. In the setting of cardiac myocyte damage or ischemia, troponin proteins will leak in to the blood stream and rise to detectable levels within the circulating blood. CK and CKMB are found in both skeletal and cardiac myocyte, with a higher concentration of CKMB in the latter. Using the ratio of CK to CKMB, higher levels of CKMB release out of proportion to CK releases in the proper clinical setting can suggest cardiac myocyte injury. Depending on an institutions' availability, utilizing troponin or CKMB levels as a sensitive marker for cardiac damage can be key to making the correct diagnosis in the correct clinical setting. Utilizing biomarkers in the appropriate setting helps to minimize false positive values and helps ensure proper utilization of resources and diagnostic tools. In using cardiac biomarkers, it is important to remember their limitations in certain clinical scenarios. For example, the use of elevated troponin T in patients with underlying renal disease decreases the sensitivity and specificity for cardiac myocyte damage.

The BNP, or brain naturetic peptide, is a protein released by the atria thought to be under increased stress from volume overload and has been shown in proper clinical scenarios to be a useful adjunct in assessing heart failure. Just like the troponin, the BNP should be utilized in the appropriate setting and used to aide in diagnosis and treatment rather than making a diagnosis. Often times, trending a BNP may be more useful than the absolute number and obtaining trends in BNP values and corresponding heart failure may be much more valuable.

Imaging modalities such as a chest x-ray in patients with chest pain is important in evaluating for other causes of chest pain aside from cardiac disease. Looking for pulmonary processes or infections, evidence for dissections, enlarged cardiac silhouettes, volume overload, or other soft tissue processes can help further direct the differential diagnosis.

Basic labs including electrolytes and renal function should be part of the initial work up. Electrolyte abnormalities, especially in the setting of suggestive ECG findings when appropriate, may be on the differential for further assessment.

With each diagnosis on the cardiac differential, a chapter covering pertinent history and physical exam findings, appropriate testing and evaluation, and treatment options are reviewed throughout the remaining chapters.

Chapter 2
Evaluation of Heart Rhythms

James Gallagher and Christine Tompkins

Introduction

The electrocardiogram (ECG) is synonymous with a cardiac evaluation, just as a chest x-ray is with a pulmonary evaluation. The ECG is inexpensive, non-invasive and easy to perform. All hospitals and most offices can perform electrocardiography and because they are so ubiquitous, being able to accurately interpret an ECG is important.

The goal of this chapter is to provide a basic understanding of the principles of how to "read" an ECG, why an ECG looks the way it does, and when to order an ECG. Because the readers of this book will likely have quite varied backgrounds and exposures to ECG interpretation, this chapter will begin with more basic principles of what an ECG is and how it is generated. We will then focus on understanding the ECG waveforms and basic rhythm diagnosis. Finally, we will

J. Gallagher (✉)
Department of Medicine, Division of Cardiology,
University of Rochester Medical Center,
Rochester, NY, USA
e-mail: james_gallagher@urmc.rochester.edu

C. Tompkins
Division of Cardiology – Electrophysiology,
University of Rochester Medical Center,
Rochester, NY, USA

J.D. Bisognano et al. (eds.), *Manual of Outpatient Cardiology*,   15
DOI 10.1007/978-0-85729-944-4_2,
© Springer-Verlag London Limited 2012

conclude with a discussion of additional ECG tests that can be performed to assess heart rhythm disturbances.

Electrocardiogram

The ECG provides a momentary picture of the electrical activity of the heart. With every beat of the heart, each heart cell depolarizes, meaning that electrolytes flow into and out of the heart cells, generating an electrical signal that provides the stimulus for the cells to contract. When enough cells depolarize together, this electrical signal becomes strong enough to be measured outside of the body. To produce an ECG, electrodes are attached to the skin and connected via wires to a machine. The machine amplifies the minute electrical signals from the heart that reach the electrodes on the skin and then filters out many unwanted signals. The machine will then display or print out a summation of the electrical activity detected by each lead. Sometimes an ECG is referred to as an EKG, which is an abbreviation of the German word *elektrokardiogram*. The standard appearance of an ECG is shown in Fig. 2.1.

When setting up an ECG, a varying number of wires can be connected to the patient. A minimum of two wires must be attached, providing a positive and negative electrode, which

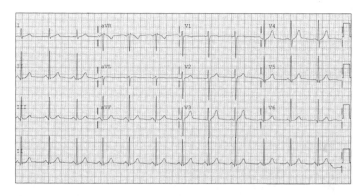

FIGURE 2.1 Standard 12-Lead ECG in sinus rhythm

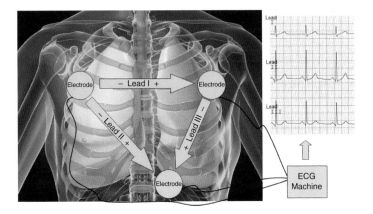

FIGURE 2.2 Einthoven's triangle. The electrode at the patient's right arm is typically always negative. The electrode towards the patient's left leg is typically always positive. The electrode at the patient's left arm can be positive or negative depending on which lead being evaluated. True bipolar leads, such as these, must always have a positive and a negative electrode

is necessary to measure changes in the electrical potential that occur with each heart beat.

The term "lead" is used to describe the electrical picture these two wires generate. While some use the term "lead" to describe the actual wire connected to the patient, technically, the correct use of "lead" is in reference to the picture that positive and negative electrodes generate together. Traditionally, three wires have been connected to the patient to form a triangle. Figure 2.2 shows what has been termed Einthoven's triangle. With these three wires, three different electrical pictures of the heart are generated, or in other words, three different "leads." These leads may show a waveform that has an upward or downward deflection depending on the direction of the electrical signal relative to that lead. By convention, a positive deflection is recorded for that lead when the electrical signal moves toward the positive electrode of that lead, and a negative deflection when electrical activity moves away from the positive electrode.

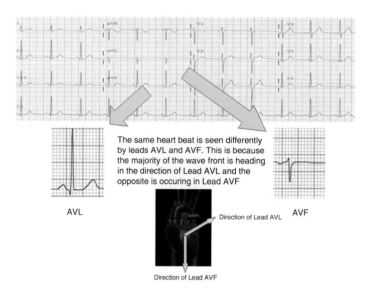

FIGURE 2.3 Different leads show a different picture of the same heart beat. Even though Lead AVL and Lead AVF are displaying the same heart beat, the waveform appears differently because in Lead AVL, the direction of electrical depolarization is away from this lead and in Lead AVF, the direction of electrical depolarization is towards this lead

Thus, it is important to realize that depending on the orientation of the electrode, the same electrical signal from the heart can be either upright or inverted as seen in Fig. 2.3. Analysis of each lead vector, therefore, provides spatial information about the electrical activity of the heart.

The heart is composed of four chambers, two upper chambers known as atria and two lower chambers know as ventricles. The sino-atrial (SA) node, which is located in the right atrium, is a group of specialized heart muscle cells whose primary function is to automatically generate an electrical signal, typically 60–100 times per minute. This signal is carried from heart cell to heart cell, thus setting the heart rate and providing the stimulus for each chamber of the heart to contract. The specialized cells of the SA node have a unique ability to spontaneously depolarize. This electrical signal then spreads throughout the heart, first traveling through both atria to the atrio-ventricular (AV) node and then to the ventricles. The wave of depolarization through the atria can be seen on the surface ECG as a p-wave. When the signal reaches the AV node, the signal slows. In a normal heart, the AV node is the sole electrical connection between the top two chambers (atria) and the two bottom chambers (ventricles) of the heart. Thus, all of the electrical signals from the atrium must travel through the AV node to reach the ventricles.

The AV node is also composed of specialized cells with slightly different electrical properties than the SA nodal cells. As a result of these differences, AV nodal cells can slow the conduction of the electrical signal. This slowing serves two purposes. First, it allows time for atrial contraction to occur prior to activation of the ventricles. Second, the slowing is a protective mechanism, limiting rapid conduction of fast impulses from the atrium to the ventricle as occurs in atrial fibrillation.

Conduction from the SA node through the AV node is seen as the PR interval on the ECG. Once the signal exits the AV node, the signal again speeds up and travels through the bundle of His to the bundle branches and into the Purkinje fibers, which are embedded in the inner lining (endocardium) of the left and right ventricles. Depolarization of the ventricles is seen as a QRS complex on the ECG.

Repolarization, which follows depolarization, is a term used to describe the recovery of heart cells back to their electrical resting state. Just as an electrical signal is generated as the heart depolarizes, a reverse electrical signal is generated when the heart repolarizes. Atrial repolarization is not seen on the ECG because the timing is coincident with ventricular depolarization (i.e. QRS complex), and the atrial mass (and hence the electrical signal) is relatively small compared to the ventricles. Conversely, ventricular repolarization is clearly evident on the ECG and is seen after the QRS as a t-wave. Occasionally u-waves are seen and the etiology of these waves is less well understood. Some have hypothesized that these are delayed after-depolarizations of the ventricles. A detailed explanation of these activities is shown in Fig. 2.4.

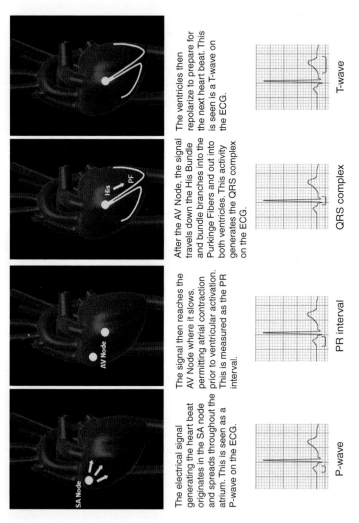

The electrical signal generating the heart beat originates in the SA node and spreads throughout the atrium. This is seen as a P-wave on the ECG.

The signal then reaches the AV Node where it slows, permitting atrial contraction prior to ventricular activation. This is measured as the PR interval.

After the AV Node, the signal travels down the His Bundle and bundle branches into the Purkinge Fibers and out into both ventricles. This activity generates the QRS complex on the ECG.

The ventricles then repolarize to prepare for the next heart beat. This is seen a T-wave on the ECG.

P-wave   PR interval   QRS complex   T-wave

FIGURE 2.4 Simplified physical and electrical structure of the heart

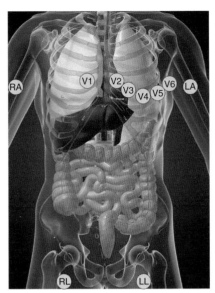

The precordial electrodes are placed on the chest. V1 and V2 are placed right and left of the sternum, respectively, in the 4th intercostal space. V4 is placed in the 5th intercostal space, mid-clavicular line, and V6 is placed in the 5th intercostal spaced, mid-axillary line. V3 and V5 are placed in between these electrodes. Electrodes are then also placed on the right arm, left arm, right leg, and left leg.

Figure 2.5 Attaching a 12-lead ECG. Reference 1: Guidelines for electrocardiography. A report of the American College of Cardiology/American Heart Association Task Force on Assessment of Diagnostic and Therapeutic Cardiovascular Procedures (Committee on Electrocardiography). JACC. 1992;19:473–81

Various forms of ECGs are routinely performed and differ mostly by the number of leads used and the duration of monitoring. Inpatient units, including cardiac care units, have patients on "telemetry." Telemetry typically involves five wires attached to the patient's chest that connect to a small transmitter. The transmitter sends the heart's electrical signals to a display monitor located at a nursing station, providing continuous tracings of the heart rate and rhythm. These monitors, which are observed by nurses and providers, are typically set up to alarm for abnormal heart rates or rhythms. Telemetry units are fully portable, allowing patients to be mobile as long as they remain within range of the monitoring station.

The most common form of the ECG is the "12-lead ECG." The 12-lead ECG typically involves attaching ten wires to the patient, as seen in Fig. 2.5. However, from these ten wires, the

ECG machine is capable of creating 12 electrical signals as shown in Fig. 2.1. Wires that are attached to the chest generate the precordial leads (V1-V6), while wires attached to the arms and legs create the limb leads (I, II, III, AVR, AVL, AVF). Each of these leads provides different spatial information about the orientation of the heart's electrical activity.

Leads I, II and III are also termed true bipolar leads because there is an actual single positive wire and single negative wire attached to the patient that is used to measure the electrical signal of the heart beat. The right arm wire is traditionally attached to the negative terminal of the ECG machine and the left arm to the positive terminal of the ECG machine. The electrical signal is then amplified and recorded as Lead I. In Lead II, the right arm wire is negative and the left leg wire is positive. Finally, in Lead III, the left arm wire is negative and the left foot wire is positive as shown in Fig. 2.2. Thus, each heart beat produces a slightly different electrical picture in each lead, depending on the direction of the electrical impulse relative to that lead. Different leads can therefore provide different information about the electrical activity of the heart. Waveforms that are not clearly evident in one lead may be quite obvious in another.

Another three limb leads seen on the 12-lead ECG are called the augmented limb leads, which are labeled as AVR, AVL, and AVF. These leads are called unipolar leads because the electrical potential of each individual wire is compared to a combined electrical potential created from the two remaining wires. In other words, the computer measures the electrical potential of the individual wire, which acts as the positive pole, and compares it to a composite negative pole calculated from the electrical signals of the two remaining wires. For example, the AVR lead, which stands for augmented vector right, compares the electrical potential of the right arm wire to that of a combined potential of the left arm wire and left leg wire. AVF compares the potential of the left leg to that of the left and right arm combined. AVL compares the potential of the left arm to the combined potential of the left leg and right arm. Again, the augmented limb leads are measured to produce a different electrical snapshot of the heart which may provide additional insight into the origin of an arrhythmia.

Lastly, in a 12-lead ECG, precordial leads are recorded. Like the augmented limb leads, these are unipolar leads. The ECG machine calculates a virtual negative pole based on the different wires attached to the patient. Each lead, V1 through V6, is then a representation of the electrical potential between the individual electrode attached to the patient's chest wall and the virtual negative pole generated by combining the potential of the remaining precordial leads.

Many clinical scenarios warrant ordering an ECG. Often, an ECG is ordered to evaluate for ischemia. Other indications include following cardiac procedures, including coronary angiography or electrophysiology studies and ablations. When administering anti-arrhythmic therapy, serial electrocardiograms should be obtained. Congenital heart disease, valvular heart disease, syncope, and conditions such as stroke which have a cardiac association warrant an ECG. In general, a 12-lead ECG should be ordered anytime further evaluation of the heart beyond the physical exam is desired. Please see the referenced guidelines (ACC/AHA Guidelines for Electrocardiography. JACC 1992) for specific indications.

Reading an ECG

The key to reading ECGs well is to be consistent, using the same method each time. This can sometimes be difficult when an obvious diagnosis is present (such as a very slow heart rhythm or a myocardial infarction), but ensures that other abnormalities will not be overlooked. A common approach is *rate*, *rhythm*, *axis*, *intervals*, and *changes*, which is described below.

When you first look at an ECG, take note of the *rate*. The heart rate is considered normal if it is between 60 and 100 beats per minute (bpm). If the rate is >100 bpm, then the rate is considered fast and the term "tachycardia" is used to describe the rate. This may still reflect a normal heart rhythm, for instance, if the subject is exercising, the heart is expected to speed up to above 100 bpm. Conversely, this may reflect an abnormal heart rhythm, which, if originating from the two top chambers (i.e. atria), would be called a supraventricular tachycardia (SVT), or if originating from the two lower chambers (i.e. ventricles) would be called a ventricular tachycardia (VT). These abnormal heart rhythms (arrhythmias) will be described further in a separate chapter of this book.

If the rate is <60 bpm, then the rate is considered slow and the term "bradycardia" is used to describe the rate. Again, this may reflect a normal heart rhythm. For instance, well-trained athletes often have slower baseline heart rates than the general population because their heart is conditioned to produce a larger stroke volume with each beat of the heart, thus allowing the heart to beat more slowly and still pump the same amount of blood. It can however reflect an abnormal heart rhythm, for which a patient may require a pacemaker. Keep in mind that the "normal" range for heart rates were decided upon in a somewhat limited manner, and many 20–30 year old people have a normal heart rate that is <60 bpm and many normal children >100 bpm. Nevertheless, these are the numbers that are typically used.

The next item to evaluate on an ECG is the *rhythm*. When looking at the ECG strips, first look to see if any atrial activity is present, as manifested by p-waves. If you do not see any p-waves specifically, that does not mean there is no atrial activity. The atria may be in atrial fibrillation, which can appear as a squiggly baseline between QRS complexes. Other causes of unapparent p-waves include sick sinus syndrome, sinus-node exit block, a junctional/ventricular rhythm or tachycardia that is obscuring the p-waves.

Once p-waves are identified, the next step is to see if each p-wave precedes the QRS and if the p-wave appears to be originating from the sinus node. Recall that the spread of atrial depolarization begins in the SA node in the right atrium and travels toward the ventricles. Thus, a p-wave that originates in the sinus node would be expected to be upright in leads I and II (i.e. signal flows toward those leads) and negative in lead AVR (i.e. signal flows away from this lead) which is shown in Fig. 2.1. The term sinus rhythm is used to describe a rhythm originating from the SA node. If the rate is

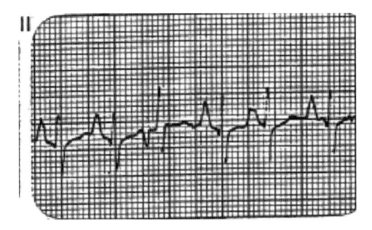

FIGURE 2.6 Multifocal atrial tachycardia. p-waves with different morphologies precede the QRS complex

>100 bpm, then the term sinus tachycardia would be applied. If the rate is <60 bpm, then the rhythm would be called sinus bradycardia.

If the p-waves are not upright in leads I and II, or negative in AVR, then it is likely that an ectopic atrial rhythm or junctional rhythm is present. An ectopic atrial focus means that the p-wave is originating from a site outside of the SA node, but still within the right or left atrium. In other words, the stimulus for the heart to beat is coming from outside the SA node but still within the atrium. If the ectopic atrial rate is >100 bpm, then the term "atrial tachycardia" is used. When three or more different p wave morphologies are seen on the ECG, meaning that three or more different sites in the atrium are causing the heart to beat, the term "wandering atrial pacemaker" is applied when the rate is <100 bpm or "multifocal atrial tachycardia" when the rate is >100 bpm (Fig. 2.6).

A junctional rhythm is considered if the PR interval is very short (i.e. <120 ms) and the p-wave appears inverted in lead II. At times, the p wave actually comes after the QRS complex. In these cases, the AV node is the source of the atrial activity. The signal that originates in the AV node travels in two directions, retrograde to the atrium resulting in atrial

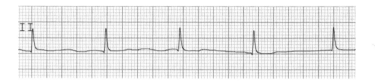

FIGURE 2.7 Junctional rhythm. No p-waves are present and the distance between each QRS complex (R-R interval) is fairly regular

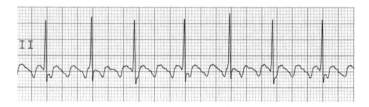

FIGURE 2.8 Atrial flutter

depolarization, and antegrade to the ventricles resulting in ventricular depolarization (Fig. 2.7).

Sometimes, the p-waves appear in a "saw tooth" pattern. These p-waves reflect continuous atrial activation and often occur at a frequency of around 300 bpm. These waves are called flutter waves, and the rhythm is known as atrial flutter (Fig. 2.8). Atrial flutter is a macro-reentrant arrhythmia in the atria, or in other words, an endless electrical loop that often circulates around the tricuspid valve. This type of flutter is called typical counter-clockwise atrial flutter and the ECG demonstrates inverted flutter waves in the inferior leads (leads II, III, and AVF) and upright flutter waves in V1. Clockwise flutter is characterized by positive flutter waves in the inferior leads and negative flutter waves in V1. Atypical flutters are flutters that do not involve the tricuspid annulus, and they often have slower flutter wave rates or mimic clockwise flutter.

If p-waves are not visible, then the next step is to determine if atrial fibrillation is present. This rhythm appears as a coarse, undulating baseline between QRS complexes, and the QRS complexes appear in an irregularly irregular pattern as shown in Fig. 2.9. Atrial fibrillation occurs when multiple areas of the

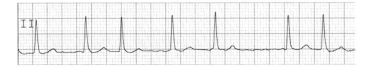

FIGURE 2.9 Atrial fibrillation

atrium are firing at the same time. This creates multiple electrical wavefronts and results in a lack of any organized electrical rhythm that would be recognized as a p-wave. Incidentally, it is this lack of organized electrical rhythm that results in loss of organized mechanical contraction of the atrium, which can result in stasis of blood and the formation of blood clots. Thus, patients with atrial fibrillation are at risk for strokes, which can occur if these blood clots form and embolize to the brain. Patients with atrial fibrillation must be evaluated for their risk of stroke using various risk assessment tools, such as the CHADS-2 score, as mentioned elsewhere in this book.

At times, however, p-waves are not present or are unapparent. Sinus node dysfunction, such as sick sinus syndrome or sinus exit block, junctional or ventricular rhythms are suspected in these instances, particularly when associated with a regular QRS pattern.

We already mentioned junctional rhythm above. Junctional rhythms can occur without visible p-waves on the ECG when the p-waves are buried in the QRS complex. The width of the QRS complex can help differentiate between a rhythm coming from the AV node, as in the case of junctional rhythms, or from the ventricles, which lie below the AV node. If the QRS complex is narrow (<120 ms), then this is likely a junctional rhythm. However, if the QRS is wide (≥120 ms), then a ventricular rhythm likely exists.

The QRS morphology is wide in ventricular rhythms because the origin of the beats is in the ventricles, not the conduction system. Since conduction of the electrical impulse through the ventricular muscle occurs more slowly outside of the conduction system, the QRS morphology is wide, as seen in Fig. 2.10. Exceptions to this include aberrantly conducted

Lead II

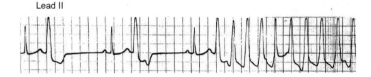

FIGURE 2.10 Ventricular tachycardia. There are two normal appearing beats, each with a wide complex early beat coming after. These single, early beats are termed premature ventricular contractions (also known as PVCs or VPCs). When these early beats sustain, this is called ventricular tachycardia

supraventricular beats. Aberrantly conducted beats mean that the rhythm is generated from the atria and conducted through the AV node; however, conduction is slowed through one of the bundle branches because of disease or drug effect, thus giving the appearance of a wide QRS complex. To differentiate ventricular rhythms from aberrantly conducted supraventricular beats, other aspects of the ECG must be examined. For instance, if the QRS is wide but the R-R intervals are irregular, atrial fibrillation may be occurring. Of note, atrial fibrillation may be suspected in Fig. 2.10 because some of the wide-complexes appear in an irregularly irregular pattern. However, p-waves can be seen in the ST/ T wave segments of the some of the beats such as the second and third wide complex beats, thus showing some organized atrial electrical activity and excluding atrial fibrillation as a diagnosis. Over the years, various criteria have been developed to distinguish ventricular tachycardia (VT) from aberrantly conducted SVT. The two most useful ones have been the Brugada criteria and the AVR (Vereckei) criteria (Fig. 2.11). It is important to learn at least one of these criteria schemes as when you are faced with a wide-complex, fast tachycardia, the treatment of VT is typically vastly different than that of an SVT as you will see later in this book.

One other very important ventricular rhythm to identify is ventricular fibrillation (Fig. 2.12). As with atrial fibrillation, ventricular fibrillation occurs when multiple areas of the ventricle fire rapidly and chaotically. This arrhythmia is life-

VT Criteria

Vereckei-Looking at Lead AVR	**Brugada**
VT if...	VT if...
• Broad monphasic R-wave in AVR	• Absence of RS complex in all precordial leads
• Initial r or q wave that is >40 msec	• R to S >100 msec in any precordial leads
• Notch on descending limb of negative QRS complex	• AV dissocaition
• Terminal electrical potential > initial electrical potential	• Morphologic VT Criteria both in V_{1-2} and V_6

FIGURE 2.11 VT criteria – AVR (Vereckei) versus Brugada

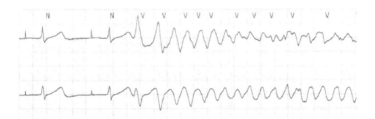

FIGURE 2.12 Ventricular fibrillation

ending if not treated. The treatment of this is direct-current, electrical defibrillation.

Axis is used to describe the overall direction of electrical current in the heart. One can evaluate the axis of p-waves, QRS complexes and t-waves. Usually, the axis of interest relates to the QRS complex, as this provides additional information including the overall orientation of the heart. For example, the electrical axis of the heart shifts leftward in the presence of increased left ventricular mass (i.e. LV hypertrophy) as occurs in chronic hypertension. Conversely, scar from a prior myocardial infarction diminishes the electrical activity in the area of scar shifting the axis in the opposite direction of the scar. If part of the conduction system is failing, such as in a hemi-block, then the axis will be shifted away from the direction of the block.

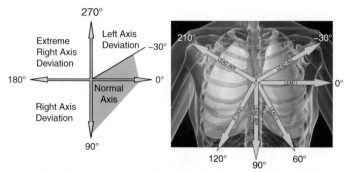

Axis of the QRS complex is determined by the direction of the QRS complex in each of the limb leads. Normal axis is between −30° to 90°, which would be a QRS complex that is positive in leads I, II, and AVF

Figure 2.13 Determining axis and normal axis

The axis of the heart that is typically evaluated is in the frontal (i.e. coronal) plane. To do this, we look at the major deflection of the QRS in different limb leads which lie in the frontal plane as shown in Fig. 2.13. The direction of the QRS deflection will be upright in leads that the electrical signal is flowing towards and negative in leads that the electrical signal is moving away. The normal axis of the heart is −30° to 90°. Left axis deviation is present when the QRS axis is −30° to −90° (Fig. 2.14). Right axis deviation is present when the QRS axis is 90°–180°, as shown in Fig. 2.15. Extreme axis or northwest axis deviation is present when the QRS axis is 180°–270° as shown in Fig. 2.16.

The next step of the evaluation is to measure the *intervals*. Basic intervals are listed in Table 2.1. The first interval to evaluate is the P-R interval. The P-R interval, a measure of the conduction time from the sinus node to the ventricles, is typically 120–200 ms. A PR-interval that is >200 ms is abnormal and suggests delay in signal conduction from the SA node to the ventricles. The term "first degree AV block" is used to describe a PR interval that is consistently >200 ms (Fig. 2.17). A short PR interval (i.e. <120 ms) can be normal, but rhythms such as a junctional rhythm or the presence of accessory pathways, as occurs in Wolf–Parkinson–White syndrome, should be considered.

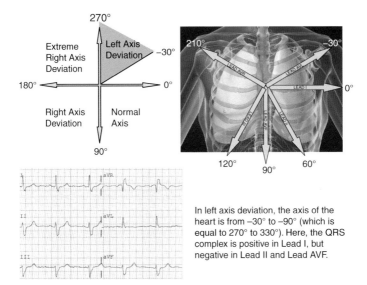

In left axis deviation, the axis of the heart is from −30° to −90° (which is equal to 270° to 330°). Here, the QRS complex is positive in Lead I, but negative in Lead II and Lead AVF.

FIGURE 2.14 Left axis deviation

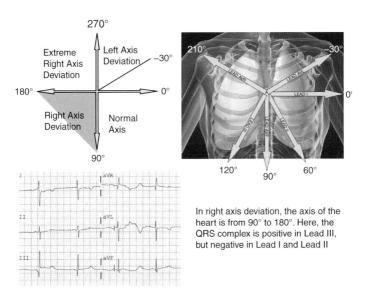

In right axis deviation, the axis of the heart is from 90° to 180°. Here, the QRS complex is positive in Lead III, but negative in Lead I and Lead II

FIGURE 2.15 Right axis deviation

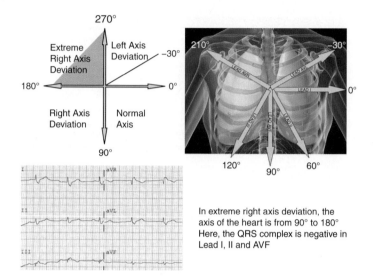

In extreme right axis deviation, the axis of the heart is from 90° to 180° Here, the QRS complex is negative in Lead I, II and AVF

FIGURE 2.16 Extreme right axis deviation

Second degree AV block is present if there is intermittent loss of conduction between the atria and ventricles. In Type I, second degree AV block, there is progressive delay in the electrical conduction from the atrium to the ventricle. Therefore, the ECG shows a gradual increase in the PR interval until there is block in the conduction within the AV node, at which point there is absence of a QRS complex following the p-wave. Figure 2.18 shows this type of block with a missing QRS complex after a p-wave that can be seen buried in the t-wave. Type II, second degree AV block occurs when there is abrupt loss of conduction between the atrium and ventricle. In this case, the PR interval is constant both before and after a non-conducted p-wave, as shown in Fig. 2.19. If there is no association between the p-waves and the QRS complexes, then atrio-ventricular dissociation is present. If there are more p-waves than QRS complexes, then complete heart block (i.e. third AV block) is present, which is a form of AV dissociation (Fig. 2.20).

TABLE 2.1 Basic intervals

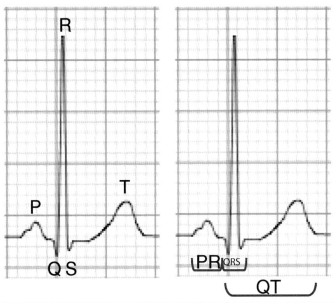

	Normal Interval
PR	120-200 msec
QRS	<100 msec
QT	Men 440 msec
	Women 460 msec

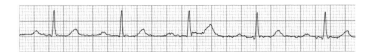

FIGURE 2.17 First degree AV block – the PR interval is prolonged

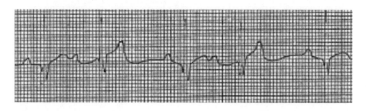

FIGURE 2.18 Second degree AV block, type I (Wenkebach) – The PR interval prolongs until the point that it no longer conducts to the ventricles and there is no QRS complex

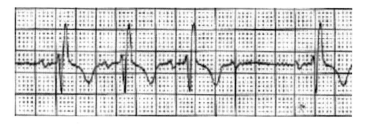

FIGURE 2.19 Second degree AV block, type II – the PR interval is fixed but intermittently the AV node does not conduct to the ventricle which results in a missing QRS complex

The next interval to evaluate is the QRS duration. This interval reflects the time it takes for electrical activation of the ventricles. Recall that when the electrical signal travels from the atrium to the ventricles, the signal travels through the AV node where it is temporarily slowed, then through the His into the left and right bundle branches to the Purkinje fibers embedded within the wall of the ventricles. The normal QRS duration is 60–100 ms. The term "incomplete" bundle branch block is used when the QRS duration is between 100 and 120 ms, suggesting conduction through one of the bundle branches is slower than normal. Complete bundle branch block is used when the QRS duration is >120 ms, suggesting absence of conduction through that bundle. Bundle branch block is further differentiated into either right or left depending on whether the right or left bundles are affected. The QRS pattern helps differentiate between right and left bundle

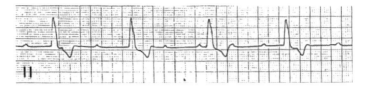

FIGURE 2.20 Third degree AV block – more p-waves than QRS complexes and no regular intervals between the p-waves and the QRS complexes

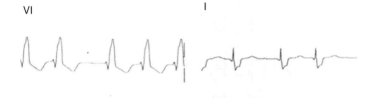

FIGURE 2.21 Right bundle branch block

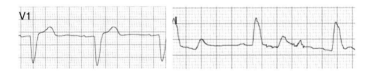

FIGURE 2.22 Left bundle branch block

branch blocks, as shown in Figs. 2.21 and 2.22. If the QRS is wide and does not appear to follow one of these two patterns, the term "non-specific inter-ventricular conduction delay" is used to describe the pattern, which suggests that there may be more than one conduction abnormality present or scar.

The easiest way to differentiate right and left bundle branch blocks is to evaluate the QRS morphology in leads V1-V2 and leads I and V6. It is important to note the position of these leads relative to the heart. V1 is positioned over the right ventricle, while V2 is positioned over the septum. Leads I and V6 are lateral leads, providing electrical information about the left ventricle. In right bundle branch blocks, conduction down the right bundle is either slowed or absent leading to delayed activation of the right ventricle. Thus, the initial deflections of the QRS reflect left ventricular activation, while the terminal portions of the QRS reflects right ventricular activation. The typical ECG pattern of RBBB is rsr', rsR' or rSR' in leads V1-V2 (often referred to as "rabbit ears" pattern) and a terminal S wave in leads I and V6. The R' and S waves in these leads reflect the electrical activity of the right ventricle.

In left bundle branch blocks, conduction down the left bundle is either slowed or absent leading to delayed activation of the left ventricle. Thus, the initial deflections of the QRS reflect right ventricular activation, and the terminal portions of the QRS reflect left ventricular activation. The typical ECG pattern of LBBB is a broad or notched r-wave in leads I and V6 and QS or S waves in V1-V2.

The last main interval to assess is the QT segment. This measures the time it takes for the ventricles to depolarize and repolarize. If the ventricle takes extra time to repolarize, then that patient has a higher risk of having a potential life-threatening arrhythmia, such as polymorphic ventricular tachycardia. This is an often overlooked, but important interval to measure. The time it takes for the ventricle to repolarize is dependent on the heart rate. When the heart beats faster, the heart will reset faster. Thus, the QT interval is often corrected for rate. Bazett's formula is often used to calculate this and is defined as corrected QT interval (QTc) = QT/square root of the R-R interval. If the QTc is >440 ms in men or >460 ms in women, it is considered prolonged. See Fig. 2.23 for an example of a long QT interval.

In the final evaluation of the ECG, we look for any morphologic changes in each waveform, specifically, the p-waves, the PR intervals, the QRS complexes, the ST segments and the t-waves. The amplitude and duration of these waves can provide information about chamber sizes. For example, the amplitude (i.e. height) of the QRS complex increases in conditions like ventricular hypertrophy because the larger tissue mass generates greater electrical signals. This is why QRS complexes are larger than p-waves.

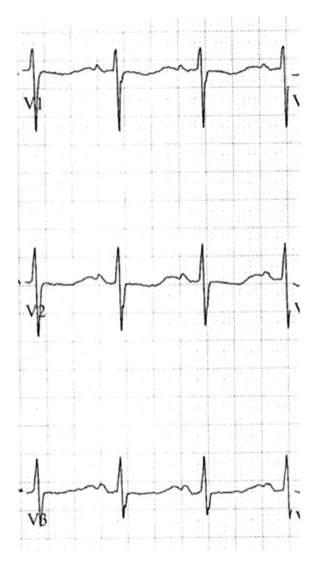

Figure 2.23 Long QT interval

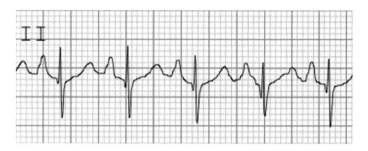

FIGURE 2.24 Right atrial enlargement – manifested by tall p-waves

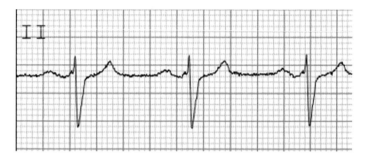

FIGURE 2.25 Left atrial enlargement – manifested by broad p-waves

The p-waves represent atrial electrical depolarization. Tall and/or broad p-waves suggest that there is likely increased atrial mass. Since the atria do not typically hypertrophy, this increased p-wave size represents increased volume. An important point to keep in mind is that right atrial activity is reflected in the initial portions of the p-wave, while left atrial activity is reflected in the terminal portions. Right atrial enlargement appears as p-waves that are >2.5 mm high in Lead II as shown in Fig. 2.24. Left atrial enlargement is seen as broad p-wave that are >120 ms in duration in Lead II and a negative deflection in the terminal portion of the p-wave in V1 that is >0.04 s wide and 1 mm deep (or 1 small box wide by 1 small box deep) as shown in Fig. 2.25.

To evaluate the PR segment, a baseline of the ECG must be established. By convention, this is the segment between the end

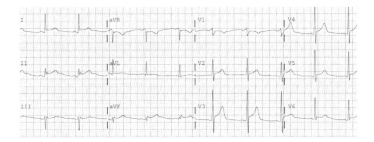

FIGURE 2.26 Pericarditis: PR depression and diffuse ST segment elevation

of the t-wave and the beginning of the p-wave. The PR segment is assessed by comparing the height of this portion to the height of the T-P segment. PR segment depression below this baseline occurs in conditions such as pericarditis as shown in Fig. 2.26.

The QRS complex is then evaluated for changes. One of the most common changes is left ventricular hypertrophy (LVH), which often occurs following years of hypertension. There are numerous ECG criteria for LVH but the most common ones to remember include the Cornell and Sokolow Lyon Criteria (Fig. 2.27). Other conditions can affect the QRS morphology including myocardial infarctions, accessory pathways in Wolff–Parkinson–White (WPW) syndrome and Brugada syndrome. WPW and Brugada syndrome will be discussed in the next chapter, Arrhythmias. As for myocardial infarctions, when a transmural (complete wall thickness) infarction occurs, q-waves can develop. Small q-waves are commonly seen, but significant and pathologic q-waves consistent with prior transmural myocardial infarctions are typically at least 0.04 s wide and 1 mm deep (i.e. a small box wide and a small box deep), or at least 1/3 the height of the QRS complex. In addition, the q-waves must be seen in at least two contiguous leads to be deemed significant. An inferior myocardial infarction manifests as q-waves in the inferior leads (Leads II, III, and AVF) as shown in Fig. 2.28. An anterior myocardial infarction will have q-waves in the anterior leads, V1-V6 (Fig. 2.29). Lateral myocardial infarctions will

LVH

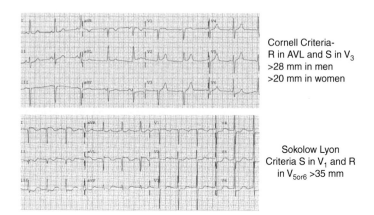

Cornell Criteria-
R in AVL and S in V$_3$
>28 mm in men
>20 mm in women

Sokolow Lyon
Criteria S in V$_1$ and R
in V$_{5or6}$ >35 mm

FIGURE 2.27 Left ventricular hypertrophy

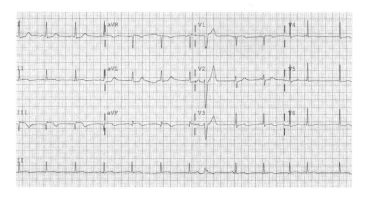

FIGURE 2.28 Inferior myocardial infarction

have q-waves in leads I and AVL (Fig. 2.30). A posterior infarct is more difficult to diagnose but can present with large R waves in Leads V1 and V2. Often, posterior wall infarcts are associated with inferior wall infarcts. Thus, q-waves in the inferior leads help diagnose a posterior wall infarct as opposed to other causes of large R waves in V1 and V2 (Fig. 2.31).

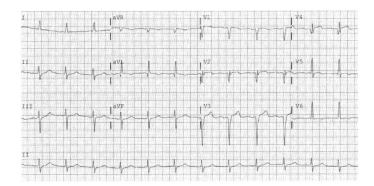

FIGURE 2.29 Anterior myocardial infarction

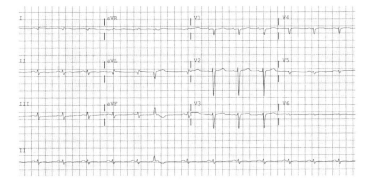

FIGURE 2.30 Lateral myocardial infarction

The next waveform to evaluate is the ST-segment. This segment is important because it shows repolarization abnormalities that can result from ischemia (inadequate blood flow to the cardiac tissue to meet the metabolic demands of the cells) or injury (inadequate blood flow to the cardiac tissue now causing cellular death), pericarditis, or electrolyte derangements. Myocardial injury is strongly suspected when there is ST-elevation in specific patterns, such as the inferior, anterior, lateral or posterior leads (Fig. 2.32). "Reciprocal changes" can be seen in leads opposite of the ST segment elevation. For example, "reciprocal changes" associated with

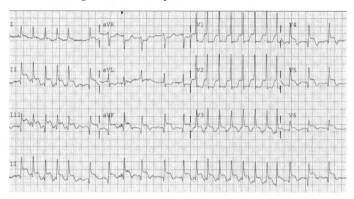

FIGURE 2.31 Posterior myocardial infarction

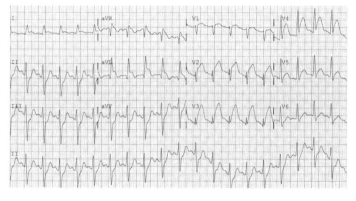

FIGURE 2.32 Acute anterior ST segment myocardial infarction – ST elevation in precordial leads and ST depression in the inferior leads (also known as reciprocal changes)

an anterior ST-segment elevation, can be seen as ST-depressions in the inferior leads, which is also shown in Fig. 2.32. When ST-depressions without ST-elevations in those same specific patterns occur, myocardial ischemia (and not necessarily injury yet) can be occurring (Fig. 2.33). Diffuse ST elevation is suggestive of pericarditis (Fig. 2.26) or electrolyte abnormalities in some cases.

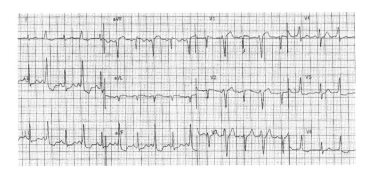

FIGURE 2.33 Inferior ST depressions

Lastly, the t-waves and u-waves can be evaluated. These tend to be less specific, but if focal t-wave inversions are seen in specific lead patterns, myocardial ischemia should be considered. Prominent u-waves can be seen in electrolyte disturbances.

Long-Term Monitoring

12-lead ECGs provide a momentary snapshot of the heart's electrical activity, but are not the only type of ECGs that can be obtained. Patients who have intermittent episodes of palpitations, syncope or near-syncope require longer periods of monitoring. In these scenarios, the patient is usually feeling fine during the office visit and the potential arrhythmia is not evident in the office 12-lead ECG. To address this, ambulatory monitoring ECGs have been developed. These ECGs can be worn for periods of up to 30 days, increasing the likelihood that an abnormal heart rhythm is captured. These include Holter monitors, event monitors and implantable loop recorders.

Holter monitors, which are named after the person that invented them, are designed to provide 24–48 hours of continuous ECG recording. Typically up to five wires are attached to the patient, similar to in-hospital telemetry monitoring, and these wires insert into a recording device that is clipped to the belt or placed in a pocket. The monitor continuously records the electrical activity of the heart for the specified 24- or 48-h period. Patients are not permitted to shower during this time. At the end of the 24 or 48 h, the Holter monitor is returned where the data is downloaded. Computer software initially analyzes the data, calculating average heart beats, the fastest and slowest heart rates, and identifies potential arrhythmias that may have occurred. Technicians then review this data and confirm or deny these arrhythmias. A report is generated and sent to the physician's office. An example of a typical tracing is shown in Fig. 2.34.

If the Holter monitor does not capture the arrhythmia or the arrhythmia is occurring infrequently but at least once monthly, an event monitor can be ordered. There are two types of event monitors: continuous looping (i.e. pre-symptom) and non-looping (post-symptom) event monitors. A continuous looping event monitor is an ECG that is worn for an entire month. Typically, two wires are attached to the patient's chest and inserted into a recording device that is attached to the belt or inserted into a pocket. These monitors continuously record the electrical activity of the heart. However, storing every heart beat for an entire month would require a significant amount of memory. Thus, the event monitor is also continuously recording new data over the old data. At the onset of symptoms, the patient presses the record button and the device stores the electrical activity present immediately prior to pressing the record button (generally up to 60 s before) and records the next 30–60 s. These events are stored in the recording device and can be transmitted over standard telephone wires or wirelessly via a cell phone. Event monitors can also be programmed to auto-detect abnormal heart rhythms. Generally, these are programmed to automatically record either very fast or very slow heart rates and do not require the patient to press the record button. This feature is particularly useful when patients are unable to press the button in the event they lose consciousness.

Non-looping monitors are intended for patients that have symptoms lasting longer than 30–45 seconds and remain conscious. The greatest advantage of non-looping monitors is

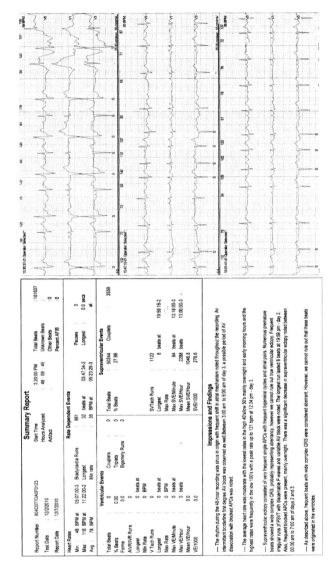

Figure 2.34 Holter monitor report

that they do not require electrodes to be attached to the patient. Rather, the patient holds the device against the chest wall and presses the record button at the onset of symptoms. The device then records 30 s of realtime ECG. The disadvantage of this device is that it cannot go back in time and capture the onset of the abnormal heart rhythm, which can often be useful in determining the type of arrhythmia present. These events are stored and can be transmitted to the event monitoring center for analysis.

Should the potential arrhythmia not occur while wearing the event monitor for a month, an implantable loop recorder can be placed. A loop recorder is the size of a "thumb" drive that is implanted under skin of the chest overlying the heart with a minor, outpatient surgical procedure. The loop recorder then continuously monitors the electrical activity of the heart. These devices are programmed to auto-detect heart rhythms that are abnormally fast or slow and can be triggered by the patient to record when symptoms occur. The patient activates the monitor to record by placing a device the size of a garage door opener over the loop monitor on the chest and pressing the record button. The loop monitor stores an ECG of the heart's electrical activity that was present several seconds before the record button is pressed and several seconds after. These devices are periodically checked, either remotely by transmitting the data over a telephone line, or by checking the device in a doctor's office. The battery on current loop monitors lasts up to 3 years. Thus, these devices are intended to provide long-term monitoring to capture abnormal heart rhythms that occur less frequently than monthly and will record abnormal heart rhythms even when a patient loses consciousness.

Other Forms of an ECG: Signal-averaged ECG

A signal-averaged ECG is a special type of ECG which averages multiple electrical signals from the heart to look for very small changes in the QRS complex. Patients who have signal-averaged ECGs must lie very still for up to 15 min because skeletal muscle contractions and movement can create noise. During this time, a continuous 12-lead ECG is recorded. Computer software then analyzes the rhythm strips and creates an average ECG appearance. By examining many QRS complexes, artifact from muscle movement can be filtered out and fine details on the ECG that persist throughout the entire recording become more apparent. At times, very low amplitude, high-frequency signals can be seen in the terminal portion of the QRS complexes, which are known as "late potentials." These "late potentials" reflect electrical abnormalities within the ventricles and may reflect an increased risk of developing life-threatening arrhythmias. Therefore, this type of ECG is performed in patients who are undergoing further risk assessment for sudden cardiac death. An example of a signal average ECG is shown in Fig. 2.35.

Electrophysiology Study

An electrophysiology study (EPS) is a procedure done by specialized cardiologists known as electrophysiologists, to help identify and potentially treat rhythm disturbances of the heart. The test is usually ordered by an electrophysiologist when work-up for an arrhythmia has not been clearly identified by ambulatory ECGs or when there is suspicion of an arrhythmia that can be treated by an ablation. An EPS typically involves bringing the patient into the cardiac catheterization lab where the patient is connected to external ECG machines. Then, usually two to four catheters are placed into the heart through sheaths placed in the femoral vein. These catheters are about the diameter of a coffee straw but much longer and more flexible. At the end of the catheters, there are smooth, round metal electrodes which can sense the electrical activity of the heart. Usually, various measurements are made to assess the intrinsic conduction properties of the heart. If an arrhythmia is not present initially, the heart is stimulated by pacing the heart (using the same catheters) at various rates and introducing premature beats in an attempt to induce an arrhythmia. If this

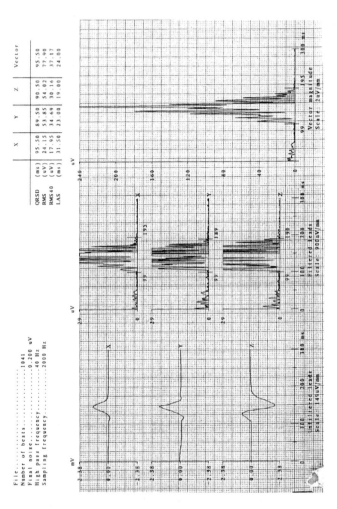

FIGURE 2.35 Signal average ECG

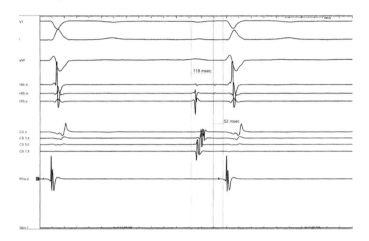

FIGURE 2.36 EPS example of sinus rhythm

does not bring out the arrhythmia, drugs that make the heart more excitable, such as isoproteronol, are administered. These procedures are usually performed with conscious sedation. Rarely, general anesthesia is implemented. Both slow and fast heart rhythm disorders can be detected by an EP study and can guide management of the arrhythmia, including the need for a pacemaker or an implantable cardioverter defibrillator (ICD). Often, an EP study identifies an abnormal heart rhythm that can be cured by ablation. An example of normal sinus rhythm seen on an EPS is shown in Fig. 2.36.

An ablation procedure is carried out by placing an ablation catheter at the site of origin of an arrhythmia. The goal of ablation is focal destruction of the offending heart tissue that is causing the arrhythmia. Ablation can occur by a variety of methods but primarily involves either heating or freezing the tissue so the heart cells will no longer conduct electrical signals. To heat the tissue, the catheter tip is designed to deliver radio frequency (RF) energy. The heart tissue absorbs this RF energy causing it to heat up and be irreversibly damaged. The damaged tissue is eventually replaced by scar, which is electrically inactive. Alternatively, cryotherapy can be applied through a specialized catheter which freezes the heart tissue around the area of the catheter tip, thereby destroying the tissue. A scar forms at this site of ablation as well. Most commonly, RF energy is used because the ablation can penetrate more deeply and is associated with better long-term success rates. Alternatively, cryotherapy is often used in higher risk situations such as AV re-entrant tachycardia where the pathologic pathway is very close to the normal electrical system. This technique allows the creation of precise lesions safely without damaging the AV node.

Conclusion

After the physical exam, an ECG is the most common method to evaluate the heart. To accurately "read" ECGs, use the same method each time. If further evaluation or treatment of a rhythm problem is deemed necessary, longer-term ECGs can be ordered or an electrophysiology study can be performed. Refer to the texts listed below for further information regarding the interpretation of ECGs.

Further Reading

For the beginner – Dubin D. Rapid Interpretation of EKG's. 6th ed. Tampa: COVER Publishing Company; 2000.

For the intermediate reader – O'Keefe J. The Complete Guide to ECG's. 3rd ed. Sudbury: Physicians' Press; 2008.

For the advanced reader – Wagner G. Marriott's Practical Electrocardiography. 10th ed. Philadelphia: Lippincott Williams & Wilkins; 2001.

For reference – Surawicz B, Knilans T. Chou's Electrocardiography in Clinical Practice. 6th ed. Philadelphia: Saunders Elsevier; 2008.

For reference – Vereckei et al. New Algorithm Using Only Lead AVR for Differential Diagnosis of Wide QRS Complex Tachycardia. Heart Rhythm. 2008;5:89–98.

For reference – Brugada et al. A New Approach to the Differential Diagnosis of a Regular Tachycardia with a Wide QRS Complex. Circulation. 1991;83:1649–59.

For practice at the intermediate and above level – Marriott HJL. Challenging ECGs. Philadelphia: Hanley & Belfus, Inc.; 2002.

For online practice at all levels – www.ekgstar.com.

Chapter 3
Cardiac Imaging

Harry E. McCrea and Michael W. Fong

The purpose of this chapter is to familiarize practitioners with the resting imaging modalities available to assess the heart. A brief technical overview of each modality will be included, but the main focus will be on the clinical indications and implications of each test. A few "pearls" will be incorporated throughout the chapter to help orient practitioners to the cardiologist's view of these tests.

Transthoracic and Transesophageal Echocardiography (TTE/TEE)

Overview

The field of echocardiography has undergone tremendous changes in the last two decades and continues to evolve at a high rate. It is likely that in 10 years the field will be virtually

H.E. McCrea (✉)
Division of Cardiology, University of Rochester Medical Center, Rochester, NY, USA
e-mail: harry_mccrea@urmc.rochester.edu

M.W. Fong
Division of Cardiology, University of Southern California, Los Angeles, CA, USA

J.D. Bisognano et al. (eds.), *Manual of Outpatient Cardiology*, 51
DOI 10.1007/978-0-85729-944-4_3,
© Springer-Verlag London Limited 2012

unrecognizable to practitioners who have not kept abreast of these changes. Additionally, the simplicity of concept behind echocardiography belies the immensely complicated technical challenges of obtaining and interpreting images.

Echocardiography relies on the Doppler effect to obtain structural and hemodynamic information. Each ultrasound transducer has tiny crystals that emit radio frequencies which are reflected by tissue bone and blood. These reflected sound waves return with different velocities and wavelengths depending on the medium of interaction. This information is then turned into visual representations of either blood flow velocity or two-dimensional gray-scale pictures. Because sound waves travel in a uniform fashion with little refraction in water, echocardiography is ideally suited for imaging heart tissue, which is mostly comprised of water. However, air, calcium and metal cause refraction, scatter and absorption of sound waves which pose technical challenges when imaging, and are particularly problematic in patients with COPD, calcific valvular disease and metallic prosthetic heart valves.

Patient size may also have an impact on image quality. Imaging can be difficult in patients with more subcutaneous tissue; however the assumption that thin patients are easy to image is a common misconception. It can often be more difficult, or even impossible, to obtain adequate images in a small, thin patient where there is very little room between rib spaces. Frequently, cardiologists refer to patients with these types of imaging impediments as having "poor acoustic windows". Ultimately, each patient is different and until imaging is actually attempted, one does not know if "good windows" exist.

Since the heart is a three-dimensional structure displayed in two dimensions, multiple views or "windows" are needed to create a complete picture. Traditionally, the heart is viewed from the parasternal, apical and sub-xiphoid locations, and the arch of the aorta can be viewed from the suprasternal location (Figs. 3.1–3.7 represent the typical TTE windows and some of the common 2-D images obtained). Because all of these views are necessary for a complete study, patients

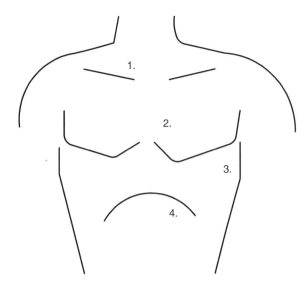

FIGURE 3.1 Location of common sites for echocardiographic evaluation. *1.* Suprasternal. *2.* Parasternal. *3.* Apical. *4.* Sub-xiphoid

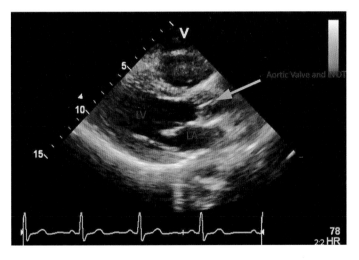

FIGURE 3.2 Long axis view from the parasternal window

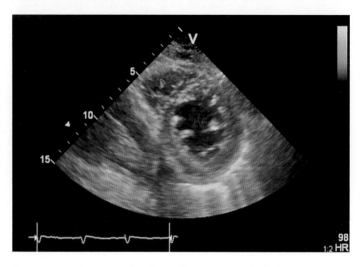

FIGURE 3.3 Short axis view from the parasternal window

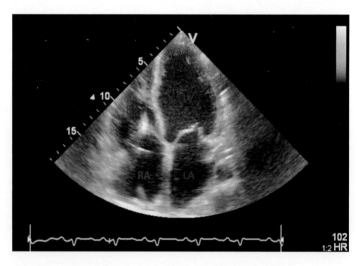

FIGURE 3.4 Four chamber view from the apical window

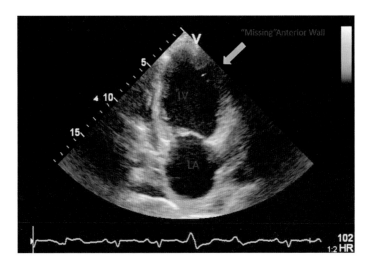

FIGURE 3.5 Two chamber view from the apical window. Note the "dropout" of the anterior wall. This artifact makes it appear as that anterior wall is "missing". In fact, the wall exists but is just not visualized. This is an example of suboptimal imaging which may result in an inconclusive study

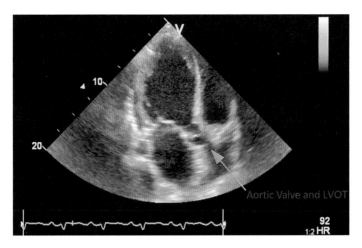

FIGURE 3.6 Three chamber view from the apical window

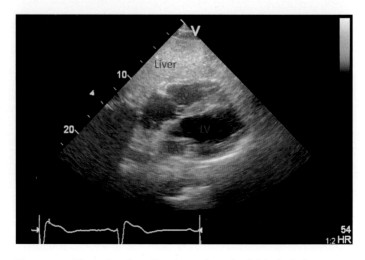

FIGURE 3.7 Four chamber view from the sub-xiphiod window

whose hearts are positioned abnormally in the thoracic cavity (e.g. vertical orientation in a COPD patient) may not be well visualized in all views. In such cases, it may not be possible to accurately assess for wall motion or valvular abnormalities. Additionally, accurate measurement of blood flow velocity as it relates to the calculation of valve area, regurgitant fraction and pressure may be impaired, since it relies on proper orientation and parallel alignment of the ultrasound beam to the flow of blood.

Given all of these limitations, it is somewhat of a challenge to obtain a complete and thorough study on every patient. If the study interpreter has incomplete clinical information regarding the patient, it may be difficult to know which information is important to the requester Therefore, it is of paramount importance for the ordering provider to have a specific question in mind, and clearly indicate the reason for the exam.

Many of the limitations seen with TTE can be overcome by performing transesophageal imaging. With TEE, the probe is placed in the esophagus of the patient and advanced to the level of the base of the heart. Because there is no subcutaneous tissue, ribs or lung tissue to obscure the views, image quality is often better. However, it is important to remember that TEE is an invasive procedure, and patients typically require moderate sedation. Any patient with a marginal respiratory status will likely not be a candidate for TEE. Patients with esophageal pathology such as stricture are also not good candidates for TEE due to the risk of perforation and bleeding. Patients with loose teeth may also be too high risk given the possibility of tooth dislodgement and aspiration. In the end, the risks of sedation, bleeding, infection and perforation must be weighed against the potential benefits of TEE in each patient. Often times, TTE may provide adequate imaging to answer the clinical question. Indeed, there are few situations where TTE should not be attempted first before referral for TEE. Finally, the time requirement, staffing requirements and cost-effectiveness can limit the overall availability of TEE.

Regardless of whether a TEE or TTE is ordered, the amount of information that can be obtained is usually extensive. While every institution is different with regards to what is routinely reported, Table 3.1 represents what may be expected/requested from a particular study.

Tables 3.2 and 3.3 represent considerations practioners should keep in mind when ordering both TTE and TEE.

Common Indications for Testing

While understanding the limitations and technical considerations of echocardiography is important, understanding when to order a study and how to interpret the results is even more important. While every indication cannot be mentioned here, the most important question remains "How will this test change my management of this patient?" Often the answer to this question reveals whether or not imaging is indicated. Finally, complete guidelines regarding the indications for echocardiographic assessment can be found on the American Heart Association website.

Table 3.1 Typical information derived from echocardiography

LV ejection fraction
RV function
Wall motion
LV/RV cavity size, mass, presence of hypertrophy
Atrial size and function
Intra-cardiac mass/clot
Valvular regurgitation/stenosis
Valve area
Valvular masses/vegetations/abscess
Pericardial effusion/thickening
Proximal aorta size/coarctation/dissection
Diastolic function
Constriction/restriction assessment
Size of IVC/respiratory variation
PA pressure/pulmonary hypertension
PFO/ASD/VSD
Cardiac output

Table 3.2 Considerations when ordering TTE

Can the heart be viewed from multiple positions on the chest wall?
Is the patient able to be rolled to the left side?
Does the patient have severe COPD?
Is the primary test indication evaluation of a structure at the base of the heart?
Is the primary test indication evaluation of intracardiac thrombus?
Does the patient have an unusual body habitus (i.e. morbidly obese or extremely petite)?

These questions may help the practitioner anticipate the need for supplemental imaging

TABLE 3.3 Considerations when ordering TEE

Can the patient lay flat without shortness of breath?
Does the patient have a history of esophageal pathology?
Does the patient have a history of difficulty swallowing?
Does the patient have sleep apnea?
Is the patient hypotensive at baseline?
Does the patient have loose or broken teeth?
Can the information be obtained with TTE?

These questions should be answered prior to ordering a TEE with the understanding that an affirmative answer may preclude TEE testing

Murmurs and Valvular Abnormalities

The evaluation of a cardiac murmur is one of the most common indications for echocardiography in the outpatient setting. Currently, recommendations underscore the importance of symptoms and auscultation in determining whom to image. Any patient with cardiopulmonary symptoms needs to be imaged. Asymptomatic patients should be referred if the murmur has characteristics making it at least a moderate probability of representing structural heart disease. Typically, soft murmurs without any other characteristics such as thrills, in young, healthy subjects should not be imaged.

Once valvular stenosis/regurgitation has been identified and imaged, the next issue that arises is how to follow the lesion. Any change/new symptom should immediately prompt referral for repeat imaging. Otherwise, any valvular abnormality classified as moderate or severe should be routinely imaged to assess for changes in the structure and function of the heart. The frequency of imaging can vary from every 3 months for severe lesions to every 3–5 years for stable, moderate lesions. Lesions deemed mild should not be routinely evaluated. Only if there is a change in symptoms or in physical exam should these patients be re-referred for imaging.

Patients who have undergone treatment or will be undergoing treatment for a stenosed or regurgitant valve represent a special population. TEE is strongly recommended for any patient being considered for valve replacement/repair. It is of the utmost importance to provide the surgeon with as much information as possible to help plan the surgery/repair. For instance, understanding the mechanism and identifying the involved segments of mitral regurgitation is needed to decide whether repair or replacement is most appropriate. Furthermore, any aortic valve lesion should have excellent imaging of the ascending aorta to help decide whether concomitant aortic arch replacement (Bentall procedure) needs to be performed. Often adequate imaging cannot be obtained using TTE. Right-sided valvular lesions, in particular, are difficult to completely image with TTE and so TEE is often needed to provide the most complete information. Once a valve has been replaced, immediate post-operative imaging should be obtained to assess the quality of the repair/replacement. Thereafter, imaging should be obtained when there is a change in either physical exam or symptoms. Additionally, when a bio-prosthetic valve nears its life expectancy, routine imaging can be instituted to detect early signs of failure.

Syncope and Arrhythmia

Patients with syncope should usually be imaged with TTE unless other testing has delineated the cause of the syncope. However, patients with classic neurogenic syncope and those without suspected cardiac disease need not be imaged. Similarly, any patient with a newly documented arrhythmia should have a TTE to evaluate for the presence of structural heart disease. Isolated ventricular premature complexes do not represent an arrhythmia and should only prompt imaging if seen in association with syncope, or when there is a suspicion of underlying heart disease. Also, patients with palpitations but no documented arrhythmia or other cardiac signs/symptoms should not be routinely imaged.

Patients with a diagnosis of atrial fibrillation/flutter being considered for non-emergent direct current cardioversion (DCCV) may need to have the diagnosis of intracardiac thrombus excluded prior to cardioversion. The most appropriate test for this is TEE. If a patient has mitral valve disease or hypertrophic cardiomyopathy, TEE prior to DCCV should be considered even if adequate, long-term anticoagulation has been documented because of the increased risk of thrombus formation in these diseases. Patients without hypertrophic obstructive cardiomyopathy (HOCM) or mitral valve disease who have been on adequate long-term anticoagulation do not need TEE prior to DCCV. Patients not on anti-coagulation but whose arrhythmia onset was within the last 48 h may or may not be imaged. No good randomized data exists to support either strategy and expert concensus opinion is mixed.

Cerebrovascular and Cardiovascular Ischemia

In general, any patient with a vascular event involving arterial occlusion thought to be of embolic origin should have a TEE performed. However, if the results of the test will not alter the course of diagnosis or treatment, then one should forego testing. TTE testing is reasonable for patients who have had neurologic events of unclear etiology or with known cerebrovascular disease. Saline contrast imaging ("bubble study") should be ordered to assess for patent foramen ovale (PFO)/atrial septal defect (ASD). Patients with suspected thoracic aortic pathology such as dissection, aneurysm and rupture should also undergo testing. TEE is usually the more valuable and appropriate test in this setting. TTE can be utilized for following aortic root dilatation and screening of first-degree relatives of patients with Marfan's syndrome or other connective tissue syndromes.

Patients presenting with signs/symptoms concerning for myocardial ischemia can undergo TTE if other testing such as ECG and cardiac biomarkers are indeterminate. In this situation, testing is ideally done during episodes of chest pain and/or immediately after resolution of symptoms to look for segmental wall motion abnormalities. TTE should also be performed in any patient diagnosed with myocardial infarction (MI) who has not had any other assessment of left ventricular (LV) function. Immediate bedside echocardiography should be performed on any patient with recent MI in whom mechanical complication such as ventricular septal defect (VSD), papillary muscle rupture, etc. is suspected. Figures 3.8–3.12 demonstrate coronary artery distributions as seen with standard TTE imaging.

Cardiomyopathy

Any patient with new onset heart failure or dyspnea that may be cardiac in origin should also undergo TTE assessment. Patients with known cardiomyopathy should be re-imaged only if a change is suspected, or the findings will alter management. Patients with a left ventricular ejection fraction (LVEF) less than 35% despite appropriate medical

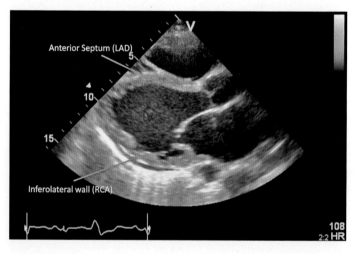

FIGURE 3.8 Parasternal long axis anatomy and coronary artery distributions

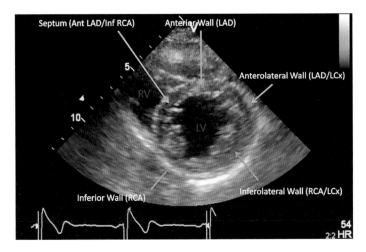

FIGURE 3.9 Parasternal short axis anatomy and coronary artery distributions

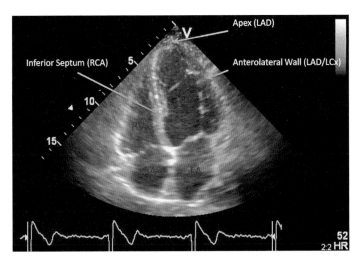

FIGURE 3.10 Apical four chamber anatomy and coronary artery distributions

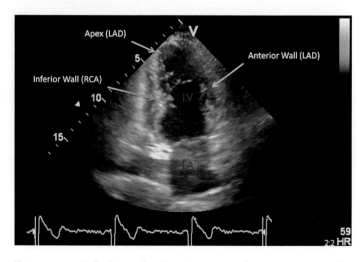

FIGURE 3.11 Apical two chamber anatomy and coronary artery distributions

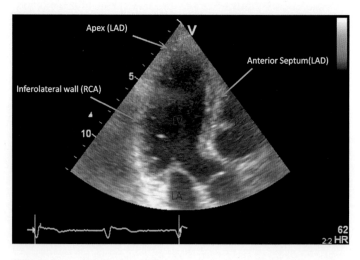

FIGURE 3.12 Apical three chamber anatomy and coronary artery distributions

therapy and/or revascularization may be candidates for AICD placement. Therefore, repeat imaging to assess the response to medical treatment and/or revascularization may be warranted. Additionally, in patients with preserved LVEF, TTE can be useful in helping to determine if dyspnea and chest pain are due to diastolic heart failure. Analysis of mitral inflow and mitral annular motion patterns can be used to help determine the presence and extent of diastolic dysfunction. Two particular populations deserve special mention: young athletes and cancer patients. While there has been appropriate media attention regarding the death of young athletes, the routine screening of young athletes for the presence of HOCM with echocardiography is not indicated in the absence of clinical cardiac disease. These recommendations are based on disease prevalence and cost-effectiveness studies. However, routine assessment of LV function is indicated in patients undergoing therapy with cardiotoxic drugs such as anthracyclines. Degradation of cardiac function in this setting has a profound impact on therapy as dosing may be limited or treatment may be altogether discontinued.

In suspected cases of infiltrative heart disease, or when trying to distinguish between ischemic and nonischemic cardiomyopathy, patients should be referred for more definitive imaging with cardiac magnetic resonance imaging (CMR).

Endocarditis

Regarding the diagnosis of endocarditis, it should be noted that the Duke Criteria forms the foundation for recommendations regarding utilization of echocardiography. As such, it is to be emphasized that endocarditis is a clinical diagnosis with echocardiography being only one component. TEE is not indicated in cases of fever without bacteremia and pathological murmur. In all cases of suspected native valve endocarditis, the initial study should be TTE. Often times, valves are imaged with enough clarity by TTE and invasive assessment with TEE is not needed.

TEE should be reserved for patients with suspected complications such as abscess or shunt, patients in whom there is a strong suspicion of culture negative endocarditis, patients with accompanying complex congenital heart disease, and patients in whom adequate imaging cannot be obtained. Patients with prosthetic heart valves represent a special population and should be treated as such. Because of the initial higher index of suspicion, only patients without bacteremia and a new murmur in the setting of transient fever should forego testing. All others should be referred for imaging with serious consideration given to TEE imaging as the initial test of choice.

Tamponade and Hypoxemia

Concern for cardiac tamponade should prompt urgent, bedside TTE imaging. Often times, "pre-tamponade" physiology can be seen before the typical, emergent clinical findings of hemodynamic compromise are present. Once the diagnosis of pericardial effusion is made, TTE can be used to routinely assess for the development of pre-tamponade physiology and also to guide pericardiocentesis. Post-pericardiocentesis imaging can be performed to assess for re-accumulation and the development of early constriction.

Patients with a variety of pulmonary issues are appropriate for echocardiography. Patients with pulmonary embolism can have TTE imaging performed to assess for right ventricular (RV) strain as part of the decision process to administer thrombolytic therapy. COPD patients can be assessed for the development of cor pulmonale and pulmonary hypertension with TTE. Certainly, unexplained hypoxia should prompt consideration of cardiac shunting and referral for TTE with saline contrast imaging.

Congenital Heart Disease

Patients with simple congenital heart disease such as ASD, PFO or VSD can usually be followed clinically. However, a change in physical exam or new onset symptoms should

TABLE 3.4 "Simple" congenital heart disease

ASD
VSD
Bicuspid AV
Coarctation of the aorta
Patent ductus arteriosus

TABLE 3.5 Complex congenital heart disease

Tetralogy of fallot
Eisenmenger's syndrome
Transposition of the great arteries
Ebstein's anomaly
Single ventricle
Pulmonary atresia

prompt referral for repeat imaging. Patients with complex congenital heart disease need more frequent monitoring and also should be imaged by specialists with expertise in the field. This often means annual referral to a more specialized center. Increasingly, adults with repaired congenital heart disease are being seen. It is important to remember that "repaired" congenital heart disease is not synonymous with "fixed". All congenital repairs are considered palliative. As such, these patients are expected to develop further cardiovascular complications. Annual imaging should be strongly considered for those patients with complicated repairs while simple repairs, such as PFO closure, can be followed every several years or if there has been a clinical change. Table 3.4 represents "simple" congenital heart defects which may be routinely followed by a general cardiologist while Table 3.5 lists more "complex" congenital heart defects that should have annual imaging performed at a center with special expertise.

Study Interpretation

The amount of data that can be obtained from a single echocardiographic study is overwhelming. Data regarding hemodynamics, structure and function make a complete overview of echo interpretation unrealistic for this text. Instead, the focus has been understanding some of the frequent terminology one may see in a report as well as some key numbers of which referring providers should be aware. Finally, because echo is one of the most frequently ordered cardiac test, a few pearls have been included to help referring providers better understand results.

One of the most common diagnoses a referring provider runs across is "hypertrophy". In the world of cardiology, not all hypertrophy is equal. Concentric hypertrophy refers to an increase in LV mass without a concomitant increase in the radius of the ventricle. This is seen in chronic pressure overload and often leads to diastolic dysfunction. This is different from eccentric hypertrophy which refers to an increase in both LV mass and chamber size as is seen in volume and pressure overload states. Eccentric hypertrophy can be seen in athlete's heart and systolic heart failure. Hypertrophy often leads to diastolic dysfunction. This disease has been divided into four classes representing a continuum of disease severity with class I diastolic dysfunction representing mild dysfunction, and class IV dysfunction representing severe disease. Unfortunately, there is very little data to help guide treatment, and certainly no recommendations exist regarding treatment based on the severity of disease.

Another common diagnosis is valvular sclerosis. Valvular sclerosis should not be confused with stenosis. Sclerosis refers to valvular thickening which is often associated with the normal aging process whereas stenosis refers to a decrease in valvular area. Finally, pericardial effusions are frequently seen. The determining factor in the development of tamponade is the time course over which the effusion accumulated. Tamponade physiology refers to the following findings: diastolic RV collapse, lack of respiratory variation of the inferior

TABLE 3.6 Echocardiography by the numbers

Abnormality being evaluated	Numbers to remember	Implication
Aortic stenosis	Valve area < 1.0 cm²	Severe AS – consider stress test if asymptomatic; surgery if symptomatic
Aortic regurgitation (chronic)	LVEF < 50% EDD > 7.5 cm ESD > 5.5 cm	Refer for valvular replacement
Mitral stenosis	Valve area < 1.5 cm² PASP > 50 mmHg	Consider further evaluation
Mitral regurgitation (chronic)	LVEF < 60% ESD > 4.0 cm	Refer for valvular repair or surgery
Dilated ascending aorta	Diameter > 5.0 cm	Surgical referral
Cardiomyopathy	LVEF < 35%	Possible AICD candidate

EDD end-diastolic diameter, *ESD* end-systolic diameter, *PAP* pulmonary artery systolic pressure

vena cava (IVC) and respiratory flow variation across the mitral valve. Many times these features will be seen before the actual development of hemodynamic compromise and should alert the provider for the need for pericardiocentesis.

While the results of each study must always be interpreted in the context of the clinical setting, there are several numbers and measurements that represent "significant" findings of which the general practitioner should be aware. These numbers should prompt the provider to refer the patient on for an intervention in some instances, or increase the frequency of follow up as patients approach the need for intervention. Table 3.6 summarizes these key numbers and what they may mean for your patient.

Finally, a few pearls that may help guide you along the way. An echocardiogram is a snapshot in time. Therefore, a wall motion abnormality may be old or new and one should not presume that this is a presentation of ACS. Furthermore, coronary anatomy varies and so inferior wall hypokinesis may be described as a right coronary artery/left circumflex (RCA/LCx) distribution abnormality. This reflects the fact that some people are right dominant and some are left dominant when it comes to the origin of the posterior descending artery (PDA). Additionally, the lateral wall can be supplied by either diagonal branches of the left anterior descending artery (LAD) or obtuse marginal branches from the LCx. Echocardiography is not suited to defining these specific anatomical structures. Similarly, a positive saline contrast study or "bubble" study often cannot define the abnormality using TTE alone. TTE reports often read "Positive for atrial level shunting" indicating this may be an ASD or a PFO. Further imaging, usually with TEE, is often needed to determine the diagnosis. However, given the risks associated with TEE, it is important to define how management will be changed before referral. Other anatomy which is often difficult to define by TTE are the RV and right ventricular outflow tract (RVOT). If right-sided information is critical to patient management consider TEE or CMR. However, a "D-sign" on TTE imaging reflects septal flattening which may be seen in cases of right-sided volume/pressure overload.

It is also important to remember that echocardiography produces gray-scale images. These pictures cannot tell whether a valvular mass is a vegetation, thrombus or other material, or whether an intracavitary mass is tumor or thrombus. Finally, assessment of LVEF is one of the most common indications listed by referring providers. It is important to remember a depressed LVEF is part of the normal physiologic response to sepsis. Therefore, utilizing echo to differentiate septic shock and acute cardiogenic shock is generally not helpful in the absence of MI. If the diagnosis is truly in doubt, a pulmonary artery catheter is more likely to provide the answer. Additionally, once a cardiomyopathy has been diagnosed there is little benefit in knowing if the ventricular function has dropped from 25% to 15%. Mortality remains unchanged, and changes in management will continue to be dictated by clinical symptoms and guidelines. Certainly, if there is new concern for valvular regurgitation or other mechanical complications, repeat imaging is warranted. However, repeating an echo for each and every heart failure admission is not necessary.

Nuclear Imaging: Multiple Uptake Gated Acquistion (MUGA)

Overview

Nuclear imaging was the first non-invasive method for evaluating cardiac function. Since its advent in the early 1970s, the principles have remained the same but the development of computer technology for image analysis has allowed the field to continue to advance. At its core, nuclear imaging involves the injection of a radioactive isotope and then capture of the decaying gamma rays using a special camera. As gamma rays are emitted, some are absorbed, some are scattered and some travel along a straight line of emission. Cameras are equipped with special filters to accept only particles traveling along a straight line. This helps with localization of emitted particles. As each particle strikes the camera it is converted into an electrical signal that generates a picture. The recording of a single particle by the camera is referred to as a "count". To create an accurate image, hundreds of thousands of "counts" are usually required.

MUGA imaging requires a patient's blood to be tagged with a radioactive isotope (usually Technitium-99m). Typical, imaging only takes 10 min. The camera is "gated" meaning it is set to receive photons in equal time increments throughout the cardiac cycle. Over the 10 min of imaging, thousands of "counts" are placed into each time increment bin. At the end of the study, each time bin's counts are averaged and placed in their appropriate position during the cardiac cycle. This creates an image of the average counts seen during a single cardiac cycle. The ratio of counts at end-systole to end-diastole represents the ejection fraction.

Advantages/Disadvantages

The major advantage of MUGA imaging is that it is based on "counts". This is in contrast to echocardiography, which bases ejection fraction on volume changes. Volumetric measurements of a three-dimensional object with two-dimensional imaging require certain assumptions regarding the shape of the ventricles. When ventricles become dysmorphic, as in heart failure, these assumptions can result in errors. MUGA avoids these volumetric issues and is highly accurate regardless of the shape of the ventricle. Furthermore, it is particularly accurate the lower the ejection fraction. Finally, it is cheaper and quicker than CMR which some consider to be the gold standard for calculation of ejection fraction. Given these advantages, MUGA is ideally suited to certain niche clinical applications. However, there are some limitations worth noting. While LVEF can be accurately quantified, the right ventricular ejection fraction (RVEF) can be difficult to assess. The problem here results from the inability to adequately isolate the RV. Regardless of the plane of imaging, there is invariably another cardiac structure overlapping a portion of the RV. This leads to extra counts from the overlapping structure contributing to what is supposed to be the RV. A clinical technique known as "First Pass Imaging" can be applied to adequately assess the RV if needed, but this is beyond the scope of discussion in this text. Another major limitation regards patients with a significant amount of ectopy or irregular rhythms. Here the variable R-R intervals create problems with accurate gating and can result in inaccurate measurements.

Clinical Applications

The two most common applications of MUGA are qualification for AICD placement and monitoring cardiotoxic side effects of chemotherapy. Many times it can be difficult to accurately determine the LVEF in a patient with a cardiomyopathy who may qualify for AICD therapy. The structural changes that define cardiomyopathies cause the assumptions regarding the shape of the ventricle to be erroneous. Furthermore, there can be inter-observer and intra-observer variability regarding ejection fraction in echocardiographic interpretation. This makes determining who is eligible for an AICD challenging. Is the LVEF 35% (AICD) or 38% (No AICD)? MUGA's reliance on counts makes it much more accurate for LVEF determination in this setting. MUGA has also found a role in cancer patients receiving cardiotoxic chemotherapy. These patients require accurate LVEF calculation as guidelines have been created regarding the amount of chemotherapy a patient is eligible for based on cardiotoxic side effects. As patients' lives may depend on completing a course of chemotherapy, accurate measurement of the LVEF is absolutely necessary. Once again, MUGA is ideally suited to this task. Serial measurements throughout a patient's treatment can cheaply and easily be performed with excellent accuracy and reproducibility.

Study Interpretation

The interpretation of MUGA scans is mostly straight forward. The LVEF will be reported as will the RVEF. It is important to remember that the RVEF may not be entirely accurate and if this is the focus of the study first pass imaging or another imaging modality such as CMR should be considered. Any technical limitations such as motion artifact or arms down positioning will be noted in the text and should alert the referring physician that the validity of the results are in question. However, given the lengthy amount of time that a patient's blood cells remained tagged and the short imaging time if these artifacts are noted imaging can be immediately repeated to ensure an accurate data set.

Cardiac Magnetic Resonance Imaging (CMR)

Overview

The field of cardiac magnetic resonance imaging (CMR) was propelled in the early 2000s with the development of ultra fast, cardiac-gated imaging sequences capable of producing high-quality cine images with spatial resolution far superior to echocardiography or nuclear imaging with single-photon emission computerized tomography (SPECT) or positron emission tomography (PET). In addition, delayed contrast enhancement imaging was used to differentiate, with a high degree of accuracy, living myocardium from fibrosis and scar. This technology has revolutionized cardiac imaging and raised our diagnostic ability to previously unimagined heights.

The physics behind MRI are complex, and beyond the scope of this chapter. Basically, MRI produces images by using radiofrequency and strong magnetic gradients to alter the orientation and spin of hydrogen atoms within the body in a static magnetic field. Gadolinium contrast, when administered, is taken up into areas of fibrosis and can pass through ruptured myocardial membranes, but is unable to penetrate living myocardial cells. This allows tissue differentiation that would otherwise be indistinguishable. Particular imaging sequences can also be used to identify intramyocardial fat and detect edema within the myocardium, which can be helpful in making certain diagnoses such as arrhythmogenic right ventricular dysplasia and myocarditis (Fig. 3.13).

Common Uses and Indications

CMR has become the gold standard for the measurement of left and right ventricular ejection fraction. This is accomplished by the acquisition of stacks of gated cardiac images, which can be measured in the end systolic and diastolic frames using post-processing software. The velocity and quantity of blood flowing through various structures like the aorta and pulmonary artery can also be measured, and is useful in detecting intracardiac shunts and measuring the degree of valvular regurgitation. As with other areas of the body, contrast imaging is used for the purpose of angiography; however, unique to the heart, contrast imaging can also be used in the detection of stress induced ischemia, to

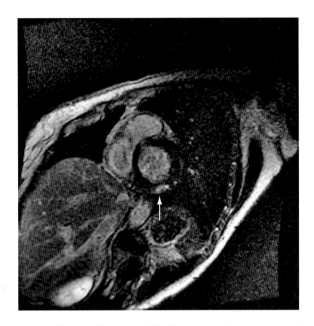

FIGURE 3.13 Short axis view of the heart showing an area of myocarditis (*arrow*) in the epicardium of the inferolateral wall of the left ventricle. Normal myocardium appears *black*

differentiate ischemic from nonischemic cardiomyopathy, and to determine extent of viability after myocardial infarction (Fig. 3.14). Edema imaging is useful in detecting myocardial inflammation, and can help identify areas at risk for further damage following acute myocardial infarction. Grid tagging can be done in the evaluation of pericardial constriction, and can also be used in the evaluation of myocardial strain. CMR can even be used to detect and quantify myocardial iron content which is useful in diseases associated with iron overload such as hemochromatosis. In this instance, the change in signal decay (known as T2*) can be followed to track disease severity and response to chelation therapy. Finally, CMR can be used to help sort out anatomy in complex congenital heart disease, and to detect and differentiate cardiac tumors from intracardiac thrombus.

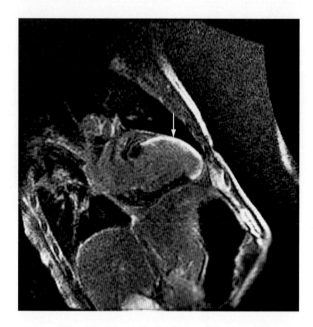

Figure 3.14 Two chamber view of the heart showing contrast enhanced transmural scar (*arrow*) of the anterior wall and apex of the left ventricle resulting from a proximal left anterior descending artery infarction. Viable myocardium appears *black*

Advantages and Disadvantages

While CMR offers more detailed imaging than echocardiography, SPECT, or PET, one must weigh the advantages of the information gleaned against the cost of the technology, its limited availability, and testing duration of often more than an hour. In addition, CMR can be difficult in patients with claustrophobia, is contraindicated in patients with ferromagnetic foreign bodies and implants, is challenging in patients with pacemakers and AICDs, and may be physically impossible in the morbidly obese. Because of the high temporal resolution needed to image fast moving structures such as heart valves, echocardiography is a more appropriate imaging modality than CMR in the evaluation of endocarditis and structural valvular abnormalities. CMR provides much of the same information as other imaging modalities, but does have the advantage of providing almost all of that information in a single test. In the detection of myocardial scar, CMR is the only technology that truly shows alive and dead myocardium and does not rely on surrogates of viability such as wall motion in echocardiography, thallium redistribution in SPECT, and metabolic activity in PET. Another distinct advantage of CMR is the ability to image in any plane. This provides views of the heart that cannot be obtained using other imaging modalities, and can be vital in certain instances such as the evaluation RV pathology, and in evaluating the relationship of extra cardiac structures or masses in relationship to the heart.

Study Interpretation

CMR is a complicated technology that requires interpretation by specially trained cardiologists and radiologists. It provides a multitude of objective measurements and data, but is also vulnerable to a degree of subjectivity due to imperfections caused by artifacts. Adequate breath holding is vital for a high quality exam, and patients who are unable to hold their breath repeatedly for periods up to 15 s, may not have adequate imaging. In rare instances where CMR is vital, exams can be performed under general anesthesia. Similar to MUGA, CMR relies on accurate cardiac gating to produce interpretable images. Abnormal heart rhythms and premature beats can cause blurring artifacts and decrease the accuracy of study interpretation.

Further Reading

Bogaert J et al. Clinical cardiac MRI. Berlin/Heidelberg: Springer; 2005. p. 99–352.

Cheitlin M et al. ACC/AHA/ASE 2003 guideline update for the clinical application of echocardiography: summary article. Circulation. 2003;108:1146–62.

Feigenbaum H et al. Feigenbaum's echocardiography. 6th ed. Philadelphia: Lippincott Williams and Wilkins; 2005.

Hendel R et al. ACCF/ASNC/ACR/AHA/ASE/SCCT/SCMR/SNM 2009 appropriate use criteria for cardiac radionuclide imaging. Circulation 2009;119;e561–87.

Iskandrian A et al. Nuclear cardiac imaging: principles and applications. 4th ed. Oxford University Press: New York; 2008. p. 31–201.

Libby P et al. Braunwald's heart disease: a textbook of cardiovascular medicine. 8th ed. Philadelphia: Elsevier Inc.; 2008. p. 227–326. 345–414.

Otto C et al. The practice of clinical echocardiography. 3rd ed. Philadelphia: Elsevier Inc.; 2007.

Sciagra R. The expanding role of left ventricular functional assessment using gated myocardial perfusion SPECT: the supporting actor is stealing the scene. Eur J Nucl Med Mol Imaging. 2007;34(7): 1107–22.

Chapter 4
Cardiovascular Stress Testing

Mohan Rao, Nicholas A. Paivanas, and James Eichelberger

Background

Establishing the anatomic presence of coronary stenosis has become increasingly important owing to the roles coronary artery bypass grafting (CABG) and percutaneous coronary interventions (PCI) have in the treatment of coronary artery disease (CAD). However, angina or myocardial infarction (MI) may occur in the absence of angiographically proven obstructive coronary lesions and, conversely, coronary obstructions may be asymptomatic and thus have uncertain prognostic significance [1–4]. Some have suggested that a functional evaluation may be more predictive of future cardiac events than anatomy alone [5, 6]. Others suggest a probabilistic model as an alternative "gold standard" [7–9]. Cardiovascular stress testing and myocardial perfusion imaging have emerged as important diagnostic tools in diagnosing coronary artery stenosis [10].

———

M. Rao • J. Eichelberger
Department of Medicine, Division of Cardiology,
University of Rochester Medical Center,
Rochester, NY, USA

N.A. Paivanas (✉)
Internal Medicine, University of Rochester Medical Center,
Rochester, NY, USA
e-mail: nicholas_paivanas@urmc.rochester.edu

J.D. Bisognano et al. (eds.), *Manual of Outpatient Cardiology*,   79
DOI 10.1007/978-0-85729-944-4_4,
© Springer-Verlag London Limited 2012

Diagnostic Accuracy of Stress Testing

The diagnostic value of a stress test for diagnosing coronary artery stenosis depends largely upon the characteristics of the patient undergoing that test. As with all tests, the diagnostic accuracy is related to sensitivity and specificity. In the case of stress testing, sensitivity is the percentage of patients with CAD (usually defined by greater than 50% occlusion of a coronary vessel) who will have an abnormal test, which is important for ruling out a disease. Conversely, specificity is defined as the percentage of normal patients who will have a negative test and is important for ruling in disease. Bayes' Theorem adds pretest probability, and is the probability of a patient having the disease prior to a test multiplied by the probability of the test providing a true result [11].

The probability of a patient having angiographic CAD can be predicted from clinical data including the patient's age, sex, traditional risk factors of diabetes, smoking, dyslipidemia, hypertension, and family history of coronary disease, characteristics of the presenting complaints, and electrocardiographic abnormalities [4, 12–17]. Diabetes, especially that associated with microalbuminuria, is increasingly being considered as an important risk factor for CAD [18, 19]. The best clinical predictor of angiographic CAD is the character of the patient's chest pain [16]. Coronary symptoms can be reliably categorized using three clinical questions [20]:

1. Is the patient's chest discomfort substernal?
2. Are the patient's symptoms precipitated by exertion?
3. Does the patient experience prompt (i.e., within 10 min) relief with rest or nitroglycerin?

If the patient's symptoms are embraced by all three of these clinical features, the symptoms can be categorized as "typical angina"; having any two of these features suggests "atypical angina"; and if the patient has only one or none of these features, the chest pain is considered nonanginal. Table 4.1 illustrates that the patient's age, sex, and symptom category can define marked differences in the probability of significant

TABLE 4.1 Pretest probability of finding coronary artery disease in males (A) and in females (B)

Age (years)	Typical angina	Atypical angina	Non-anginal pain	No chest pain
(A) *Males*				
30–39	Intermediate	Intermediate	Low	Very low
40–49	High	Intermediate	Intermediate	Low
50–59	High	Intermediate	Intermediate	Low
>60	High	Intermediate	Intermediate	Low
(B) *Females*				
30–39	Intermediate	Very low	Very low	Very low
40–49	Intermediate	Low	Very low	Very low
50–59	Intermediate	Intermediate	Low	Very low
>60	High	Intermediate	Intermediate	Low

Source: Adapted from Gibbons et al. [55]
High indicates >90%; intermediate 10–90%; low <10%; very low <5%

CAD, assuming average levels of risk factors [15,21]. Integrating data from additional cardiovascular risk factors yields similar results [16, 17] but does not significantly refine probabilities of CAD for individual patients [22]. In general, exercise stress electrocardiography has an average sensitivity of 66% and specificity of 80% for diagnosing CAD in a patient with intermediate pretest probability [23].

These principles help to guide selection of appropriate patients for stress testing. In a patient with low pretest probability of CAD, a positive test result would be more likely to be false, and you would be less inclined to pursue further studies. Conversely, in a patient with high pretest probability, a negative stress test is more likely to be false, and you would still be inclined to pursue definitive testing with angiography. The most useful scenario is a patient who has an intermediate probability of having CAD prior to the test being performed so that your management would change depending on the result of the test.

Exercise Stress Electrocardiography

The most basic stress test currently performed is exercise stress electrocardiography. It is performed in an ambulatory subject who is able to walk on a treadmill at baseline. Although exercise electrocardiography may be performed for a variety of indications, it is commonly used in the diagnosis of CAD [24, 25]. The Bruce protocol is the most commonly utilized exercise protocol for exercise electrocardiography. The Bruce protocol consists of four stages, each 3 min long with increasing speed and grade of incline. The protocol starts at a treadmill speed of 1.7 mph and is gradually increased every 3 min to 3.4 mph, 5.0 mph and 5.5 mph with corresponding increase in the treadmill incline grade from 10% to 14%, 18% and 20% [11]. The subject is monitored in each stage until he or she completes the protocol or is unable to continue due to symptoms. In subjects with reduced exercise capacity, the Bruce protocol can be modified by starting with two 3-min stages at 1.7 mph at 0% grade and 1.7 mph at 5% grade incline. The test relies mainly on symptoms and electrocardiographic changes that may occur during exercise due to ischemia. In addition, other parameters including maximal work capacity, heart rate achieved, blood pressure response and the heart rate-systolic blood pressure product (rate-pressure product) that are measured may provide additional information that can provide insight into the patient's cardiac function.

Electrocardiographic Response

ST segment depression or elevation during exercise or in the recovery phase typically indicates ischemia, although several factors other than ischemia may cause ST changes [26]. In addition, the location of electrocardiographic changes can help localize the coronary vascular territory that is ischemic (e.g. ST depression in leads V1-V4 may suggest LAD territory ischemia). ST segment depression is usually measured 80 ms from the J point. Up sloping of the ST segment with less than 1.5 mm ST depression after the J point is considered a normal electrocardiographic response to exercise. Ischemic ST segment changes include J point depression and flattening or down sloping of the ST segment by >1 mm when measured 80 ms from the J point during three consecutive beats. Table 4.2 summarizes "average" operating characteristics for

TABLE 4.2 Operating characteristics of exercise electrocardiography for angiographic coronary artery disease

ST segment depression (mm)	Sensitivity (%)	Specificity (%)	Likelihood ratio for result
0.5–0.99	86	67	**2.60**
1.0–1.49	65	79	**3.09**
1.5–1.99	42	88	**3.50**
2.0–2.49	33	89	**3.0**
>2.5	20	99	20

different degrees of ST-segment depression [14]. T wave abnormalities during exercise are less specific in diagnosing CAD. In normal subjects, pseudo normalization of the T wave may be a normal response but in rare cases may be a sign of ischemia and requires further substantiation.

Maximal Exercise Capacity

The amount of exercise capacity at each stage can be quantified and compared to routine activities by using metabolic equivalents (MET). One MET is defined as 3.5 mL/O2/kg/min of body weight and is equivalent to resting in a seated position. Stage 1 of the Bruce Protocol is roughly equivalent to 5 METs, which is similar to walking at 3–4 mph or golfing. Stage 2 is roughly 7 METs, which is similar to backpacking or playing tennis. Stage 3 is roughly 10 METs, similar to heavy labor or running at 6–7 mph. Stage 4 is 13 METs or higher, similar to high-intensity exercise. The peak exercise capacity measured in METs has been shown to be a strong predictor of the risk of death in patients with and without coronary artery disease with a 12% improvement of survival for each one MET increase in exercise capacity [27].

Heart Rate

Reaching 85% of the age-predicted maximal heart rate is the physiologic target during the stress test. The age-predicted heart rate is calculated using the formula: (220 − age). The accuracy of detecting CAD depends on the ability to reach the target heart rate. The sensitivity decreases if patients are unable to reach 85% of their maximum predicted heart rates, usually due to poor functional capacity or medication effect [28]. Failure to reach the target heart rate with maximal exercise, also called chronotropic incompetence, indicates an adverse prognosis and may itself be a sign of myocardial ischemia. An abnormal heart rate recovery following cessation of exercise has been shown to predict worse prognosis with respect to future mortality compared to subjects with a normal heart rate recovery [29].

Blood Pressure

Blood pressure should increase with exercise and decrease to resting levels following the cessation of exercise. A drop in blood pressure or failure to increase blood pressure can be a sign of multi-vessel coronary disease, severe left ventricular dysfunction and left ventricular outflow obstruction such as severe aortic stenosis and hypertrophic obstructive cardiomyopathy. A hypertensive response with sub-maximal exertion has also been shown to increase the risk of future cardiac events and death [30].

Heart Rate: Systolic Blood Pressure Product

The heart rate–systolic blood pressure product is utilized as a surrogate measure of myocardial oxygen demand. Peak rate–pressure product can be used to measure cardiovascular performance. Normally if a subject attains a rate pressure product of more than 20,000 mmHg/beats/min, the stress test is considered adequate response to exercise for evaluating cardiac performance.

Duke Treadmill Score

The Duke Treadmill Score is a validated prognostic tool that can help to further risk stratify patients based on their performance during a Bruce protocol stress test. The treadmill score is equal to (exercise time) – (5 × ST deviation) – (4 × angina index) where the angina index is 0 for no angina, 1 for non-limiting angina, and 2 for exercise limiting angina. A score of +5 or more correlates with 'low risk' and predicts a 4-year survival of 98–99%. Moderate risk (score −10 to +4) predicts a 4-year survival of 92–95%. High risk (score less than –10) predicts a 4-year survival of 71–79% [31].

Augmented Stress Testing

During stress electrocardiography, the cardiologist reviews the electrocardiographic data for evidence of ischemia. The addition of cardiac imaging allows the visualization of regions of poor perfusion. In addition, cardiac imaging can help characterize the severity and extent of ischemia, as well as localize the vascular territory that may be the culprit [11]. Imaging can also enhance the accuracy, sensitivity, and specificity of a stress test. The imaging modalities used currently include echocardiography, nuclear perfusion (SPECT), and cardiac MRI (CMR). Cardiac MRI is discussed separately (Chap. 3).

Echocardiography

Echocardiography compares images of wall motion and thickening obtained at rest with those during or immediately after exercise or pharmacologic stress [13]. Unlike myocardial perfusion imaging, echocardiography relies on regional dysfunction of a myocardial segment to make the diagnosis of coronary disease (Fig. 4.1). The hallmark of coronary ischemia is characterized by a qualitative deterioration of regional function with stress. Infarction may be identified if a segment is dysfunctional at rest. The extent and severity, time of onset, and duration of stress-induced wall motion abnormalities are indicative of the severity of CAD [32]. Current sensitivity and specificity of echocardiographic imaging in diagnosing CAD are approximately 80% and 90%, respectively, having improved with technologic advances including digitization techniques, harmonic imaging, and microbubble contrast agents to help delineate endocardial borders. The sensitivity and specificity of the different stress echocardiography are shown in Table 4.3. Limitations of echocardiography include

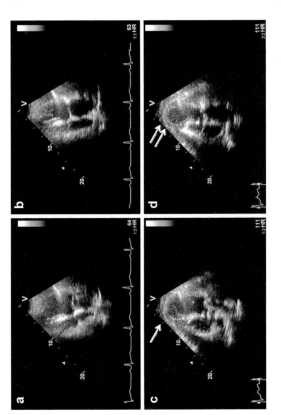

Figure 4.1 Stress echocardiogram images showing the apical four chamber view showing normal diastolic (a) and systolic wall motion evidenced by a normal contraction of the ventriculalr walls (b) during rest. (c) shows abnormal diastolic and (d) systolic wall motion during stress evidenced by ballooning of the apex (*single arrow*) that is exaggerated with (d) systole (*double arrows*) due to ischemia of the apex likely due to stenosis in the left anterior descenging artery

TABLE 4.3 Sensitivity and specificity[a] of diagnosing coronary artery disease across various stress tests

	Exercise stress (%)	Dobutamine echo (%)	Dipyridamole echo (%)	Nuclear stress (%)
Sensitivity	66	78	81	87
Specificity	80	88	90	70
Accuracy	70	82	86	81
PPV	91	92	96	85
NPV	49	69	73	72

[a]Compared to angiographical finding of at least 50% reduction in lumen diameter of a major vessel or its branches
Source: Adapted from San Roman et al. [23]
PPV Positive predictive value, *NPV* negative predictive value

the high level of operator and interpreter dependence and difficulties in obtaining adequate windows for viewing all left ventricular segments [33].

Myocardial Perfusion Imaging

Myocardial perfusion imaging (MPI) couples standard electrocardiography data with planar or single photon emission computed tomographic (SPECT) cardiac images obtained at rest and during exercise or pharmacologic stress. Cardiac images are constructed by quantifying photons released through decay of radiotracer taken up in the myocardium after intravenous injection. Thallium-201 has a longer history of use with MPI, but technetium-99 m sestamibi (MIBI) confers the advantages of attenuation reduction and left ventricular function assessment. The hallmark of myocardial ischemia is a deficit in perfusion during stress, indicated by an area of diminished tracer uptake, relative to perfusion at rest (Fig. 4.2). An inducible perfusion abnormality indicates impaired perfusion reserve that usually corresponds to epicardial coronary obstruction [28]. Although this classic "reversible" perfusion defect improves the accuracy for

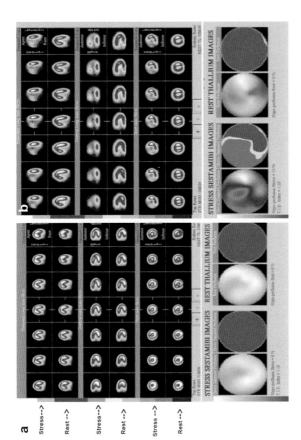

FIGURE 4.2 Nuclear SPECT images. (a) shows normal perfusion at rest and stress. (b) shows mild resting perfusion defect in the inferior and inferolateral segments at rest with worsening of perfusion in the anterior wall, apex and septum indicating ischemia in these regions that is likely due to left anterior descending artery stenosis

diagnosing CAD, other patterns of abnormalities may occur, including irreversible defects suggestive of previous myocardial injury.

The value of MPI in detecting CAD and in prognostic assessment has been well established [34–42]. The sensitivity and specificity of exercise SPECT imaging in diagnosing CAD are approximately 84% and 87%, respectively [67] Operating characteristics vary across studies, depending on demographic and methodologic factors such as the proportion of patients with previous infarctions, the percentage of men, the extent of blinding of the interpretations, and the presence of workup bias [43]. The number of perfusion defects and the finding of increased pulmonary uptake can be used to estimate the risk of future cardiac events [44].

Pharmacological Stress Testing

Patients who are unable to adequately exercise due to physical inactivity at baseline, poor effort on a treadmill, joint problems, neurological disease, or anything that would limit a patient's mobility require pharmacologic stress testing [11, 45]. Pharmacologic stress testing is coupled with cardiac imaging for a more accurate noninvasive evaluation of coronary ischemia. Pharmacologic options for this increasingly large group of patients include inotropes such as dobutamine (+/– atropine) [46] and vasodilators such as dipyridamole, adenosine or regadenoson infusion [47]. Dipyridamole, adenosine and regadenoson cause coronary vasodilation, leading to heterogeneous flow in zones with significant stenosis compared to normal zones, without necessarily causing true ischemia. Thus vasodilator infusion is generally reserved for use with perfusion imaging, since echocardiography requires true ischemia for the development of regional dysfunction. Dobutamine (+/– atropine) increases myocardial oxygen demand by increasing heart rate and contractility, leading to ischemia when significant coronary stenosis is present. Dobutamine (+/– atropine) infusion can therefore be used with either perfusion imaging or echocardiography. Dobutamine infusion is started at a rate of 5 mg/kg/min and increased, until 85% of the age-estimated maximum heart rate is achieved, up to a maximal dose of 40–50 mg/kg/min [11]. If the maximum dobutamine dose is reached and the heart rate is still below target, 1 mg of atropine can be given to try to reach the target heart rate.

Diagnostic Strategy for Stress Testing to Evaluate Coronary Artery Disease

The first step in diagnosis is to determine the pretest probability of CAD by deciding the likelihood that the patient's symptoms are attributable to coronary ischemia. If the pretest probability is very low (<10%) or very high (>90%), noninvasive testing offers little additional diagnostic information, because neither a positive nor a negative test result will greatly change the probability of CAD. In patients with pretest probabilities greater than 10% and less than 90%, noninvasive testing can lead to a meaningful revision of the probability of CAD, and is most helpful diagnostically when the pretest probability is in an intermediate (30–70%) range. Table 4.4 illustrates the ACC/AHA guidelines and appropriateness criteria for stress testing based on the pretest probability of diagnosing coronary artery disease with exercise electrocardiography, stress echocardiography and myocardial perfusion imaging. Table 4.5 shows the ACC/AHA guidelines and appropriateness criteria for choosing a stress test for risk stratification in patients with suspected or documented CAD.

Once a decision has been made to perform a stress test for evaluation of coronary ischemia, choosing among several types of readily available stress testing techniques can be difficult. This decision should be based on integrating institutional experience and expertise, functional capacity of the patient, operating characteristics of the test, baseline electrocardiographic parameters, cost, risk, and the ability of the test to evaluate additional potential clinical concerns.

TABLE 4.4 Recommendation class and/or appropriateness criteria for the detection/diagnosis of CAD

	Exercise stress	Stress echocardio-graphy	Cardiac radionuclide imaging
(A) *Symptomatic*			
Low pretest probability	Class IIB	Class I; appropriate (if ECG uninterpretable or unable to exercise)	Appropriate (if ECG uninterpretable or unable to exercise)
Intermediate pretest probability	Class I	Class I; appropriate	Class I; appropriate
High pretest probability	Class IIB	Class I; appropriate	Class I; appropriate
(B) *Acute chest pain*			
Possible ACS	No recommendation	Class I; appropriate	Class I; appropriate
Definite ACS	Class III	Class III; inappropriate	Class III; inappropriate
(C) *Asymptomatic*			
Low CHD risk	Class III	Class III; inappropriate	Inappropriate
Moderate CHD risk	Class IIB	Class IIB; inappropriate	Uncertain
High CHD risk	Class IIB, or class IIA only for DM	Class IIB; uncertain	Class IIA; appropriate

Source: Adapted from ACC/AHA guidelines [55] (Cheitlin et al. [61]; Cheitlin et al. [62]; Klocke [63]) as well as ACCF appropriateness criteria: (Douglas et al. [64]; Hendel et al. [65]; Douglas and Patel [66])

TABLE 4.5 Recommendation class and/or appropriateness criteria for risk assessment and prognosis

	Exercise stress	Stress echocardiography	Cardiac radionuclide imaging
(A) *Symptoms new or worsening*			
Post-revascularization with PCI or CABG	Class I	Class I (typical symptoms) or IIa (atypical); appropriate	Class I; appropriate
Previously abnormal stress test or known CAD	Class I	Appropriate	Class I; appropriate
Previously normal stress test	No specific recom-mendation	Appropriate (when previous test was stress ECG)	Class I; uncertain
(B) *Asymptomatic or stable symptoms*			
Post-revascularization with PCI	Class III (stress imaging is recommended)	Class III; inappropriate if <2 years, uncertain if >2 years	Class IIa (at 3–5 years); inappropriate if <2 years, uncertain if >2 years
Post-revascularization with CABG	No specific recom-mendation	Class III; inappropriate if <5 years, uncertain if >5 years	Class IIa (at 3–5 years); uncertain if <5 years, appropriate if >5 years
Previously abnormal stress test or known CAD	Class IIB	Class IIA; inappropriate (uncertain if previous study >2 years earlier)	Class IIB (at 1–3 years); inappropriate (uncertain if previous study >2 years earlier)

(continued)

TABLE 4.5 (continued)

	Exercise stress	Stress echocardiography	Cardiac radionuclide imaging
Previously normal stress test	IIA for Diabetics prior to vigorous exercise, IIB for non-diabetics to guide risk reduction therapy or certain populations prior to vigorous exercise	Inappropriate (uncertain if high-risk patient with previous study >2 years earlier)	Inappropriate (uncertain if high-risk patient with previous study >2 years earlier)

Source: Adapted from ACC/AHA guidelines [55] (Cheitlin et al. [61]; Cheitlin et al. [62]; Klocke [63]) as well as ACCF appropriateness criteria: (Douglas et al. [64]; Hendel et al. [65]; Douglas and Patel [66])

A standard exercise test without imaging should be considered in all patients who are able to exercise and who have an interpretable electrocardiogram (including patients with RBBB). In this group, if clinical risk is low and if coronary ischemia is the main concern, standard exercise testing without imaging is appropriate. In higher-risk patients, coupling imaging with standard treadmill data has independent prognostic value, even in the setting of low-risk treadmill results [48]. Meta-analyses comparing myocardial perfusion imaging with stress echocardiography generally show higher sensitivities (83–85% vs. 78–80%, respectively) and lower specificities (77–83% vs. 86–91%, respectively) with perfusion imaging when performed in institutions experienced in both techniques [49, 50]. Therefore, when imaging is desired, stress echocardiography may be more appropriate in circumstances where the likelihood of a false-positive test is increased, as in lower risk groups or when perfusion artifacts (mainly attenuation) are more likely. Exercise echocardiography also may be preferred in patients with additional concerns (pericardial, aortic, valvular) that can be simultaneously evaluated by echo imaging. Higher sensitivities with myocardial perfusion imaging may make this imaging modality preferable in higher-risk patients. Perfusion imaging also may be preferred in patients with known coronary disease and preexisting ventricular dysfunction, since interpretation of stress-induced wall motion changes by echocardiography may be difficult in this group. Perfusion imaging is also a more established technique in quantifying ischemia and may be advantageous when this information is desired. If the above considerations do not decisively influence test choice, then incremental cost, test time, and necessary radiation exposure associated with stress perfusion imaging may favor stress echocardiography.

The diagnostic accuracy of standard treadmill testing without imaging in detecting coronary ischemia is significantly reduced when electrocardiographic abnormalities are present [51]. These include patients with conduction defects, left ventricular hypertrophy, preexcitation, unexplained baseline repolarization changes, and patients on digoxin, even if the baseline electrocardiogram appears normal. In these patients, coupling imaging with standard electrocardiographic data is recommended in most circumstances for the diagnosis of coronary ischemia, using the general guidelines described above.

When some form of pharmacologic stress testing is necessary, usually due to inability to adequately exercise, it is useful to first consider potential adverse effects of specific pharmacologic agents. Dobutamine infusion may induce dysrhythmias (atrial fibrillation, ventricular tachycardia) in patients predisposed, and may be less effective in patients who are unable to augment heart rate (e.g. pacemaker dependency). Dipyridamole (or adenosine) infusion can induce bronchospasm and is relatively contraindicated in patients with this condition. However, newer specific adenosine receptor agonists do not cause significant bronchospasm and can be used in patients with reactive airway diseases. Dipyridamole (or adenosine or regadenoson) infusion coupled with perfusion imaging is advantageous when dobutamine (+/– atropine) is contraindicated, whereas perfusion or echo imaging can be considered in cases where dobutamine (+/– atropine) infusion is preferred. The comparative value of perfusion imaging versus echocardiography in this group mirrors that in patients who are able to adequately exercise.

Certain patient subgroups warrant special consideration. Standard exercise testing without imaging in women has been demonstrated to show a high false-positive rate, partly caused by the lower prevalence of coronary disease in women and partly because the criteria for a positive test are based on data obtained in men [52, 53]. Since myocardial perfusion imaging has overall lower specificity compared to stress echocardiography, and in this group specificity may be further reduced due to a higher prevalence of (breast) attenuation with perfusion imaging, exercise echocardiography may be preferred.

Patients with LBBB pose a particular problem, as reversible or fixed septal defects can be seen when combining nuclear perfusion imaging with exercise or dobutamine infusion, even in the absence of coronary stenoses [54]. Abnormal septal motion in the presence of a LBBB may also interfere with echo interpretation [55], so dipyridamole (or adenosine or regadenoson) nuclear perfusion imaging may be preferred in this subgroup.

Patients with cardiomyopathies are most problematic when noninvasively evaluating for coexisting coronary ischemia. Baseline electrocardiographic abnormalities are more likely, reducing the accuracy of standard treadmill exercise techniques. Preexisting ventricular dysfunction is more likely, making interpretation of stress-induced wall motion changes by echocardiography difficult. In addition, all forms of cardiomyopathies can be associated with perfusion defects in the absence of epicardial coronary stenosis, likely due to varying degrees of myocyte inflammation and necrosis, reducing the accuracy of perfusion imaging in these disorders [56]. Therefore, when high clinical risk and baseline ventricular dysfunction are present in patients with cardiomyopathy, invasive evaluation using coronary angiography may be the preferred initial diagnostic approach. When baseline ventricular systolic function is normal, as in most cases of hypertrophic cardiomyopathy, stress echocardiography may be preferred, especially if evaluation of associated abnormalities (outflow tract obstruction, mitral regurgitation) is needed.

Newer Diagnostic Techniques

Additional noninvasive techniques to evaluate for coronary stenosis have been developed in recent years and warrant brief discussion. On a cautionary note, while diagnostic characteristics of newer technologies exist, often relative to coronary angiography as a 'gold standard', there is presently little outcomes data comparing newer technologies to conventional stress testing modalities. Moreover, incremental value of newer technologies over a combination of current clinical risk indices and conventional stress testing has not been convincingly demonstrated. Therefore, the relative value and appropriate use of newer technologies are yet to be defined.

Positron emission tomography (PET) is a validated technique to assess for coronary stenosis. Advantages of PET over nuclear imaging are higher energy of the photon signal released from positron decay yielding enhanced count statistics and the ability to provide attenuation-corrected images, thereby increasing specificity. Disadvantages are more costly equipment and operations as well as limited availability. Prospective comparisons with quantitative angiography and with nuclear imaging demonstrate sensitivities and specificities in the range of 90% [57].

Electron-beam computerized tomography (also known as ultrafast CT or EBCT) uses an electron gun rather than a standard x-ray tube, permitting very rapid scanning, and thereby reducing artifact related to cardiac motion. EBCT is able to noninvasively detect and quantify coronary calcium, serving a marker for coronary atherosclerosis. Taking advantage of the predictable attenuation that calcium causes on x-ray beams, a calcium score is generated based on the measured plaque area and the degree of attenuation in an area of interest. The higher the calcium score, the greater the likelihood of occlusive coronary disease. Pooled data using a cutoff calcium score of >400 demonstrate a sensitivity and specificity in detecting coronary disease of roughly 90% and 50%, respectively [58]. Relatively low specificity has limited the widespread use of this technique. Moreover, coronary calcium measured by EBCT correlates poorly with stenosis on coronary angiography in groups prone to calcific vasculopathy, such as patients with renal failure [59].

Direct visualization of coronary stenosis using rapid CT scan techniques are now widely available and continue to develop. Technical limitations with respect to cardiac motion, particularly at higher heart rates, and artifacts due to coronary calcification currently limit this technology. Hybrid techniques incorporating simultaneous CT scanning to quantify calcium and detail anatomic stenosis along with PET imaging to assess for functional impairment are in development.

Cardiac magnetic resonance imaging is an emerging noninvasive modality that is now able to assess myocardial perfusion at rest and during pharmacologic vasodilation by analyzing the first pass of a contrast agent through the myocardium. An index of myocardial perfusion reserve is determined to assess for coronary stenosis. In one study, after 7% of patients were excluded, the sensitivity and specificity for detecting ≥70% coronary stenosis were 88% and 90%, respectively [60]. The technique is limited mainly by breathing artifacts in those patients that can tolerate imaging. In addition, different technical approaches by different vendors preclude comparison of results and multicenter trials. Before magnetic resonance perfusion measurements can be routinely used in clinical practice, further improvements in technique are needed.

References

1. Dagenais G et al. Survival of patients with a strongly positive exercise electrocardiogram. Circulation. 1982;65:452–6.
2. McNeer J et al. The role of the exercise test in the evaluation of patients for ischemic heart disease. Circulation. 1978;57:64–70.
3. Podrid P, Graboys T, Lown B. Prognosis of medically treated patients with coronary artery disease with profound ST-segment depression during exercise testing. N Engl J Med. 1981;305:1111–6.
4. Fisher L et al. Diagnostic quantification of CASS (Coronary Artery Surgery Study) clinical and exercise test results in determining presence and extent of coronary artery disease. A multivariate approach. Circulation. 1981;63:987–1000.
5. Kaul S et al. Superiority of quantitative exercise thallium-201 variables in determining long-term prognosis in ambulatory patients with chest pain: a comparison with cardiac catheterization. J Am Coll Cardiol. 1988;12:25–34.
6. Wackers F et al. Prognostic significance of normal quantitative planar thallium-201 stress scintigraphy in patients with chest pain. J Am Coll Cardiol. 1985;6:27–30.
7. Diamond G et al. A model for assessing the sensitivity and specificity of tests subject to selection bias: application to exercise radionuclide ventriculography for diagnosis of coronary artery disease. J Chronic Dis. 1986;29:343–55.
8. Pryor D et al. Estimating the likelihood of severe coronary artery disease. Am J Med. 1991;90:553–62.
9. Pryor D et al. Value of the history and physical in identifying patients at increased risk for coronary artery disease. Ann Intern Med. 1993;118:81–90.
10. Passamani E et al. A randomized trial of coronary artery bypass surgery. Survival of patients with a low ejection fraction. N Engl J Med. 1985;312:1665–71.
11. Fletcher GF et al. Exercise standards for testing and training: a statement for healthcare professionals from the American Heart Association. Circulation. 2001;104(14):1694–740.
12. Pashkow F. Diagnostic evaluation of the patient with coronary artery disease. Cleve Clin J Med. 1994;61:43–8.
13. Patterson R, Horowitz S, Eisner R. Comparison of modalities to diagnose coronary artery disease. Semin Nucl Med. 1994;24:286–310.
14. Diamond G, Forrester J. Analysis of probability as an aid in the clinical diagnosis of coronary artery disease. N Engl J Med. 1979;300:1350–8.
15. Diamond G et al. Computer assisted diagnosis in the noninvasive evaluation of patients with suspected coronary artery disease. J Am Coll Cardiol. 1983;1:444–55.

16. Pryor D et al. Estimating the likelihood of significant coronary artery disease. Am J Med. 1983;75:771–80.
17. Goldman L et al. Incremental value of the exercise test for diagnosing the presence or absence of coronary artery disease. Circulation. 1982;66:945–53.
18. Wachtell K et al. Albuminuria and cardiovascular risk in hypertensive patients with left ventricular hypertrophy: the LIFE study. Ann Intern Med. 2003;139(11):901–6.
19. Gerstein H et al. Albuminuria and risk of cardiovascular events, death, and heart failure in diabetic and nondiabetic individuals. JAMA. 2001;286(4):421–6.
20. Diamond G. A clinically relevant classification of chest pain. J Am Coll Cardiol. 1983;1:574–5.
21. Diamond G. Bayes' theorem: a practical aid to clinical judgment for diagnosis of coronary artery disease. Pract Cardiol. 1984;10:47–77.
22. Vliestra R et al. Risk factors and angiographic coronary artery disease: a report from the Coronary Artery Surgery Study (CASS). Circulation. 1980;62:254–61.
23. San Román JA et al. Selection of the optimal stress test for the diagnosis of coronary artery disease. Heart. 1998;80:370–6.
24. Goldschlager N. Use of the treadmill test in the diagnosis of coronary artery disease in patients with chest pain. Ann Intern Med. 1982;97:383–8.
25. American College of Cardiology/American Heart Association Task Force on Assessment of Cardiovascular Procedures: Guidelines for exercise testing. J Am Coll Cardiol. 1986;8:725–38.
26. Friesinger G et al. Exercise electrocardiography and vasoregulatory abnormalities. Am J Cardiol. 1972;30:733–40.
27. Myers J et al. Exercise capacity and mortality among men referred for exercise testing. N Engl J Med. 2002;346:793–801.
28. Libby P et al. Braunwald's heart disease: a textbook of cardiovascular medicine. 8th ed. Philadelphia: Saunders; 2008.
29. Vivekananthan D et al. Heart rate recovery after exercise is a predictor of mortality, independent of the angiographic severity of coronary disease. J Am Coll Cardiol. 2003;42:831–8.
30. Weiss SA et al. Exercise blood pressure and future cardiovascular death in asymptomatic individuals. Circulation. 2010;121(19):2109–16.
31. Mark DB et al. Prognostic value of a treadmill exercise score in outpatients with suspected coronary artery disease. N Engl J Med. 1991;325(12):849–53.
32. Marwick T. Current status of stress echocardiography in the diagnosis of coronary artery disease. Cleve Clin J Med. 1995;62:227–34.
33. Iliceto S et al. Clinical use of stress echocardiography: factors affecting diagnostic accuracy. Eur Heart J. 1994;15:672–80.
34. Berman D et al. Clinical applications of exercise nuclear cardiology studies in the era of healthcare reform. Am J Cardiol. 1995;75:3D–13.

35. Nallamothu N et al. Comparison of thallium-201 single-photon emission computed tomography and electrocardiographic response during exercise in patients with normal rest electrocardiographic results. J Am Coll Cardiol. 1995;25:830–6.
36. Pollock S et al. Independent and incremental prognostic value of tests performed in hierarchical order to evaluate patients with suspected coronary artery disease. Validation of models based on these tests. Circulation. 1992;85:237–48.
37. Beller G. Myocardial perfusion imaging with thallium-201. J Nucl Med. 1994;35:674–80.
38. Mahmarian J, Verani M. Exercise thallium-201 perfusion scintigraphy in the assessment of coronary artery disease. Am J Cardiol. 1991;67:2D–11.
39. Brown K. Prognostic value of thallium-201 myocardial perfusion imaging. A diagnostic tool comes of age. Circulation. 1991;83:363–81.
40. Hachamovitch R et al. Exercise myocardial perfusion SPECT in patients without known coronary artery disease: incremental prognostic value and use in risk stratification. Circulation. 1996;93:905–14.
41. Nallamouthu N et al. Prognostic value of simultaneous perfusion and function assessment using technetium-99m sestamibi. Am J Cardiol. 1996;78:562–4.
42. Hachamovitch R et al. Effective risk stratification using exercise myocardial perfusion SPECT in women: gender-related differences in prognostic nuclear testing. J Am Coll Cardiol. 1996;28:34–44.
43. Detrano R et al. Factors affecting sensitivity and specificity of a diagnostic test: the exercise thallium scintigram. Am J Med. 1988;84:699–710.
44. Allison T et al. Subspecialty clinics: cardiology-cardiovascular stress testing: a description of the various types of stress tests and indications for their use. Mayo Clin Proc. 1996;71:43–52.
45. Beller G. Pharmacologic stress imaging. JAMA. 1991;265:633–8.
46. Gunalp B et al. Value of dobutamine technetium-99m-sestamibi SPECT and echocardiography in the detection of coronary artery disease compared with coronary angiography. J Nucl Med. 1993;34:889–94.
47. Leppo J. Dipyridamole myocardial perfusion imaging. J Nucl Med. 1994;35:730–3.
48. Poornima I et al. Utility of myocardial perfusion imaging in patients with low risk-treadmill scores. JACC. 2004;43:194–9.
49. Geleijnse ML, Elhendy A. Can stress echocardiography compete with perfusion scintigraphy in the detection of coronary artery disease and cardiac risk assessment? Eur J Echocardiogr. 2000;1:12–21.
50. Sckinkel A et al. Noninvasive evaluation of ischemic heart disease: myocardial perfusion imaging or stress echocardiography? Eur Heart J. 2003;24:789–800.

51. Patel D, Baman T, Beller G. Comparison of the predictive value of exercise induced ST depression versus exercise technetium-99m sestamibi single photon emission computed tomographic imaging fro detected of coronary disease in patients with left ventricular hypertrophy. Am J Cardiol. 2004;93(3):333–6.

52. Detry J et al. Diagnostic value of history and maximal exercise electrocardiography in men and women suspected of coronary heart disease. Circulation. 1977;55:756–61.

53. Guiteras P et al. Diagnostic accuracy of exercise ECG lead systems in clinical subsets of women. Circulation. 1982;65:1465–74.

54. Caner B et al. Dobutamine thallium-201 myocardial SPECT in patients with LBBB and normal coronary arteries. J Nucl Med. 1997;38:424–7.

55. Gibbons R, et al. ACC/AHA 2002 guideline update for exercise testing: a report of the American College of Cardiology/American Heart Association Task Force on Practice Guidelines (Committee on Exercise Testing). American Collegeof Cardiology Web site. Available at: www.acc.org/clinical/guidelines/exercise/dirIndex.htm Accessed on 1/16/2011 (2002).

56. Iskandrian A, Hakki A, Kane S. Resting thallium-201 myocardial perfusion patterns in patients with severe left ventricular dysfunction: differences between patients with primary cardiomyopathy, chronic coronary artery disease or acute myocardial infarction. Am Heart J. 1986;111:760–7.

57. Demer L et al. Assessment of coronary artery disease severity by positron emission tomography: comparison with quantitative coronary arteriography in 193 patients. Circulation. 1989;79:825–35.

58. Mahamadu F et al. Does electron beam computer tomography provide added value in the diagnosis of coronary artery disease? Curr Opin Cardiol. 2003;18:385–93.

59. Sharples E et al. Coronary artery calcification measure with electron-beam computerized tomography correlates poorly with coronary artery angiography in dialysis patients. Am J Kidney Dis. 2004;43:313–9.

60. Nagel E et al. Magnetic resonance perfusion measurements for the noninvasive detection of coronary artery disease. Circulation. 2003;108:432–7.

61. Cheitlin, M, J. Alpert et al. ASS/AHA guidelines for the clinical application of echocardiography: executive summary. A report of the American College of Cardiology/ American Heart Association Task Force on Practice Guidelines (Committee on Clinical Application of Echocardiography). Journal of the American College of Cardiology. 1997;29:862–879.

62. Cheitlin, M. D, W. F. Armstrong et al. ACC/AHA/ASE 2003 guideline update for the clinical application of echocardiography: summary articlea report of the American college of cardiology/American

heart association task force on practice guidelines (ACC/AHA/ASE committee to update the 1997 guidelines for the clinical application of echocardiography)." Journal of the American College of Cardiology. 2003;42(5):954–970.

63. Klocke FL. ACC/AHA/ASNC Guidelines for the Clinical Use of Cardiac Radionuclide Imaging--Executive Summary: A Report of the American College of Cardiology/American Heart Association Task Force on Practice Guidelines (ACC/AHA/ASNC Committee to Revise the 1995 Guidelines for the Clinical Use of Cardiac Radionuclide Imaging). Circulation. 2003;108(11):1404–1418.

64. Douglas PS, B. Khandheria et al. ACCF/ASE/ACEP/AHA/ASNC/ SCAI/SCCT/SCMR 2008 Appropriateness Criteria for Stress Echocardiography: A Report of the American College of Cardiology Foundation Appropriateness Criteria Task Force, American Society of Echocardiography, American College of Emergency Physicians, American Heart Association, American Society of Nuclear Cardiology, Society for Cardiovascular Angiography and Interventions, Society of Cardiovascular Computed Tomography, and Society for Cardiovascular Magnetic Resonance: Endorsed by the Heart Rhythm Society and the Society of Critical Care Medicine." Circulation. 2008;117(11):1478–1497.

65. Hendel RC, DS. Berman et al. ACCF/ASNC/ACR/AHA/ASE/ SCCT/SCMR/SNM 2009 Appropriate Use Criteria for Cardiac Radionuclide Imaging: A Report of the American College of Cardiology Foundation Appropriate Use Criteria Task Force, the American Society of Nuclear Cardiology, the American College of Radiology, the American Heart Association, the American Society of Echocardiography, the Society of Cardiovascular Computed Tomography, the Society for Cardiovascular Magnetic Resonance, and the Society of Nuclear Medicine: Endorsed by the American College of Emergency Physicians." Circulation. 2009;119(22): e561–e587.

66. Douglas PS, G. M., Haines DE, Lai WW, Manning WJ, and P. M. Patel AR, Polk DM, Ragosta M, Ward RP, Weiner RB. (2010). "ACCF/ ASE/AHA/ASNC/HFSA/HRS/SCAI/SCCM/SCCT/SCMR 2011 appropriate use criteria for echocardiography." Journal of the American College of Cardiology.

67. Chou, Tony; Amidon, Thomas. Evaluating Coronary Artery Disease Noninvasively – Which Test for Whom? West J Med. 1994;161:173–180.

Chapter 5
Coronary Artery Evaluation

Michael Katz, Blake Gardner, and John P. Gassler

Introduction

For centuries the coronary arteries have been known to medical practitioners only from cadaveric anatomic evaluations while in training. In living patients with chest pain syndromes they remained hidden, protected like "crown jewels", akin to that from which their names derives from the Latin "corōnārius" meaning "belonging to a wreath or crown". Though the understanding of the dual circulation of the body had been unraveled over the preceding centuries, the main use of catheters had been in animal experiments to understand pressure and volume issues of the circulatory system.

The first cardiac catheterization in a human was performed in 1929 by a young German physician in training, Werner Forssmann [1]. At the time, the standard thought was that putting anything in the heart would be fatal. Dr. Forssmann felt that placing a catheter into the heart would aid in such applications as directly delivering drugs in patients with acute shock, injecting radio-opaque dyes, or measuring blood

M. Katz (✉) • B. Gardner • J.P. Gassler
Department of Medicine, Division of Cardiology,
University of Rochester Medical Center, Rochester, NY, USA
e-mail: michael_katz@urmc.rohester.edu

J.D. Bisognano et al. (eds.), *Manual of Outpatient Cardiology*,   105
DOI 10.1007/978-0-85729-944-4_5,
© Springer-Verlag London Limited 2012

pressure. Though he received some opposition to the idea, he decided to try it out on himself. After anesthetizing his arm, he inserted a catheter into his antecubital vein and advanced the catheter 65 cm. He then walked up two flights of stairs in order to take an x-ray for which he found the catheter in his right atrium.

It was 27 years later that Forssmann, along with Andre F. Cournand and Dickinson W. Richards, received the Nobel Prize in Physiology or Medicine for their work in utilizing cardiac catheterization in elucidating the inner workings of cardiac physiology. As Dr. Cournand famously stated in his Nobel lecture "the cardiac catheter was only the key in the lock" [2], it still required men of courage and conviction to turn the key and start in motion the evolution of invasive cardiology. Up to this point in the history of invasive cardiology, the focus was upon hemodynamics and the right sided chambers of the heart. The data garnered by these studies are still valuable today in the assessment of congestive heart failure and valvular heart disease, but these topics are the focus of other chapters within this book.

The evolution of invasive cardiology shifted from the right heart to the left, and next step was the first retrograde approach to the left ventricular cavity reported by Zimmerman [3] and others in 1950. Seldinger reported his percutaneous approach to intravascular access in 1953 [4]. The next major step forward occurred when fortune smiled on Mason Sones, MD. While performing aortography on a 26-year-old male with rheumatic heart disease, the catheter tip migrated into the right coronary artery and the dye was directly injected before it could be removed. The patient survived, and thus began Sones interest in further the evaluation of the anatomy of coronary artery disease [5].

Today cardiac catheterization is a term used to describe a procedure whereby a small plastic tube (catheter) is inserted into a peripheral artery or vein and then advanced to the heart to obtain important diagnostic information from the heart. The diagnostic information can be obtained from two different modalities: (1) Angiography and (2) Hemodynamics. In this chapter, we will discuss both the original invasive assessment of coronary anatomy and the more recent evolution of non invasive assessment by Coronary CT angiography.

Invasive Coronary Angiography

General Concepts/Examples

Coronary angiography is a technique performed by a trained cardiologist in a specialized cardiac catheterization lab. The purpose of coronary angiography is to define the coronary anatomy and to determine the presence and extent of obstructive coronary artery disease (CAD). Additionally, the operator can assess the feasibility and appropriateness of various forms of therapy, such as revascularization by percutaneous or surgical interventions. It is also used when the diagnosis of coronary disease is uncertain and coronary disease cannot be reasonably excluded by noninvasive techniques. There is a wide array of data that can be gathered from cardiac catheterization, including right and left heart hemodynamics and filling pressures, cardiac output and index measurements, and quantification of intracardiac shunting. However, the most common indication is to establish the epicardial coronary anatomy, the presence and extent of CAD, and the function of the left ventricle. The combination of the coronary angiogram with the left-sided hemodynamic measurements is routinely termed a left heart catheterization. It is very helpful if the patient has had prior coronary artery bypass grafting or previous percutaneous coronary intervention that those records be reported to the physician performing the upcoming procedure, as this saves time and contrast in performing a complete study.

Coronary angiography is performed in many clinical scenarios. The majority are performed in elective situations for stable angina patients, who are not able to be controlled on medical therapy. Prior to the procedure labwork and a basic history and physical are performed. Specific labwork includes coagulation studies, blood counts including platelet counts, serum electrolytes and creatinine. Abnormalities in any of these tests should be taken into consideration and corrected, if possible, prior to the procedure. If the patient has an elevated INR, the cardiologist performing the procedure should be contacted to see what level would be acceptable for the procedure. If the patient has signs or symptoms of an acute infection, the procedure may be delayed until the infection can be treated.

The history and physical are geared toward symptoms of heart failure, obstructive sleep apnea and allergies to agents that might be used during the angiogram (IV contrast dye, narcotics, benzodiazepines). Most institutions successfully use IV contrast dye in allergic patients by using a steroid protocol starting the day before the procedure. The dose varies from 20 to 50 mg oral Prednisone every 6 h starting 13 h before the intended procedure. H2 antagonists, such as Cimetidine, may be utilized as well, along with Benadryl at the time of the procedure [6]. It is recommended to contact the institution performing your patient's procedure, if your patient has such an allergy so that they can be appropriately prepared.

Since the patient is required to lie flat for the duration of the procedure, congestive heart failure should be aggressively treated prior to performance of the procedure. Not only is this important for patient comfort, but also to reduce the chance of sudden movements during the procedure that could lead to serious complications. Ideally the patient is made NPO for greater than 12 h. The labwork and H&P should be performed by the referring physician a few days prior to the procedure and then communicated to the cardiologist performing the procedure.

Two other common clinical questions relate to diabetic patients and those on chronic Coumadin therapy [6]. Diabetic patients on insulin should have there insulin adjusted to their NPO status before their procedure. In addition, they should be scheduled early to minimize their duration without caloric intake. Patients on Glucophage are requested to hold the AM dose on the day of their procedure and not to restart the agent for at least 48 h afterwards, and only after documenting a stable creatinine post procedure. This is due to the risk of severe lactic acidosis if they should have a worsening of their renal function, while still on the drug.

Coumadin anticoagulation becomes an issue in patient chronically on the drug, both before and after cardiac catheterization. The recommendation is to stop taking the Coumadin 3 days before the procedure with an INR drawn to demonstrate that the value is below 1.7 or 1.8 [6]. Above that value the risk of bleeding is generally considered to be too high to safely perform invasive angiography. If the patient is considered to be high risk from a thromboembolic perspective, consideration of covering the patient with Lovenox or admitted for IV heparin can be discussed with their primary cardiologist. Finally, if the patient is being considered for PCI based upon the results of the angiogram, it is beneficial for the patient to be initiated on aspirin and Clopidogrel, with a 300 or 600 mg load on the day before the procedure [7].

In emergent and urgent situations such as STEMIs, NSTEMIs, new onset heart failure or malignant arrythmias, the previous workup and precautions may not be able to be fully performed. Still, for patient safety, the patient should be as thoroughly performed as the situation allows, especially related to contrast allergies, and advanced knowledge of the patient's hematocrit, platelet counts, and degree of renal insufficiency. In these situations the benefit of the emergent or urgent angiogram typically outweighs the potential risks.

There are known risks to cardiac catheterization and coronary angiography which have been defined over the history of the procedure. The Society of Cardiac Angiography and Intervention has performed several registry analyses since the beginning of coronary intervention. The most recent in 1990 [8] performed on 58,332 patients worth of data, demonstrated the following complication risks: cardiac death (0.08%), myocardial infarction (0.05%), cerebrovascular accident (0.07%), and any access site event, such as bleeding, dissection, or pseudoaneurysm (0.5–0.6%). Overall, any complication occurred in 1.5% of cases and included other less common events such as air embolism, contrast reactions ranging from hives up to anaphylactoid reactions (<1%), pyretic reactions, and emergent coronary artery bypass surgery.

Contrast induced nephropathy (CIN) in all comers, defined as an increase in serum creatinine of >0.5 mg/dL or an increase of >25% from baseline, occurred in 5% of patients transiently. The need for dialysis was much less common. N-Acetylcysteine, which had been a mainstay for years based upon small trials [9, 10], was refuted at the AHA meetings of 2010, by the ACT trial investigators, who determined in over 2,000 patients that oral administration of 1,200 mg of N-Acetylcysteine pre- and post-catheterization had no bene-fit on reducing CIN in a high-risk population. Sodium Bicarbonate administration immediately pre- and into the post-procedural period [11] has merit as does Theophylline administration [12] immediately before the procedure in the holding area.

Technical/Procedural Overview

On the day of an elective angiogram the patient will usually arrive to the cath lab an hour or two before the procedure. This allows for a review of the patients labwork and a history and physical by both the nursing staff and physicians per-forming the procedure. The patient typically will wait in a pre-cath holding area. When the patient arrives in the cath lab they will be transferred to a special radiolucent table which allows the X-rays to pass unaltered through to the patient and the image intensifier (film) beyond. The patient is then cleansed at the access site in a typical sterile fashion and then covered from neck to the end of the table in a sterile drape. The brachial artery was the original access point uti-lized, but the femoral artery, accessed through a percutane-ous arteriotomy, has been the most common site for the last 30 years. Over the last 10 years there has been a surge, slow but steady, moving toward using the right Radial artery for access if appropriate. There is evidence that patient comfort may be improved and that procedure completion and safety do not seem to be affected, but at a possible cost of slightly greater radiation exposure. The physicians perform surgical grade sterile preparation on their hands and full sterile garb is donned. Moderate levels of conscious sedation are preferred over general sedation for hemodynamic reasons and because the cooperation of the patient is needed at times during the procedure. If the patient has sleep apnea a CPAP machine is typically used.

Regardless of the access site, a 0.035 in guide wire is advanced first, with the angiography catheters following to the level of the sinuses of the aorta. The wire is removed, and the catheter attached to a contrast injection system with removal of any air in the system, to avoid air embolism to the myocardium or other areas of the body. Numerous catheter shapes and sizes are available to the operator, but the goal is the same regardless of the access site or catheter used, to carefully insert the tip of a catheter into the right and left coronary artery ostia. A small amount of radio-opaque contrast dye is then injected under fluoroscopy (continuous x-ray) and subsequent pictures are taken with standardized views. This allows the physician to visualize the anatomy of the main epicardial coronary arteries and side branches. Contrast dye is also routinely injected into the left ventricle so that the physician can estimate the left ventricular ejection fraction and any wall motion abnormalities that may be present (Figs. 5.1–5.4).

After the procedure, the patient may need to be monitored overnight depending on what occurred during the procedure, in particular if they underwent percutaneous coronary angioplasty and/or stenting. If the patient underwent a diagnostic study alone, they can return home later that evening after the requisite time of monitoring post-procedure. If the femoral artery is accessed during the procedure, the patient is asked to not lift over 10 lb for 3–5 days so as to prevent bleeding of the access site. Otherwise, most patients are able to return to

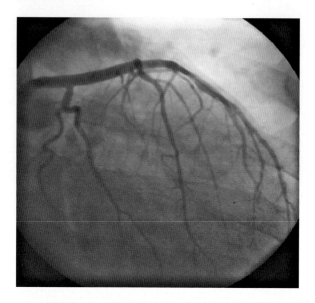

FIGURE 5.1 This image demonstrates a right anterior oblique (image intensifier (II) at the patient's right side) caudal (II toward the patient's feet) view of the left coronary system. The left main trunk is the large caliber vessel at the end of the catheter to the *top left* of the screen. The left circumflex vessel is the branch that drops *down* on the screen. The left anterior descending travels from where the left circumflex drops *down* out to the *right* of the screen

pre-procedural activity within 24–36 h. If the patient had an elevated baseline creatinine, they will often be asked to have a repeat serum creatinine checked in 48–72 h to ensure that there has been no undocumented increase above baseline.

Indications

The indications for coronary angiography have been well studied and general recommendations and guidelines have been developed by the American Heart Association and

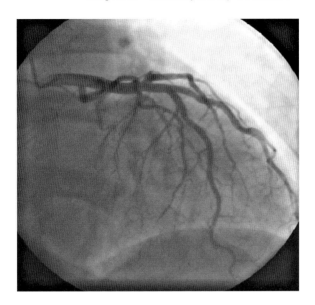

FIGURE 5.2 This image demonstrates an anterio-posterior (II directly over the patient's midline) projection with cranial angulation (II tilted toward the patient's head) view of the patient's left coronary system. Again, the left main trunk is seen to arise in the *top left* of the screen from the catheter tip. The left anterior descending travels from 11 o'clock in this view to 5 o'clock. The branches arising *above* the LAD are diagonal branches, while the vessels arising *below* are septal branches. The left circumflex artery is running behind the LAD and mostly obscured in this view

American College of Cardiology. For a more detailed list of indications for coronary angiography, please refer to the ACC/AHA guidelines on coronary angiography [13]. Below, we will list the more common clinical scenarios regarding class I indications adapted from the ACC/AHA guidelines. Class I is defined by the American College of Cardiology and American Heart Association as appropriate use for a study with an expectation of beneficial outcomes.

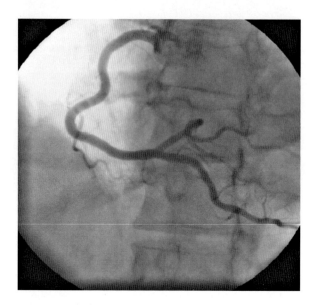

FIGURE 5.3 This image demonstrates a left anterior oblique (II at the patient's left side) view of the patient's right coronary artery. The vessel comes to the *left* of the screen as it travels around the right ventricle and branches in the 6 o'clock position to the posterior descending artery running straight *down* and posterolateral branches

Recommendations for Coronary Angiography in Patients with Known or Suspected CAD Who Are Currently Asymptomatic or Have Stable Angina

Class I
1. CCS class III and IV angina on medical treatment. (Level of Evidence: B)
2. High-risk criteria on noninvasive testing regardless of anginal severity. (Level of Evidence: A)
3. Patients who have been successfully resuscitated from sudden cardiac death or have sustained (>30 s) monomorphic ventricular tachycardia or nonsustained (<30 s) polymorphic ventricular tachycardia. (Level of Evidence: B)

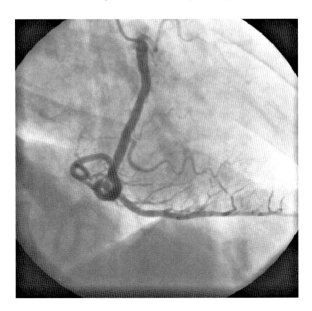

FIGURE 5.4 This image demonstrates a right anterior oblique (II to the patient's right) view of the right coronary artery which is coming at you at the *top* of the screen and then runs into the screen after the halfway mark. The vessel projecting to the *bottom right* of the screen is the posterior descending artery running along the inferior ventricular septum

Recommendations for Coronary Angiography in Patients with Nonspecific Chest Pain

Class I
   High-risk findings on noninvasive testing. (Level of Evidence: B)

Recommendations for Coronary Angiography in Unstable Coronary Syndromes

Class I
1. High or intermediate risk for adverse outcome in patients with unstable angina refractory to initial adequate medical

therapy, or recurrent symptoms after initial stabilization. Emergent catheterization is recommended. (Level of Evidence: B)
2. High risk for adverse outcome in patients with unstable angina. Urgent catheterization is recommended. (Level of Evidence: B)
3. High- or intermediate-risk unstable angina that stabilizes after initial treatment. (Level of Evidence: A)
4. Initially low short-term–risk unstable angina that is subsequently high risk on noninvasive testing. (Level of Evidence: B)
5. Suspected Prinzmetal variant angina. (Level of Evidence: C)

Recommendations for Coronary Angiography in Perioperative Evaluation Before (or After) Noncardiac Surgery (further definition in alternative chapter)

Class I: Patients with suspected or known CAD
1. Evidence for high risk of adverse outcome based on noninvasive test results. (Level of Evidence: C)
2. Angina unresponsive to adequate medical therapy. (Level of Evidence: C)
3. Unstable angina, particularly when facing intermediate or high-risk noncardiac surgery. (Level of Evidence: C)
4. Equivocal noninvasive test result in a high-clinical-risk patient undergoing high-risk surgery. (Level of Evidence: C)

Recommendations for Use of Coronary Angiography in Patients with CHF

Class I
1. CHF due to systolic dysfunction with angina or with regional wall motion abnormalities and/or scintigraphic evidence of reversible myocardial ischemia when revascularization is being considered. (Level of Evidence: B)
2. Before cardiac transplantation. (Level of Evidence: C)

3. CHF secondary to postinfarction ventricular aneurysm or other mechanical complications of MI. (Level of Evidence: C)

Contraindications

There are no absolute contraindications for coronary angiography except for a competent patient's refusal to undergo the procedure, though many other relative contraindications exist. Please see the ACC/AHA guidelines [13] for a more detailed list of contraindications. Listed below are a few common scenarios:

Coagulopathy
Decompensated congestive heart failure
Poorly controlled hypertension
Acute CVA
Refractory arrhythmia
GI hemorrhage
Anemia
Pregnancy
Poor patient cooperation
Active infection
Chronic or acute renal failure
Contrast medium allergy

Limitations

Technical limitations are primarily related to obtaining access to the patient's vasculature. Many patients sent for coronary angiography also have coexistent peripheral vascular disease of the lower extremities, making femoral access difficult. Also, very obese patients have deeper femoral arteries, making access difficult as well. In both of these circumstances radial access is a particularly important option. An additional limitation is that catheterization tables and equipment have limits on the weight they can support. Also, very large patients increase the need for X-ray output by the equipment. Especially with older, equipment the image quality degrades rapidly with severely obese patients, making it difficult to determine coronary anatomy, and particular the decision to attempt an intervention on these patients.

Computed Tomography Angiography (CTA) and Coronary Artery Calcification (CAC)

General Concepts

CTA is a diagnostic modality that provides the ability to document and grade the severity of coronary atherosclerosis. The coronary artery lumen and vessel wall can be visualized after intravenous injection of contrast agent. Recent technical improvements in CT imaging, specifically the development of 64 slice multidetector computed tomography (MDCT), allow for the necessary spatial and temporal resolution, as well as short acquisition time, required for the accurate detection of coronary artery stenosis. The ability to detect obstructive disease may be useful in the outpatient setting to evaluate chest pain symptoms in patients with an equivocal stress test, demonstrate anomalous coronary arteries, to differentiate ischemic from non-ischemic cardiomyopathy and eventually to evaluate bypass graft patency.

Numerous studies have compared the accuracy of CTA to traditional coronary angiography. Although these studies vary by technique and patient population, data examining accuracy of per vessel and per patient identification of coronary stenosis are available. Overall, the strength of CTA is its high negative predictive value, or ability to accurately rule out obstructive coronary artery disease in those patients that test negative, ranging from 93% to 100%. The positive predictive value has been found to be lower, ranging from 50% to 100% per patient and 36–97% per vessel segment [14–17]. Therefore, CTA tends to overestimate disease severity in comparison to traditional invasive angiography.

As a point of clarification, CT determination of coronary calcification (CAC scoring), as opposed to CTA, provides an estimation of artherosclerotic disease burden, which may be helpful for risk stratification, not anatomic evaluation. Measuring CAC may be useful for documenting the general presence and extent of atherosclerosis, but not as a site-specific marker [18]. The absence of CAC does not rule out the presence of obstructive coronary artery disease. An important corollary to this is that CAC is not necessarily associated with hemodynamically relevant stenoses. Therefore, the presence of CAC alone does not require invasive coronary angiography.

CAC is typically reported as a score developed by Agatston [19]. There are five risk stratified subgroups: low (CAC 0–10), mild (CAC 11–100), moderate (CAC 101–399), high (400–999), and very high (CAC > 1,000), based upon registry data [20]. A given patient's score must be interpreted within the context of their age and gender [21]. Normative standards are available and percentile scores for men and women are generally reported.

To reconcile the rapid growth of cardiac imaging with emerging data and evidence, representatives from eight professional societies have written appropriateness criteria to clarify prior recommendations [22]. Ninety-three clinical scenarios are covered in the guidelines. It should be emphasized that many of the indications are further broken down according to the patients' pretest probability of coronary disease. From these scenarios, a series of algorithms to determine the appropriateness of CTA were developed. *In general, the writing group found that cardiac CT angiography is usually appropriate for diagnosis or risk assessment in patients with an otherwise low or intermediate risk of coronary artery disease, but it is usually inappropriate for patients at high risk for significant coronary artery disease*. Figures 5.5–5.9 are all taken from the 2010 appropriate use criteria [22] and used with permission.

Advantages/Disadvantages

The advantages of Coronary CT Angiography arise from its non invasive nature. There is no extensive preparation required and no need for surgical levels of sterility. Studies are completed within 15 min in most centers. There is no risk

Age	Asymptomatic	Nonanginal Chest pain	Atypical/Probable Angina	Typical Angina
Men				
< 39	Very low	Low	Intermediate	Intermediate
40–49	Low	Intermediate	Intermediate	High
50–59	Low	Intermediate	Intermediate	High
> 60	Low	Intermediate	Intermediate	High
Woman				
< 39	Very low	Very low	Very low	Intermediate
40–49	Very low	Very low	Low	Intermediate
50–59	Very low	Low	Intermediate	Intermediate
> 60	Low	Intermediate	Intermediate	High

Very low: < 5% pretest probability; low: between 5 and 10% pretest probability; intermediate: between 10 and 90% pretest probability; high > 90% pretest probability.

FIGURE 5.5 Pretest probability of CAD by age, sex, and symptoms. Adapted from J Am Coll Cardiol 2010;56(22):1864 and J Am Coll Cardiol 2002;40:1531

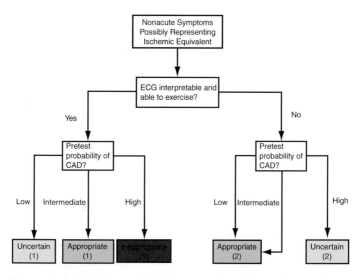

FIGURE 5.6 Detection of CAD in symptomatic patients without known heart disease: symptomatic – non-acute presentation. Adapted from J Am Coll Cardiol 2010;56(22):1864. With permission from Elsevier

of a study related myocardial infarction, coronary dissection, or CVA, nor is there any risk for access site complications, such as hematomas or retroperitoneal bleeds.

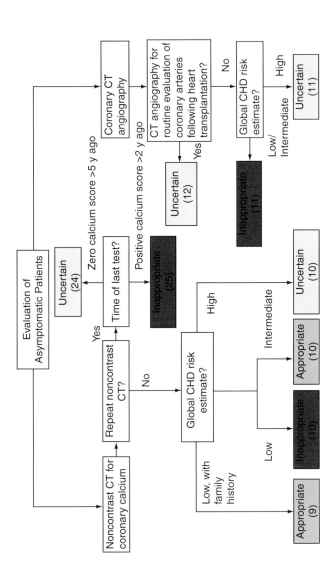

FIGURE 5-7 Detection of CAD/Risk assessment in asymptomatic individuals without known coronary artery disease. Adapted from J Am Coll Cardiol 2010;56(22):1864. With permission from Elsevier

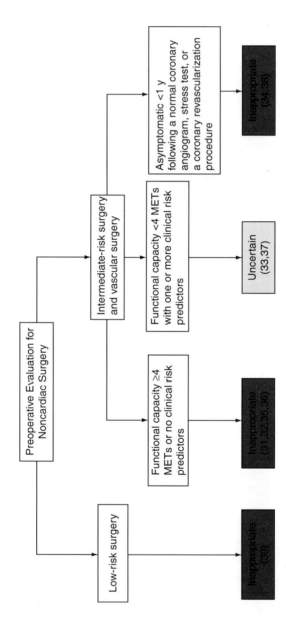

FIGURE 5.8 Risk assessment preoperative assessment for noncardiac surgery. Adapted from J Am Coll Cardiol 2010;56(22):1864. With permission from Elsevier

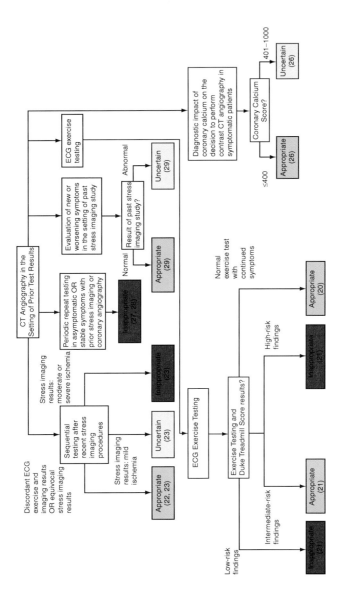

FIGURE 5.9 Use of CT angiography in the setting of prior test results. Adapted from J Am Coll Cardiol 2010;56(22):1864. With permission from Elsevier

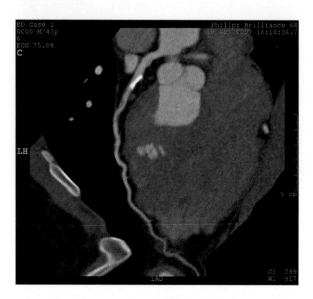

FIGURE 5.10 Curvilinear reconstruction of a left anterior descending artery travelling from 12 o'clock to 6 o'clock across the image. There is evidence of significant calcium located in the LAD immediately beyond the distal left main trunk

Additionally, the vast amounts of data collected during a brief Coronary CTA allow for generation of a coronary calcium score and measure of left ventricular function, as well as generation of multiple different methods of viewing the coronary arteries, from curvilinear planar images to linear rotating images to three-dimensional reconstructions of the coronary arteries. Where invasive angiography has been noted to be lumenography, only outlining the lumen characteristics as depicted by filling the vessel with contrast, CT angiography allows us to look both at the lumen and at the appearance of the vessel wall. In this way, we can see soft and hard plaque in greater detail than could ever have been imagined with invasive angiography (Figs. 5.10–5.16).

The major disadvantages of the technology include the greater radiation exposure per evaluation, greater contrast load per study, inability to perform studies with patients in atrial fibrillation or with frequent ectopy, and the inability to

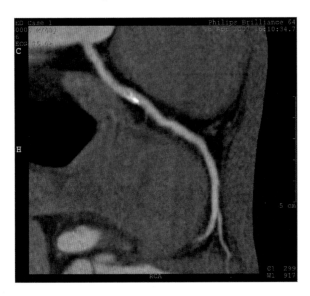

FIGURE 5.11 Curvilinear reconstruction of a right coronary artery travelling from 11 o'clock to 5 o'clock across the screen. The bright area is a calcified lesion in the mid vessel

perform ad hoc angioplasty if a severe lesion is demonstrated on the study. Another disadvantage of CTA is the higher radiation exposure administered during a study. During an uncomplicated normal coronary angiogram, the patient is exposed to between 4 and 10 mSv of radiation. The same patient will be exposed to between 9.6 and 15 mSv Even with dose modulation (restricting high dose radiation to certain phases of the cardiac cycle) the dose is higher than for an invasive angiogram. While there are no long term data yet available quantifying the risks involved, some investigators who have modeled the risk from such exposure have determine that young females are at the highest risk of cancer related to such a CT scan [23].

Technical and Procedural Overview

In computed tomography (CT), images are created by rotating a source of emitted x-rays around the patient. While some x-rays

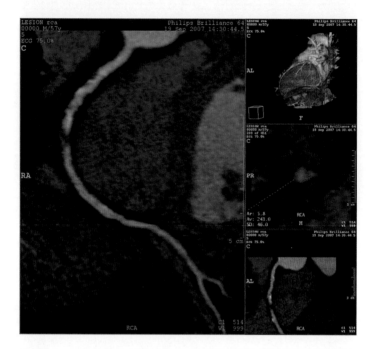

Figure 5.12 Curvilinear reconstruction of a right coronary artery with milddisease in the proximal vessel. The apparent discontinuation of the vessel is due to a severe, subtotal occlusive lesion of the mid vessel

are absorbed or scattered, the transmitted x-rays are sensed by detectors surrounding the patient. Different structures attenuate the x-ray beam to differing extents. These data are interpreted by computer algorithm to create a set of axial images.

MDCT, most commonly used for CTA and CAC scoring, uses an x-ray tube mounted on a gantry opposite multiple detectors, which is physically rotated around the patient. Meanwhile, the patient is moved through the scanner. The time of a 360° rotation is extremely rapid which allows for high temporal resolution. Thin collimation allows for the high spatial resolution needed to adequately image such small structures. Currently, the ability to acquire 64 slices simultaneously is considered a prerequisite for the high-resolution required for cardiac imaging.

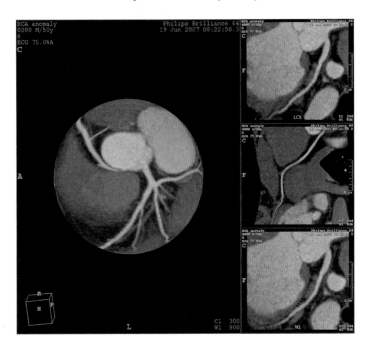

FIGURE 5.13 Globe view 3D reconstruction of the aorta with coronary vessels arising from it. The left main trunk arises at 5 o'clock and travels straight out. The left anterior descending arises at the trifurcation and travels toward the 7 o'clock position, while the Ramus intermedius travels to 5 o'clock and the left circumflex travels to 3 o'clock. The right coronary artery arises at 8 o'clock and takes a sharp angulated position after arising from the anterior aorta

It is important to note that both CTA and CAC scoring require contiguous cross-sectional imaging of the heart. As the heart is nearly constantly in motion, every image must be of the same cardiac phase. Data acquisition must be triggered by the patient's electrocardiogram or, when images are acquired continuously, retrospectively correlated to simultaneous electrocardiogram data. Additionally, the motion of breathing also causes the heart to move within the chest cavity. To reduce motion artifact, an attempt is made to acquire all CT imaging within a single breath hold.

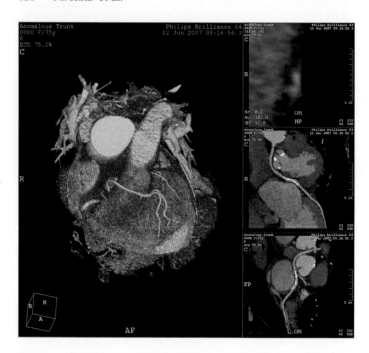

FIGURE 5.14 3D reconstruction of the cardiac structures as if looking down from the base of the heart. The aorta is readily apparent is *white*, as is the pulmonary artery (*PA*) arising anterior to the aorta, with a small left anterior descending arising posterior to the PA and travelling over it to the anterior wall

Patients are instructed to remain NPO for at least 3 h prior to their study. They are also asked to avoid agents such as Sildenafil, or others of its ilk, due to the profound hypotension seen when those agents are in the patients system and the sublingual Nitroglycerine is administered to maximally vasodilate the patient's coronary arteries. In addition, patients are provided a single dose of beta blocker to take at home the morning of the study to begin to lower their resting heart rate to the ideal target rate of 60–65 beats per minute to obtain the best quality study. Additional doses of IV beta blocker are often administered in the pre procedural holding area. It is important that the patient understand and be able to hold their breath for at least 10 s.

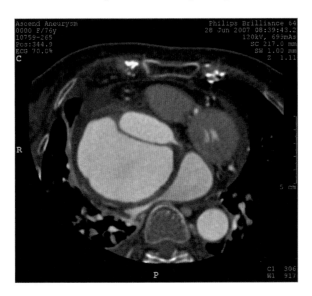

FIGURE 5.15 Usual CT view of an ascending aortic dissection with a true lumen (smaller, anterior in the picture) and false lumen (larger and posterior in the picture) present

During CTA, to visualize the coronary artery lumen, large, uniform dye loads of 80–100 cc of iodinated contrast agent are utilized. If there is concern for these dye loads and the risk of CIN, then invasive angiography should be entertained, due to the ability to obtain a complete study with significantly less contrast volume. Patients with mild allergic reactions to contrast (rash, hives) may require premedication with diphen-hydramine and steroids over the 13 h leading up to the study. Anaphylactoid reactions to contrast are generally considered an absolute contraindication to CTA by most institutions.

Additional relative contraindications to performing Cardiac CTA include Atrial fibrillation or frequent ectopy, which make the gating process suboptimal, and the inability for the patient to hold their breath for more than 10 s. Active hyperthyroidism is also considered a relative contraindica-tion due to the potential risk of thyrotoxicosis with the iodine load.

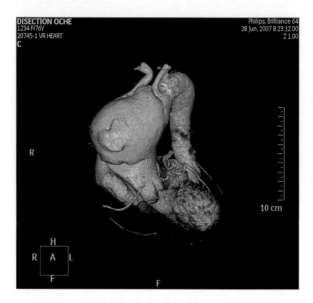

FIGURE 5.16 3D reconstruction of the same chronic ascending aortic dissection, utilizing gated coronary protocol. The coronary CT allowed definition of the coronary anatomy clearly eliminating the need for invasive angiography though the dissection plane to demonstrate whether there was a need for CABG at the time of aneurysm/dissection repair

Limitations and Special Considerations

Several imaging artifacts are inherent to the current state of CT technology. Motion of the body or heart itself will typically blur the contours of the heart and coronary arteries. Errors or inconsistency in electrocardiogram gating due to atrial fibrillation or ectopic beats may cause misalignment of adjacent slices of coronary arteries, thereby creating artifacts that can be mistaken as coronary lesions. Areas of very high CT density, such as metal from implantable cardiac devices (AICD, pacemakers, coronary stents, etc) or severe calcification, can cause "beam hardening" which causes the image to "bloom". This bright area around the high density object makes interpretation of the surrounding soft tissue structures extremely difficult.

References

1. Forssmann, W. Die Sondierung des rechten Herzens. Klin Wochenschr. 1929;8:2085.
2. Cournand, AF. Nobel lecture, December 11, 1956. In: Nobel Lectures, Physiology and Medicine 1942–1962. Amsterdam: Elsevier, 1964:529.
3. Zimmerman HA, Scott RW, Becker ND. Catheterization of the left side of the heart in man. Circulation. 1950;1:357.
4. Seldinger SI. Catheter replacement of the needle in percutaneous arteriography: a new technique. Acta Radiol. 1953;39:368.
5. Sones FM Jr, Shirey EK. Cine coronary arteriography. Mod Concepts Cardiovasc Dis. 1962;31:735–38.
6. Bayshore TM, et al. ACC/SCA&I Expert Consensus Document on Cath Lab Standards. JACC. 2001;37:2170–214.
7. King III et al. Focused Update of the ACC/AHA/SCAI 2005 Guideline Update for Percutaneous Coronary Intervention. JACC. 2008;51:172–209.
8. Noto TJ, et al. Cardiac Catheterization 1990: a report of the registry of the Society of Cardiac Angiography and Interventions. Cathet Cardiovasc Diagn. 1991;24:75.
9. Birck R, Krzossok S, Markowetz F, et al. Acetylcysteine for prevention of contrast nephropathy: meta-analysis. The Lancet. 2003;362: 598–603.
10. Marenzi G, Assanelli E, Marana I, et al. N-acetylcysteine and contrast-induced nephropathy in primary angioplasty. N Engl J Med. 2006;354:2773–82.
11. Brigouri C, Airoldi F, D'Andrea D, et al. Renal Insuffiency Following Contrast Media Administration Trial (REMEDIAL): A randomized comparison of 3 preventive strategies. Circulation. 2007;115: 1211–217
12. Bagshaw SM, Ghali WA. Theophylline for prevention of contrast-induced nephropathy: a systematic review and meta-analysis. Arch Int Med 2005;165:1087–93.
13. Scanlon PJ, et al. ACC/AHA Guidelines for coronary angiography: executive summary and recommendations. Circulation. 1999;99: 2345–57.
14. Mollet NR, Cademartiri F, Krestin GP, et al. Improved diagnostic accuracy with 16-row multi-slice computed tomography coronary angiography. J Am Coll Cardiol 2005;45:128.
15. Garcia MJ, Lessick J, Hoffmann MH, CATSCAN Study Investigators. Accuracy of 16-row multidetector computed tomography for the assessment of coronary artery stenosis. JAMA. 2006;296:403.
16. Leschka S, Alkadhi H, Plass A, et al. Accuracy of MSCT coronary angiography with 64-slice technology: first experience. Eur heart J. 2005;26:1482.

17. Raff GJ, Gallagher MJ, O'Neill WW, Goldstein JA. Diagnostic accuracy of noninvasive angiography using 64-slice spiral computed tomography. J Am Coll Cardiol. 2005;46:552.

18. Rumberger JA, Simons DB, Fitzpatrick LA, et al. Coronary artery calcium area by electron-beam computed tomography and coronary atherosclerotic plaque area: a histopathologic correlative study. Circulation 1995;92:2157–62.

19. Agatston AS, Janowitz WR, Hildner FJ, et al. Quantification of coronary artery calcium using ultrafast computed tomography. J Am Coll Cardiol. 1990;15:827–32.

20. Budhoff M, Shaw L, et al. Long term prognosis associated with coronary calcification: observation from a registry of 25,253 patients. JACC. 49:18;2007:1860–70.

21. McClelland RL, Chung H, Detrano R, et al. Distribution of coronary artery calcium by race, gender, and age: results from the Multi-Ethnic Study of Atherosclerosis (MESA). Circulation. 2006;113: 30–37.

22. Taylor AJ, Cequeira M, Hodgson JM, et al. Appropriate use criteria for cardiac computed tomography: A report of the American College of Cardiology Foundation Appropriate Use Criteria Task Force, the Society of Cardiovascular Computed Tomography, the American College of Radiology, the American Heart Association, the American Society of Echocardiography, the American Society of Nuclear Cardiology, the Society for Cardiovascular Angiography and Interventions, and the Society for Cardiovascular Magnetic Resonance. J Am Coll Cardiol. 2010; 56:1864–94.

23. Einstein AJ et al. Estimating risk of cancer associated with radiation exposure from 64-slice computed tomography coronary angiography. JAMA. 2007;198:317–23.

Part II
Common Cardiac Diseases

Chapter 6
Hypertension

**Melissa Gunasekera, John D. Bisognano,
and G. Ronald Beck**

With an estimated 50 million Americans diagnosed with hypertension, it is the most common medical condition in the United States. Patients with hypertension and no identifiable cause are said to have essential or primary hypertension, which is the type of hypertension for 90% of hypertensive patients. A number of factors have been implicated in the development of hypertension including dietary salt intake, obesity, alcohol intake, occupation, and stress. Patients with hypertension have an increased risk of developing a morbid cardiovascular event and will likely benefit from medical therapy. Their evaluation should be directed at identifying correctable forms of hypertension, the presence of target organ damage, and other risk factors for cardiovascular

———

M. Gunasekera (✉)
Department of Medicine, University of Rochester Medical Center,
Rochester, NY, USA
e-mail: melissa_gunasekera@gmail.com

J.D. Bisognano
Division of Cardiology, Department of Internal Medicine,
University of Rochester Medical Center, Rochester, NY, USA
e-mail: john_bisognano@urmc.rochester.edu

G.R. Beck
Division of Cardiology, Department of Internal Medicine,
University of Rochester Medical Center,
Rochester, NY, USA

J.D. Bisognano et al. (eds.), *Manual of Outpatient Cardiology*,   135
DOI 10.1007/978-0-85729-944-4_6,
© Springer-Verlag London Limited 2012

disease. Risk factors of an adverse prognosis in hypertension include male sex, smoking, diabetes mellitus, obesity, hypercholesterolemia, and African-American race. This chapter focuses on target blood pressure guidelines, lifestyle modifications, and the medical management of hypertension.

Proper Techniques for Measuring

The most common method of measuring blood pressure in the outpatient setting is through use of a manometer, which is a mercury or aneroid instrument calibrated to the nearest 2 mmHg. To obtain the best blood pressure measurement, the patient should be seated in a quiet room at an ideal temperature. After 5 min of rest, locate the patient's brachial artery at the midpoint of the upper arm by palpating between the biceps and triceps muscles on the inner surface. An appropriately sized cuff should encircle at least 80% of the arm, and be smoothly secured with the manometer bladder centered directly over the palpated artery with the lower edge of the cuff 2.5 cm above the antecubital fossa. A stethoscope bell is placed where the brachial artery is strongest using light pressure to avoid artery occlusion. The cuff is rapidly inflated and slowly deflated while listening for Korotkoff sounds. Systolic pressure is determined at the pressure level of the first Korotkoff sound, also known as K1, which is described as the pressure level at which the first, faint consistent tapping sounds are heard. Diastolic pressure is determined at the last pressure level of the last Korotkoff sound, also known as K5, which is the pressure level when the last regular blood pressure is heard and all sounds disappear. A second reading should be obtained approximately 5–10 min later and the results averaged.

A valuable measurement in evaluating hypertensive patients and their response to therapy is a set of blood pressures measured at home or outside of the clinical setting. Patients should be advised to measure their blood pressure after sitting quietly for at least 5 minutes in a chair with their legs uncrossed, feet on the floor, and with their body positioned for support by the chair. Recording 8–10 readings, measured at varying times of the day, and within 2 weeks of the initial evaluation or during the interval between evaluations will provide an adequate set of blood pressures.

For patients using a wrist cuff instead of an upper arm cuff, consideration to the patient's positioning of the monitor, which ideally should be level with the heart, will contribute to the reliability of the readings. When patients bring their monitor to the evaluation, the health care provider has an opportunity to observe their skill in using the monitor as well as to determine if the cuff size is appropriate, and to measure a simultaneous blood pressure using a calibrated clinical manometer for comparison. After calculating the range and mean of a patient's blood pressure readings, those values can then be compared to the patient's blood pressure goal to evaluate the effectiveness of his or her current medical therapy and guide changes to it.

Guidelines for BP Goals

While there is no singular definition for hypertension, it is conventionally defined as the presence of a blood pressure that increases the risk for target organ damage in vascular beds including the brain, retina, heart, and kidney, and the large arteries. The US guidelines are based on periodic reports from the Joint National Committee on the Prevention, Detection, Evaluation and Treatment of High Blood Pressure (JNC), which first reported in 1976. At the time of this publication, JNC 7 guidelines are the most recent US guidelines available and are summarized below. The JNC 7 algorithm risk stratifies by blood pressure based on the presence of compelling indications including ischemic heart disease, heart failure, diabetes mellitus, chronic kidney disease, and a prior stroke or transient ischemic attack.

BP classification	Systolic BP (mmHg)		Diastolic BP (mmHg)[a]	Lifestyle modification	Without compelling indications	With compelling indications
Normal	<120	And	<80	Encourage	No therapy	No therapy
Prehypertension	120–130	Or	80–89	Yes	No therapy indicated	Therapy for compelling indications[b]
Stage I hypertension	140–159	Or	90–99	Yes	Thiazide-type diuretic for most; may consider ACE-I, ARB, b-blocker, CCB or combination[c]	Other antihypertensive drugs (diuretics, ACE-I, ARB, b-blocker, CCB) as needed
Stage II hypertension	≥160	Or	≥100	Yes	Two-drug combination for most	Other antihypertensive drugs (diuretics, ACE-I, ARB, b-blocker, CCB) as needed

ACE-I Angiotensin-converting enzyme inhibtor, *ARB* Angiotensin receptor blocker, *CCB* Calcium channel blocker

[a] Treatment determined by highest BP category

[b] Treat patients with chronic kidney disease or diabetes to BP goal of <130/80 mmHg

[c] Initial combined therapy should be used cautiously at risk for orthostatic hypotension

Lifestyle Modifications and Expected Results

Blood pressure is affected by body weight and diet composition. Lifestyle modifications for reduction in blood pressure include weight loss, reduction in alcohol, salt restriction, tobacco cessation, and physical exercise.

Modification	Recommendation	Approximate SBP reduction range
Weight reduction	Maintain normal body weight (BMI 18.5– 24.9 kg/m^2)	5–20 mmHg per 10 kg weight loss
DASH diet	Diet rich in fruits, vegetables and low-fat dairy products with reduction in saturated and total fat	8–14 mmHg
Reduction of dietary sodium	Reduce dietary sodium intake to <2.4 g sodium	2–8 mmHg
Physical activity	Regular aerobic physical activity ≥5 times per week	4–9 mmHg
Reduction of alcohol consumption	Limit ETOH consumption to <2 drinks per day in men and <1 drink per day for women	2–4 mmHg

General Medical Treatment Guidelines and Expected Results

Patient education prior to starting medical therapy is an integral part of hypertension management to ensure adherence to antihypertensive therapy. Using educational materials, providing reinforcement, and promoting social support are key strategies in educating patients for antihypertensive adherence. Regular home blood pressure monitoring should be encouraged in motivated patients. Medical providers starting patients on antihypertensive therapy should titrate the medications on a regular basis to achieve goal blood pressure targets as underdosing and inadequate titration of medications contributes to failure of therapy.

Thiazides

Thiazide diuretics are useful, low-cost first-line agents in the treatment of systolic and diastolic hypertension, which also reduce cardiovascular morbidity and mortality. Thiazide diuretics increase urinary excretion of sodium by inhibiting the sodium-chloride reabsorption pump in the distal convoluted tubule. All thiazides can be given once daily with good effect at low doses. As monotherapy in low doses, diuretics control blood pressure in approximately 50% of patients with stage I or early stage II hypertension. In combination with other drugs, diuretics can control up to 70% of patients. Although hydrochlorothiazide is commonly used, chlorthalidone may be a better choice in many patients.

The Antihypertensive Lipid-Lowering Treatment to Prevent Heart Attack (ALLHAT) Trial randomized more than 42,000 individuals with stage I or II hypertension to chlorthalidone, doxazosin, lisinopril or amlodipine as initial treatment demonstrating that chlorthalidone was superior to doxazosin with respect to the incidence of heart failure. The Systolic Hypertension in the Elderly Program (SHEP) studied the effect of chlorthalidone compared to placebo on the incidence of stroke and other cardiovascular events over 5 years and demonstrated an overall reduction in BP of 27/8 mmHg compared to 12/2 mmHg in placebo group.

Drug	Daily dosing (mg)	Frequency	Comments
Thiazide-type diuretics			
Chlorthalidone	12.5–50.0	Once daily	Longer acting effect compared to HCTZ
Hydrocholorthiazide (HCTZ)	12.5–50.0	Once daily	
Indapamide	1.25–5.0	Once daily	
Metolazone	2.5–10.0	Once daily	Effective at GFR <40 mL unlike other thiazides; poor bioavailability
Loop diuretics			
Furosemide	40–240	BID-TID	Multiple daily dosing to avoid rebound sodium retention
Bumetanide	0.5–4.0	BID-TID	Multiple daily dosing to avoid rebound to avoid Na retention
Torsemide	5.0–100.0	Once daily – BID	Longer duration of action
Ethacrynic acid	25.0–100.0	BID-TID	Ototoxicity

Side effects of thiazide use include volume depletion, hyponatremia, hypokalemic alkalosis, and hyperuricemia.

Potassium-Sparing Diuretics

Potassium-sparing diuretics such as amiloride and triamterene selectively block sodium transport channels in the distal tubules, which indirectly leads to increased urinary sodium excretion. Both are considered weaker diuretic compounds compared to thiazide and loop diuretics as these agents are relatively ineffective when used as monotherapy for hypertension. As a result, both amiloride and triamterene are often used with HCTZ for effective treatment of hypertension. Common adverse effects of amiloride include: hyperkalemia, orthostatic hypotension, headache, diarrhea, loss of appetite, nausea and vomiting. Common adverse effects of triamterene include: photosensivity, hyperkalemia, hyperuricemia, diarrhea, nausea and vomiting.

Loop Diuretics

Loop diuretics act on membrane ion transport mechanisms in the thick ascending limb of loop of Henle to prevent reabsorption of chloride and sodium. Loop diuretics are also venodilators allowing for their immediate preload-reducing effects in pulmonary edema. There is little arteriolar dilator effect so these agents are relatively ineffective in reducing blood pressure in most individuals with hypertension. The initial diuresis occurs during the first 2 h post-administration followed by a period of sodium retention that can result in neutral or occasionally positive sodium balance despite initial diuresis; therefore, multiple daily dosing is necessary for diuresis unless one of the longer-acting loop diuretics such as torsemide is used.

β-Adrenergic Blockers

The current JNC 7 guidelines allow β-adrenergic blockers as an appropriate first-line alternative treatment for hypertension based on the reduction of morbidity and mortality in several clinical trials. β-adrenergic blockers are appropriate for treatment of hypertension, especially in patients who also have concomitant ischemic heart disease, heart failure and/or arrhythmias. Multiple large clinical trials demonstrate a decrease in the incidence of stroke, myocardial infarction, and heart failure.

The mechanism of action is competitive inhibition of the effects of catecholamine at the β-adrenergic receptor causing a decrease in heart rate and cardiac output. β-adrenergic blockers also reduce plasma renin, increase circulating vasodilatory prostaglandins, and decrease plasma volume, which all contribute to the reduction of blood pressure. β-adrenergic antagonists can be subdivided into two classes; β_1-blockers, which are primarily cardioselective, and non-selective agents with β_1- and β_2-blocking effects. Alternatively, β-adrenergic antagonists can be categorized according to the presence or absence of intrinsic sympathomimetic activity (ISA) as β-adrenergic blockers with ISA cause less bradycardia compared to those without it. Common adverse effects of β-adrenergic antagonists include: bradyarrhythmia, heart block, heart failure, hypotension, pruritus, rash, diarrhea, dizziness, fatigue, depression, and Raynaud's phenomenon.

Commonly Used β-Adrenergic Antagonists

Medication	Properties	Initial dose	Usual dosage range (mg)
Atenolol	β_1 selective	50 mg daily – BID	25–100
Acebutolol	β_1 selective, ISA	400 mg daily, 200 mg daily	200–1,200
Betaxolol	β_1 selective	10 mg daily	5–40
Bisoprolol	β_1 selective	5 mg daily	2.5–20
Carteolol	ISA	2.5 mg daily	2.5–10
Carvedilol	α and β-antagonist	6.25 mg BID	12.5–50
Labetolol	α and β-antagonist	100 mg BID	200–1,200
Metoprolol	β_1 selective	50 mg BID	50–450
Metoprolol XL	β_1 selective	50–100 daily	50–400
Nadolol	Nonselective	40 mg daily	20–240
Penbutolol	ISA	20 mg daily	20–80
Pindolol	ISA	5 mg daily	10–60
Propanolol	Nonselective	40 mg daily	40–240
Timolol	Nonselective	10 mg BID	20–40

Selective α₁-Adrenergic Antagonists

Selective α_1-adrenergic antagonists block postsynaptic vasoconstrictor effects of norepinephrine causing a reduction in blood pressure. As a balanced arterial and venous dilator, there is little or no change in cardiac output. Based on the ALLHAT trial, selective α_1-adrenergic antagonists appear to be less efficacious in blood pressure lowering effects compared to ACE inhibitors, calcium channel blockers, and diuretics. Common adverse effects include: headache, fatigue, orthostatic hypotension, dizziness, and syncope associated with the "first dose effect." That results from a greater decrease in blood pressure with the first dose compared to subsequent doses.

These agents can be effective as monotherapy or as a multi-drug regimen though in clinical practice, selective α_1-adrenergic antagonists are often used to reach target goals in stage II hypertension as part of a multi-drug regimen. The effects are additive in combination with beta-blockers, ACE-inhibitors, ARBs, calcium channel blockers and diuretics. Race, age or gender has not been shown to significantly influence medication response. Selective α_1-adrenergic antagonists such as alfuzosin and tamsulosin, which are not indicated for hypertension, are used to treat benign prostatic hyperplasia and bladder outlet obstruction.

Commonly used selective α_1-adrenergic antagonists

Medication	Initial dose	Usual dosage range (mg)
Doxazosin	1 mg daily	1–16
Prazosin	1 mg BID-TID	1–20
Terazosin	1 mg QHS	1–20

Centrally Acting Adrenergic Agents

Centrally acting α_2-sympathetic agonists reduce blood pressure by decreasing sympathetic nervous outflow, systemic vascular resistance, and heart rate. These agents are not particularly effective as monotherapy due to salt and water retention and therefore should be paired with a thiazide diuretic. These agents can be useful to treat hypertensive patients with anxiety; however, common adverse effects include: headache, dizzinesss, somnolence, fatigue, constipation, dry mouth, and contact dermatitis or erythema with use of the transdermal patch.

Medication	Initial dose	Usual dose range (mg)	Comments
Clonidine	0.1 mg BID	0.1–1.2	May experience rebound HTN if used w/ β-blockers
Clonidine patch	0.1 mg transdermal patch Q weekly	0.1–0.3	
Guanfacine	1 mg daily	1–3	
Guanabenz	4 mg BID	4–64	
Methyldopa	250 mg BID – TID	250–2,000	Safe in pregnancy-induced HTN

Calcium Channel Antagonists

Calcium channel antagonists effectively treat all forms of hypertension in both monotherapy and combination therapy. These agents block the transmembrane influx of calcium ions into cardiac and vascular smooth muscles. It also reduces peripheral vascular resistance and lowers blood pressure by causing direct vasodilatation in the peripheral arteries of the vascular smooth muscle. The three main subclasses of calcium channel antagonists include phenylalkylamines such as verapamil, benzothiazepines including diltiazem and 1,4-dihydropyridines such as nifedipine. A negative inotropic effect occurs in the nondihydropyridine class of calcium channel antagonists. Other indications for use include diastolic dysfunction, variant angina, cerebral vascular disease, and cyclosporine hypertension. In the ALLHAT trial, the rates of coronary events and death were similar in amlodipine, chlorthalidone, and lisnopril.

Many of the calcium channel antagonists have been reformulated into sustained-release preparations, allowing for the convenience of once-a-day dosing. All agents are metabolized by the liver; therefore, patients with cirrhosis or using other medications that inhibit hepatic metabolism should be dose adjusted. Calcium channel antagonists can be used in patients of all ages and races and remain effective over a wide range of dietary salt intake.

ACE Inhibitors

Angiotensin converting enzyme inhibitors (ACE inhibitors) are effective antihypertensive agents that decrease the production of angiotensin II, which indirectly increases bradykinin levels. This stimulates the production of endothelium-derived relaxing factor, nitric oxide and induces prostacyclin release causing vasodilatation. ACE inhibitors slow the progression of target organ damage such as a reduction in proteinuria in nephropathy, while decreasing mortality in both high-risk coronary artery disease and post-myocardial infarction (post-MI). A lower response rate to ACE inhibitor monotherapy has been noted in certain patient populations including the elderly, African-Americans, and diabetics. In the post-MI population, initiation of a low-dose ACE inhibitor within 24 h of the infarction significantly reduced the risk of stroke, cardiovascular death, and another infarction as well as prevention of left ventricular remodeling.

The co-administration of a diuretic or calcium antagonist enhances the antihypertensive effect of an ACE inhibitor. The combination of a diuretic and ACE inhibitor depletes sodium, which activates the renin-angiotensin system and sensitizes the patient to ACE inhibition. Common adverse effects of ACE inhibitors include: hypotension, dizziness, syncope, hyperkalemia, headache, cough, and abnormal renal function tests. An infrequent, but serious response is angioedema of the head and neck.

Commonly used calcium channel antagonists

Medication	Properties	Initial doses	Usual dose range (mg)	Side effects	Notes
Amlodipine	Dihydropyridine	5 mg daily	2.5–10	LE edema, flushing, HA, rash	Longer plasma half life and more vasoselective compared to nifedipine
Diltiazem	Benzothiazepine	30 mg QID	90–360	Nausea, HA and rash	Negative cardiac inotrope and chronotropic effect
Diltiazem SR	Benzothiazepine	60–120 mg BID	120–360	Nausea, HA and rash	Negative cardiac inotrope and chronotropic effect
Diltiazem CD	Benzothiazepine	180 mg BID	180–360	Nausea, HA and rash	Negative cardiac inotrope and chronotropic effect
Diltiazem XR	Benzothiazepine	80 mg daily	180–480	Nausea, HA and rash	Negative cardiac inotrope and chronotropic effect
Isradipine	Dihydropyridine	2.5 mg BID	2.5–10	LE edema, flushing, HA, rash	Longer plasma half life and more vasoselective compared to nifedipine
Nicardipine	Dihydropyridine	20 mg TID	60–120	LE edema, flushing, HA, rash	Longer plasma half life and more vasoselective compared to nifedipine

(continued)

Medication	Properties	Initial doses	Usual dose range (mg)	Side effects	Notes
Nicardipine SR	Dihydropyridine	30 mg BID	60–120	LE edema, flushing, HA, rash	
Nifedipine	Dihydropyridine	10 mg TID	30–120	LE edema, flushing, HA, rash	
Nifedipine XL	Dihydropyridine	30 mg daily	30–90	LE edema, flushing, HA, rash	
Nisoldipine		20 mg daily	20–40		
Verapamil	Diphenylalkylamine	80 mg TID	80–480	Constipation, nausea, HA and orthostatic hypotension	Negative cardiac inotrope and chronotropic effect
Verapamil ER	Diphenylalkylamine	80 mg daily	180–480	Constipation, nausea, HA and orthostatic hypotension	Negative cardiac inotrope and chronotropic effect
Verapamil SR	Diphenylalkylamine	120–140 daily	120–480	Constipation, nausea, HA and orthostatic hypotension	Negative cardiac inotrope and chronotropic effect

Commonly used ACE-inhibitors

Medication	Initial dose	Usual dose range (mg)	Comment	Fixed-dose combination
Benazepril	10 mg BID	8–32		Benazepril/HCTZ (Lotensin HCT)
Captopril	25 mg BID-TID	50–450	Generic available	Captopril/HCTZ (Capozide)
Enalapril	5 mg daily	2.5–40	Generic and IV	Enalapril/HCTZ (Vaseretic)
Fosinopril	10 mg daily	10–40	Hepatic and renal elimination	Fosinopril/HCTZ (monopril-HCT)
Lisinopril	10 mg daily	5–40	Generic available	Lisinopril/HCTZ (Prinzide, Zestoretic)
Moexipril	7.5 mg daily	7.5–30		Moexipril/HCTZ (Uniretic)
Quinapril	10 mg daily	5–80		Quinapril/HCTZ (Accuretic)
Ramipril	2.5 mg daily	1.25–20	Indicated in high-risk pts	
Trandolapril	1–2 mg daily	1–4	Hepatic and renal elimination	

Angiotensin Receptor Blockers

Angiotensin receptor blockers (ARBs) selectively bind to angiotensin AT_1 receptors, which mediate vasoconstriction. Several clinical trials including ARBs such as losartan have reported outcome benefits demonstrating a reduction in systolic hypertension in the Lorsartan Intervention for Endpoint Study (LIFE). ARBs may be used as an alternative agent for patients with heart failure who are unable to tolerate ACE inhibitors. Other positive outcome benefits with ARBs have been seen in patients with diabetic nephropathy, ischemic heart disease, heart failure, and stroke. The common adverse effects of ACE inhibitors are less common with the use of ARBs. The serious response of angioedema of the head and neck is also less common.

Medication	Initial dose	Usual dosage range (mg)	Half-life	Comments
Candesartan	8 mg daily	8–32	9–13 h	
Irbesartan	150 mg daily	150–300	11–15 h	Labeled indication in DM II nephropathy
Losartan	25 mg daily	25–100	2 h	Labeled indication in DM II nephropathy
Olmesartan	20 mg daily	20–40	13 h	
Telmisartan	20 mg daily	20–80	24 h	Dose dependent bioavailability of 42–58%
Valsartan	80 mg daily	80–320	6 h	Labeled indication in CHF

Direct Arterial Dilators

Direct arterial dilators directly relax vascular smooth muscle cells allowing for arterial dilation. Initially they are effective in lowering blood pressure; however, over time their effects decline. Direct arterial dilators are rarely used as monotherapy for hypertension due to many intolerable side effects including flushing, headaches, and palpitations. As a result, direct arterial dilators are often used in triple therapy combination with diuretics and anti-adrenergic agents to control these side effects.

Hydralazine is absorbed by the gastrointestinal tract and has a half-life of 4 h with clinical action lasting 8–12 h with maximum effect occurring 15–75 min after administration. The adverse effects profile of hydralzine is extensive and not limited to inducing a lupus-like syndrome, nausea, vomiting, peripheral neuropathy, and edema. Hydralazine-induced lupus can present with arthralgias, malaise, weight loss, pericardial effusion, and skin rash.

Minoxidil, a more potent vasodilator, acts on potassium channels to limit calcium entry into certain cells. It is rapidly absorbed from the GI tract and is metabolized by the liver. The half-life is approximately 3–4 h though duration of action lasts from 12 to 72 h. This agent is useful in patients with renal insufficiency and refractory hypertension. Minoxidil should be administered with a potent diuretic and an adrenergic inhibitor to control minoxidil-induced tachycardia and edema. Common adverse effects include: hypotension, body fluid retention, hypernatremia, and hypertrichosis. Serious adverse effects include: cardiac effusion, occasionally with tamponade, and an abnormal electrocardiogram (e.g. change in the direction and magnitude of T waves).

Novel Treatment: Direct Renin Inhibitors

Aliskiren, FDA approved in 2007 for the treatment of primary hypertension in adults, is the first direct renin inhibitor on the market. Aliskiren binds to the $S3^{bp}$ binding pocket of renin, which prevents the conversion of angiotensinogen to angiotensin II. Common adverse effects include: diarrhea, dizziness, headache, and increased serum blood urea nitrogen and creatinine values. Serious adverse effects of hyperkalemia and angioedema have respective incidences of 0.9% and 0.06%.

Aliskiren is contraindicated in pregnancy and breast-feeding women.

Combination Antihypertensive Therapy

Monotherapy in the treatment of hypertension is often inadequate to maintain long-term blood pressure reduction as physiologic counterregulatory mechanisms activate, limiting the effectiveness of the primary agent. Combination therapy improves long-term efficacy, tolerability of treatment, and adherence. There are more than 25 combination single pill antihypertensive formulations on the market with many generic formulations available making them convenient and cost-effective for patients.

Special Populations

Elderly Populations

Hypertension is found in 75% of elderly patients defined as individuals >60 years old. The most common form of hypertension in this group is isolated systolic hypertension likely due to age-related changes including aortic stiffness. There is an increased risk of left ventricular hypertrophy, increased vascular resistance, and decreased plasma renin activity compared to younger patients. The JNC 7 guidelines recommend a SBP goal of less than 140 mmHg and a DBP goal of less than 90 mmHg when no other comorbid conditions exist. If an elderly patient has diabetes mellitus, chronic kidney disease, or ischemic heart disease, the guidelines recommend a SBP goal of less than 130 mmHg and a DBP goal of less than 80 mmHg. The Systolic Hypertension in the Elderly Program (SHEP) study reported that initial treatment for hypertension with a diuretic was associated with a lower incidence of fatal MI, stroke, and overall mortality. Combination therapy using diuretics, calcium channel blockers, ACE inhibitors, and ARBs is often necessary to achieve patient-specific goal values.

Consideration of a systolic blood pressure goal of less than 145 mmHg may be given to patients 80 years of age or older who: (a) are free of diabetes mellitus or vascular or renal disease; (b) have blood pressures refractory to intensive medical therapy; or (c) have developed adverse side effects or laboratory abnormalities to intensive therapy (e.g. light-headedness, fatigue, declining renal function values, hypokalemia, or hyponatremia). This consideration is based on the results of the Hypertension in the Very Elderly Trial and recent AHA guidelines. An international, multi-centered, randomized double-blind placebo controlled trial. It enrolled patients 80 years old or older with a systolic blood pressure in the range of 160–199 mmHg and diastolic blood pressure less than 110 mmHg to receive a placebo or to be treated with either indapamide SR 1.5 mg daily or indapamide SR 1.5 mg daily and perindopril 2 mg or 4 mg daily to achieve a targeted blood pressure of 150/80 mmHg. After 4 years, the group treated with either indapamide or indapamide with perindopril decreased their systolic blood pressure by 15 mmHg and decreased their diastolic blood pressure by 6 mmHg resulting in a 30% reduction in all strokes, a 39% reduction in fatal strokes, a 64% reduction in heart failure, and a 21% reduction in total mortality compared to the group receiving a placebo. After 2 years there were no significant differences between the groups with regard to their potassium, creatinine, glucose, and uric acid values.

Minority Populations

In African-Americans, the use of ACE inhibitors, ARBs, and β-blockers has been shown to be less effective in lowering blood pressure as this population group generally has lower plasma renin levels, higher plasma volume, and higher vascular resistance compared to Caucasians. Initial therapy with diuretics and in combination with calcium-channel antagonists is most effective for hypertension management. There is an increased risk of cough and flushing in Asian-Americans and angioedema in African Americans from ACE inhibitors.

Obesity

A large number of longitudinal studies, such as the Framingham study, have demonstrated a relationship between obesity and hypertension with increased vascular resistance, higher cardiac output, and lower plasma renin activity. While weight loss, changes in diet, and increased activity are lifestyle modifications that have successfully reduced blood pressure, medications are often needed to control hypertension until a reduction in body weight by at least 10–15% from baseline is achieved. There is no difference in the management of hypertension in the obese patient compared to the nonobese population. Practitioners should be aware that β-blockers may induce worsening fatigue and reduced exercise intolerance while ACE-inhibitors and α-adrenergic receptor blocking agents may increase insulin sensitivity.

Diabetes Mellitus

Hypertensive diabetic patients are at higher risk for cardiovascular disease, and medications should be optimized to achieve blood pressure control with a goal blood pressure of less than 130/80 mmHg. Lifestyle modifications, including weight loss if the BMI is greater than 30, and dietary changes, are essential to overall management. Combination therapy often requiring a diuretic, ACE inhibitor or ARB, and calcium channel blocker will be necessary to achieve control. Multiple large clinical trials have shown that ARBs and ACE inhibitors are effective in lowering blood pressure as well as protecting against proteinuria, heart failure, systolic dysfunction, and mild renal insufficiency.

Chronic Renal Insufficiency

Hypertensive patients with renal insufficiency should maintain a blood pressure of less than 130/80 mmHg or lower to prevent and treat the advancement of renal disease. The management of these patients often requires three or more agents to achieve this goal. Loop diuretics are an essential part of management in non-dialysis patients as the retention of sodium and water can exacerbate the hypertensive state. The use of an ACE inhibitor or ARB to block the renin-angiotensin-aldosterone system is efficacious in slowing chronic kidney disease. In patients with advanced renal disease with a serum creatinine greater than 5 mg/dL, there is no evidence that continued use of ACE inhibitors or ARBs has additional benefit to lowering blood pressure. The addition of α-adrenergic agents and β-blockers as third- or fourth-line agents can be helpful to achieve target blood pressure.

Coronary Artery Disease

Patients with hypertension and known coronary artery disease are at higher risk for future cardiovascular events including unstable angina and myocardial infarction. β-blockers should be first-line agents as they decrease mortality, subsequent reinfarction, and unstable angina as well as secondary prevention of future cardiac events and increase long-term survival after myocardial infarction. ACE inhibitors should be started within 24 h after a myocardial infarction, if the patient is hemodynamically stable, to decrease mortality and reduce left ventricular remodeling.

Heart Failure

Heart failure and hypertension increase the risk of left ventricular dilation and sudden death. ACE inhibitors, hydralazine, and nitrates are often used irrespective of hypertension as they decrease mortality in heart failure patients. Calcium channel antagonists should be used cautiously due to negative inotropic effects, which may worsen heart failure.

Resistant Hypertension

Hypertensive patients present a challenge after multiple agents have been initiated and titrated to control blood pressure. Patient noncompliance, inappropriate blood pressure cuff size, and pseudohypertension due to noncompressibility of severely arterioscelertoic or calcified arteries should be considered in the approach to the resistant hypertension patient. Home blood pressure monitoring with journaling should be considered for patients with white coat hypertension, which is defined by blood pressures greater than 140/90 mmHg on two or more clinical readings that are not consistent with those measured at home. Drug interference such as concomitant non-steroidal anti-inflammatory drug use may reduce antihypertensive efficacy. Most often, volume overload resulting from sodium and water retention can cause persistent elevations in blood pressure and can be discovered through diet analysis. Anxiety, new weight gain, and excessive alcohol intake can also increase blood pressure. Bilateral renal artery stenosis, pheochromocytoma, and primary hyperaldosteronism, though rare, should also be considered if the patient is resistant to multiple drug therapy and all other causes of resistant hypertension have been eliminated.

Further Reading

ACCF/AHA 2011 Expert consensus document on hypertension in the elderly. a report of the American College of Cardiology Foundation Task Force on Clinical Expert consensus documents developed in collaboration with the American Academy of Neurology, American Geriatrics Society, American Society for Preventive Cardiology, American Society of Hypertension, American Society of Nephrology, Association of Black Cardiologists, and European Society of Hypertension. Aronow WS, et al. J Am Coll Cardiol. 2011 May 17;57(20)2037–114. Epub April 25, 2011.

ALLHAT Collaborative Research Group. The Antihypertensive and Lipid Lowering Treatment to Prevent Heart Attack Trial (ALLHAT). Major outcomes in high-risk hypertensive patients randomized to angiotensin converting enzyme inhibitor or calcium channel blockers vs. diuretic. JAMA. 2002;288:2981.

Beckett NS, Peters R, Fletcher AE, et al. Treatment of hypertension in patients 80 years of age or older. N Engl J Med. 2008;358:1887–98.

Chobanian AV, Bakris GL, Black HR, et al. The seventh report of the Joint National Committee on the Prevention, Detection, Evaluation and Treatment of High Blood Pressure (JNC VII). JAMA. 2003; 289(6):2560–72.

Kaplan N. Systemic hypertension: mechanisms and diagnosis. In: Zipes D et al., editors. Braunwald's heart disease. 7th ed. Philadelphia: Saunders; 2005.

Pickering TG, Hall JE, Appel LJ, et al. Recommendations for BP measurement in humans and experimental animals; part 1: BP measurement in humans: a statement for professionals from the subcommittee of Professional and Public Education of the American Heart Association Council on High BP Research. Hypertension. 2005;45:142–61.

Sacks FM, Svetkey LP, Vollmer WM, et al. Effects on blood pressure of reduced dietary sodium and the dietary approaches to stop hypertension (DASH) diet. N Engl J Med. 2001;344:3–10.

SHEP Cooperative Research Group. Prevention of stroke by antihypertensive drug treatment in older persons with isolated systolic hypertension. JAMA. 1991;265:3255–64.

Stampfer MJ, Hu FB, Manson JE, et al. Primary prevention of coronary heart disease in women through diet and lifestyle. N Engl J Med. 2000;343:16–22.

Wachtell K, Lehto M, Gerdts E, et al. Angiotensin II receptor blockade reduces new onset atrial-fibrillation and subsequent stroke compared to atenolol: the losartan intervention for end point reduction in hypertension (LIFE) study. J Am Coll Cardiol. 2005;45(5):712–9.

Chapter 7
Dyslipidemia

Kevin J. Woolf and Robert C. Block

Introduction

Dyslipidemia is a common disorder of abnormal metabolism or levels of one or more of various triglyceride or cholesterol molecules. Based on the most recent guidelines established by the National Cholesterol Education Program (NCEP) Adult Treatment Panel III, approximately 23% of the United States population requires treatment for a cholesterol abnormality with either lifestyle modification or administration of medications [1]. Hypercholesterolemia is a well established risk factor for the development of coronary artery disease (CAD) [2], and is a strong marker for mortality in patients with CAD [3]. There is an ever increasing body of evidence that suggests aggressive treatment of dyslipidemia in an at-risk population (primary prevention) as well as in patients with established CAD (secondary prevention) is essential in the prevention of CAD and its complications.

K.J. Woolf (✉)
Division of Cardiology, University of Rochester Medical Center, Rochester, NY, USA
e-mail: kevin_woolf@urmc.rochester.edu

R.C. Block
Department of Community and Preventive Medicine,
The University of Rochester School of Medicine and Dentistry,
Rochester, NY, USA

J.D. Bisognano et al. (eds.), *Manual of Outpatient Cardiology*,   159
DOI 10.1007/978-0-85729-944-4_7,
© Springer-Verlag London Limited 2012

Lipid Metabolism and Pathophysiology

Lipids are utilized by peripheral tissues for cell membrane composition and function, metabolism, hormone production, and bile acid formation [4]. They are insoluble in plasma and are transported via lipoproteins, which are made up of cholesterol, triglycerides, protein, and phospholipids. There are five lipoprotein subtypes, each classified by the relative amount of each of these substances in the particle. Chylomicrons are large particles that carry dietary lipid, primarily triglycerides but also cholesterol and vitamins. Very low density lipoprotein (VLDL) and intermediate density lipoprotein (IDL) carry cholesterol esters and triglycerides. Low density lipoprotein (LDL) and high density lipoprotein (HDL) carry ApoB and ApoA cholesterol esters, respectively. Chylomicrons and VLDL are the primary transporters of triglycerides, while HDL and LDL are the primary transporters of cholesterol. Apolipoproteins, such as Apo B and ApoA are associated with lipoproteins, and are required for lipoprotein assembly and function.

Lipid metabolism occurs through two pathways, classified as endogenous and exogenous. In the exogenous pathway, dietary lipids are absorbed by the intestine. Free fatty acids combine to form triglycerides, and cholesterols are esterified. These particles are transported by chylomicrons and enter the cholesterol pool in the tissues, particularly the liver. The chylomicrons progressively shrink in size due to transfer of cholesterol esters to HDL and lipolysis, and ultimately form chylomicron remnants, which are rapidly cleared from the circulation. As a result of this, few chylomicrons should be present after a 12-h fast.

In the endogenous pathway, VLDL particles are synthesized by the liver. The VLDL particles are converted to IDL particles via lipolysis of their triglyceride core by lipoprotein lipase. The liver removes roughly half of the circulating IDL; the remaining IDL is converted to LDL via remodeling by hepatic lipase. Ultimately, the cholesterol in LDL accounts for more than half of the cholesterol in most individuals.

Cholesterol contained in LDL is removed from the circulation via LDL receptor-mediated endocytosis as well as by HDL mediated transfer to the liver.

Cholesterol can only be effectively excreted from the body via enteric tissues into the gut lumen, or via hepatic tissues as bile. Cholesterol found within peripheral tissues is transported to the liver and intestine via reverse cholesterol transport, which is mediated by HDL. HDL particles are synthesized by the intestine and liver and acquire cholesterol and phospholipids from their site of origin, as well as from chylomicrons as indicated previously. The HDL particles then undergo extensive remodeling which enables them to more effectively take up cholesterol from the periphery. Cholesterol contained in HDL can be transferred to hepatocytes either by direct uptake via a specific receptor, or by indirect transfer to LDL lipoproteins via cholesteryl ester transport protein (CETP). LDL is then removed from the circulation as mentioned previously.

The most common and morbid condition which is promoted by abnormal levels of lipoproteins is atherosclerosis. Clinically, atherosclerosis is the most common direct cause of coronary, peripheral, and neurological vascular disease. Atherosclerosis is a complex process involving not only lipoproteins but inflammatory cells as well [5]. The formation of an atherosclerotic plaque is either initiated by or greatly exacerbated by elevated levels of LDL cholesterol. This promotes accumulation of LDL particles in the intima of the artery, forming a "fatty streak" which is the precursor to an atherosclerotic plaque. This sequestration of LDL from the bloodstream within the vessel serves to remove the particles from antioxidants, promoting oxidation of the lipoproteins. This appears to trigger an inflammatory response and the expression of leukocyte adherent receptors in the intima as well as the release of cytokines. Monocytes adhere to and ultimately some migrate into the intima. These monocytes exhibit expression of receptors for the oxidized lipoproteins, and they are incorporated into cells via phagocytosis. These monocytes create "foam cells" in which their cytoplasm contains a large amount of lipid droplets. Smooth muscle cells then begin to migrate from the artery's media and accumulate throughout the intima. These form the collagenous matrix within the intima that will make up the largest mass of the plaque. The presence and rupture of these atherosclerotic plaques causes the vast majority of CAD, as well as peripheral and cerebrovascular disease. Atherosclerosis is also a major cause of chronic renal disease [6].

Dyslipidemia and Coronary Artery Disease

There are two broad categories of disorders of lipid metabolism: Inherited (primary) disorders and secondary disorders. The treatment goals and general approach in all types of dyslipidemia is essentially the same; however, patients with inherited disorders may be more refractory to medical treatment because of severe abnormalities in cholesterol metabolism. Numerous familial disorders of abnormal lipid metabolism have been identified [7, 8]. These disorders have been classified by the type of lipoprotein that is elevated (see Table 7.1). Many of these disorders may result in collections of LDL in the skin and tendons known as xanthomas. Pancreatitis is also common in Fredrickson classes I and V where the triglycerides are most prominently elevated. However, the most important cardiovascular clinical manifestation in this group of patients is premature coronary artery disease.

The most common secondary causes of dyslipidemia are type II diabetes and obesity. Lipid levels can also be elevated by cigarette smoking, hypothyroidism, chronic kidney disease, nephrotic syndrome, or cholestatic liver disease. Lipid levels in secondary dyslipidemia may be improved with treatment of the inciting factor; however, additional therapy is often indicated.

Hypercholesterolemia has long been recognized as a risk factor for CAD. Multiple studies have shown a direct relationship between cholesterol levels and the risk of coronary disease [2, 3]. In particular, elevated levels of total cholesterol and LDL are associated with an increased risk of CAD. There

TABLE 7.1 Fredrickson classification of familial (primary) hyperlipidemia

Class	I	IIa	IIb	III	IV	V
Elevated lipoprotein	Chylomicrons	LDL	LDL and VLDL	Chylomicrons and VLDL remnants	VLDL	Chylomicrons and VLDL
Total cholesterol	normal	↑↑	↑↑	↑	normal to ↑	↑
LDL	↓	↑	↑	↓	↓	↓
HDL	↑↑	↑	↑↑	↑↑	↑↑	↑↑
Triglycerides	↑↑	normal	↑	↑	↑↑	↑↑
Xanthomas	+	+	–	+	–	+
Pancreatitis	+	–	–	–	–	+

is an inverse relationship between CAD and HDL, i.e. a decreased level of HDL raises the risk of CAD. Abnormal levels of cholesterol are predictive of morbidity and mortality in the presence of CAD, with up to a 12-fold increased risk of death between the lowest LDL and the highest LDL groups [3]. The risk of CAD is most strongly correlated with LDL levels as opposed to other lipoproteins, and a risk association with total cholesterol is most likely present because LDL makes up the majority of the total cholesterol levels. Thus, total cholesterol is essentially a surrogate marker for LDL levels, and its use has been superseded by measurement of other markers, including LDL. Non-HDL is another excellent marker for adverse cardiovascular outcomes [9].

Hypertriglyceridemia is more loosely associated with CAD risk. It is strongly associated with other CAD risk factors such as diabetes, obesity, smoking, and decreased HDL levels which have been difficult to control for to evaluate the contribution of triglycerides as a risk factor. In a meta-analysis of observational data, hypertriglyceridemia contributed an increase in relative risk of 14% in men and 37% in women [10].

Hyperlipidemia has also been associated with non-coronary cardiovascular disease. For example, it has been demonstrated to be a risk factor for non-hemorrhagic stroke [11] and carotid stenosis. There is also an association between hyperlipidemia and kidney disease, with low HDL levels appearing to be a particular risk for developing chronic kidney disease [12]. The evidence behind treatment of hyperlipidemia in neurologic and kidney disease is much less robust than in CAD, however, and this is reflected in the NCEP treatment guidelines.

Treatment Options

Lifestyle Modification

Once the diagnosis of dyslipidemia has been made, an initial approach to treatment should include dietary modification and the initiation of an exercise regimen. Dietary modification should target weight loss and should include a reduction in the intake of saturated fat and cholesterol. Various foods such as fish oil, soy, red yeast rice, plant sterols, and fiber have a beneficial effect on LDL levels and patients should be advised to increase the intake of these items. Exercise levels should be increased, and in general patients should be counseled to exercise for a minimum of 30 min at a moderate intensity at least 5 days a week. In one study, diet and exercise together reduced LDL by 14.5 mg/dL in women and 20.0 mg/dL in men [13]. The effects of either diet or exercise alone were not significant.

HMG CoA Reductase Inhibitors (Statins)

HMG (3-hydroxy-3-methyl-glutaryl) CoA reductase inhibitors (statins) act on the enzyme HGM CoA reductase to reduce cholesterol biosynthesis. These medications have a strong effect on reducing LDL levels, and a more modest effect on increasing HDL and decreasing triglycerides [14]. The degree of effect on LDL, HDL, and triglycerides is variable by medication within this class. The most common side effect of statins is myalgia, which is relatively common. Rhabdomyolysis, on the other hand, is relatively uncommon. Other unusual complications include actual hepatic dysfunction, which is rare, and elevated transaminase levels which is much more common but only rarely associated with hepatic dysfunction. There has been no proven difference in side effect profiles of the various statins available, though higher doses are associated with more liver toxicity and myalgias. Also, female gender, increased age, and the presence of diabetes mellitus are associated with increased risk for these side effects.

Statins are, by far, the best studied medications in terms of cardiac outcomes, and have become the recommended first line agent for pharmacological treatment of hyperlipidemia. In terms of primary prevention, the AFCAPS/TexCAPS [15] (lovastatin) and ASCOT-LLA [16] (atorvastatin) trials showed improvement in cardiac events in patients with no

TABLE 7.2 Relative effects of various statins

Medication	Dose range (mg)	LDL decrease at starting dose (%)	LDL decrease at maximal dose (%)	HDL increase (%)	Triglyceride decrease (%)
Pravastatin	10–40	20	30	3–6	8–13
Simvastatin	10–80	28	46	5–7	12–18
Atorvastatin	10–80	37	51	2–6	20–28
Rosuvastatin	10–40	46	55	8–10	20–26

Adapted from Jones et al. [20]

prior CAD and elevated cholesterol. The earlier WOSCOPS [17] trial used pravastatin in men with no prior CAD, and also showed a reduction in cardiovascular events, including a 32% risk reduction in cardiovascular death. The most recent NCEP guidelines recommend statins as the first line agent in primary prevention when medications are indicated.

There are numerous statin medications available currently, with modestly differing effects on lipoprotein concentration as well as potency (see Table 7.2) [18–20]. The most potent statins are rosuvastatin and atorvastatin, and these medications have been shown to achieve the NCEP LDL goals at the starting dose more frequently than some of the older statins. However, similar reductions in LDL can be achieved with higher doses of simvastatin, pravastatin, or lovastatin. Rosuvastatin also raises HDL levels (8–10%), and atorvastatin and rosuvastatin both have a modest beneficial effect in terms of triglyceride lowering.

Statins have also been extensively studied in patients with pre-existing CAD (secondary prevention). In the 4S trial [21], patients with CAD and hyperlipidemia who were given simvastatin showed a significant reduction in cardiac events, including total mortality. In this trial, the number needed to treat to prevent one cardiac event was only six. The LIPID trial showed similar effects with pravastatin [22]. Several trials have shown benefit in patients with normal or low LDL levels. The Heart Protection Study enrolled patients with documented CAD or diabetes mellitus, and randomized to simvastatin 40 mg or placebo. The simvastatin group showed a significant reduction in cardiac events, as well as total mortality. Interestingly, 33% of those enrolled had a baseline LDL less than 116 mg/dL [23]. Another trial specifically evaluated statin use in patients with documented CAD but with normal LDL levels, and found benefit [24]. This evidence has led to the accepted use of statins in all patients with CAD, irrespective of serum LDL.

The current NCEP guidelines recommend initiating statins at a dose that is anticipated to achieve the recommended LDL level based on risk (see below). However, there is some evidence that treating CAD patients with more potent doses irrespective of LDL levels is beneficial. The IDEAL study randomized post-myocardial infarction (MI) patients to atorvastatin 80 mg or simvastatin 20 mg, and found a modest reduction in non-fatal MI with atorvastatin [25]. The TNT study showed a significant reduction in cardiovascular events with use of atorvastatin 80 mg vs. atorvastatin 10 mg [26]. In both of these trials, the rates of side effects were significantly higher in the group receiving the more potent statin. These trials demonstrate that patients that are at the highest risk of coronary events, such as those with uncontrolled co-morbid risk factors or a recent acute coronary syndrome (ACS), should have their hyperlipidemia treated with a more aggressive regimen. The NCEP has adjusted its LDL goal for the highest risk patients to reflect this approach [27].

Because of the extensive volume of evidence supporting mortality benefit with use of statins in prevention and treatment of CAD, they are the recommended first line agents in the treatment of hyperlipidemia. Patients who are intolerant of one statin due to side effects may be perfectly tolerant of a lower dose of the same medication or another statin. Data also exist supporting the use of extended release fluvastatin or every other day statin use to alleviate myalgia side effects [28]. If a patient is truly intolerant of the medication class, or additional lipid control (i.e. increasing HDL or further

TABLE 7.3 Pharmacologic management of hyperlipidemia with relative effect on lipoproteins

Medication class	Examples	LDL	HDL	Triglycerides	Side effects
Statins	Simvastatin, atorvastatin	↓↓	↑	↓	Myopathy, elevated LFTs
Fibric acid derivatives	Gemfibrozil, fenofibrate	↓	↑↑	↓↓	Dyspepsia, myopathy, gallstones
Bile acid sequestrants	Cholestyramine	↓	↑	No change	Bloating, cramping, nausea
Cholesterol absorption inhibitors	Ezetimibe	↓↓	No change to slight ↓	↓	Diarrhea, arthralgia
Nicotinic acid	Niacin	↓	↑↑↑	↓	Flushing, hyperglycemia, hyperuricemia, elevated LFTs

decrease in LDL) is desired, additional classes of lipid-modifying drugs can be substituted or added to a patient's regimen. Table 7.3 summarizes the effects of medications for hyperlipidemia [29].

Fibric Acid Derivatives

The fibric acid derivatives gemfibrozil and fenofibrate reduce the hepatic secretion of VLDL, facilitate clearance of triglyceride-bearing lipoproteins, and stimulate HDL synthesis. Their effect is to decrease triglyceride levels and increase HDL levels. Their main side effect is muscle toxicity, which is more common with gemfibrozil. Because of this, and renal excretion differences, fenofibrate is the preferred agent by many physicians when used in combination with statins. However, disappointing results from the FIELD Study using fenofibrate and more promising and consistent effects in the Helsinki Heart

Study [30], and VA-HIT studies with gemfibrozil [31] have lead many providers to favor gemfibrozil in many patients.

Bile Acid Sequestrants

Bile acid sequestrants bind bile acids in the intestine. As a result, the most common side effects include nausea, bloating, and cramping; elevated liver enzymes are also a recognized side effect. It is important that these drugs not be prescribed for patients with hypertriglyceridemia as they can worsen this lipid disorder. Medications in this class include cholestyramine, colestipol, and colesevelam. These medications result in an overall decrease in LDL. Cholestyramine showed a modest benefit in cardiovascular events in a primary prevention trial [32].

Cholesterol Absorption Inhibitors

There is currently one cholesterol absorption inhibitor, ezetimibe. Ezetimibe impairs dietary and biliary absorption of cholesterol at the brush border of the intestine. This has the effect of a reduction in LDL levels, and when combined with a statin will lead to greater LDL reduction than with an increase in the statin dose [33]. This has the theoretical benefit of keeping statins at a lower dose. Although clinical trials [34, 35] have suggested no benefit from ezetimibe with respect to clinical outcomes, via the measurement of carotid intimal media thickness (CIMT), these studies were not statistically powered to carefully examine effects on clinical events. Their use of the surrogate outcome of CIMT also creates doubt on whether these so-called "negative" results are clinically important and should drive the use of this cholesterol absorption inhibitor, particularly in light of the fact that the numbers of subjects enrolled in these studies are tiny compared to those enrolled in clinical trials of statins. The ongoing IMPROVE-IT study is designed to test the hypothesis that taking ezetimibe reduces cardiovascular disease events [36].

Nicotinic Acid

Nicotinic acid, or niacin, inhibits the hepatic formation of VLDL and subsequently its metabolite LDL. It also inhibits the transfer of HDL to VLDL and slows HDL clearance. This has the effect of an increase in HDL, and, at higher doses, modest reductions in triglyceride and LDL concentrations. The most common side effect is flushing, which is often severe enough that patient compliance with niacin becomes an issue. This side effect can be minimized by timing aspirin administration shortly prior to niacin, ingesting niacin prior to taking a hot shower, taking niacin with a meal, and avoiding hot beverages within about 2 h of the niacin dose. Other potential side effects include elevated liver enzymes, hyperglycemia, and hyperuricemia. Niacin has been demonstrated to reduce adverse cardiovascular events [37] vs. placebo and was superior to ezetimibe in improving serial carotid intima-media thickness measurements [35].

Screening Recommendations and Goals of Therapy

The high prevalence of hyperlipidemia in the population amplifies the importance of identification and treatment of the disease from a public health standpoint. The trials referenced above have demonstrated significant benefit in both prevention and treatment of CAD. A meta-analysis estimated a 15% reduction in cardiovascular mortality for each 10% lowering of cholesterol [38]. The risk of development of CAD is dependent upon other risk factors, and the relatively short-term benefits in the prevention of events obtained through treatments for hyperlipidemia is greatest in patients at higher risk. As such, the NCEP has established evidence-based criteria for screening, risk-stratifying, and treatment goals for hyperlipidemia based on an individual patient's risk. The NCEP is currently working on updated recommendations that should be available in 2011.

Screening for Hyperlipidemia

The NCEP recommends that all people 20 years and over should have screening at least once every 5 years. The recommended test is a fasting lipid panel performed after a 9–12 h fast to eliminate post-prandial elevations in LDL or triglycerides. Patients with optimal results (see Table 7.4) who have 0–1 risk factors and no known CAD can be rescreened in 5 years. Patients with borderline results should be rescreened in 1–2 years.

TABLE 7.4 NCEP ATP III classification of LDL, total, and HDL cholesterol

LDL cholesterol	
<100	Optimal
100–129	Near optimal/above optimal
130–159	Borderline high
160–189	High
≥190	Very high
Total cholesterol	
<200	Desirable
200–239	Borderline high
≥240	High
HDL cholesterol	
<40	Low
41–59	Normal
≥60	High

Adapted from Third Report of the National Cholesterol Education Program (NCEP) [1]

Identifying Cardiovascular Risk

An individual's risk in the NCEP guidelines is determined by the presence of CAD or CAD "equivalents," the presence of risk factors for CAD, and the Framingham 10-year risk for developing CAD. A patient is considered to be in the CAD risk equivalence category if they have documented CAD, diabetes mellitus, symptomatic carotid artery disease, peripheral arterial disease, or an abdominal aortic aneurysm. Next, a patient's risk factors are identified: cigarette smoking, hypertension (BP≥140/90 or on antihypertensive medication), HDL cholesterol less than 40 mg/dL for men and less than 50 mg/dL for women, family history of premature CAD (first generation male with CAD at age<55 or first generation female with CAD at age<65), or age (≥45 years in men, 55 years in women). The existing risk factors present will determine the 10-year Framingham CAD risk; if the risk is >20%, the patient is considered to be in the CAD risk equivalent category. These data allow for stratification by the NCEP's risk categories (see Table 7.5).

Determining LDL Goal

Each risk category is associated with an LDL goal, an LDL level at which to initiate therapeutic lifestyle changes, and an LDL level at which to consider drug therapy (see Table 7.5). The ATP III goal for lower risk patients is an LDL of less than 160 mg/dL. For patients in the moderate or moderately high-risk categories, the LDL goal is less than 130 mg/dL, with an optional goal of 100 mg/dL in the moderately high-risk category. Patients in the CAD equivalent category have an LDL goal of less than 100 mg/dL, and have the consideration of a goal of 70 mg/dL in very high-risk patients. Very high-risk patients are those with a recent MI or ACS or those with poorly controlled risk factors. Although this is not reflected in the NCEP guidelines, there are data to support the use of statins in patients with documented CAD irrespective of starting LDL (i.e. in patients with normal or low LDLs) [23].

TABLE 7.5 NCEP/ATP III modified risk categories and LDL targets

Risk Category	Characteristics	LDL goal	LDL level at which to initiate therapeutic lifestyle changes	LDL level at which to initiate pharmacologic therapy
High risk	CAD, CAD equivalent[a], 2+ risk factors[b] with Framingham 10-year risk >20%	<100 mg/dL; <70 mg/dL in very high risk patients	≥100 mg/dL	≥100 mg/dL; consider <100 mg/dL
Moderately high risk	2+ risk factors[b] with Framingham 10-year risk 10–20%	<130 mg/dL	≥130 mg/dL	≥130 mg/dL; consider in 100–129 mg/dL
Moderate risk	2+ risk factors[b] with Framingham 10-year risk <10%	<130 mg/dL	≥130 mg/dL	≥160 mg/dL
Lower risk	0–1 risk factor	<160 mg/dL	≥160 mg/dL	≥190 mg/dL; consider in 160–189 mg/dL

[a]Documented CAD, diabetes mellitus, symptomatic carotid artery disease, peripheral arterial disease, or abdominal aortic aneurysm

[b]Cigarette smoking, hypertension (BP ≥140/90 or on antihypertensive medication), HDL cholesterol <40 mg/dL (men) or <50 mg/dL (women), family history of premature CAD (first generation male with CAD at age <55 or first generation female with CAD at age <65), or age (≥45 years in men, 55 years in women)

Adapted from Third Report of the National Cholesterol Education Program (NCEP) [1] and Grundy et al. [27].

Secondary Goals

While the LDL goal outlined above should be the primary target for lipid-lowering therapy, in certain circumstances treatment directed at elevated triglycerides or low HDL may be appropriate. In patients with elevated triglycerides (>150 mg/dL), treatment should first be directed at achieving the LDL goal. Once that is achieved, weight management and physical exercise intensification may result in additional lowering of the triglyceride level. The NCEP guidelines suggest that a secondary goal in patients with elevated triglycerides be non-HDL cholesterol (total cholesterol − HDL cholesterol), and that this goal be set at the patient's LDL goal+30. In patients with a triglyceride level of 200–499 mg/dL who have achieved their LDL goal, consideration may be given to adding nicotinic acid or a fibrate to lower triglyceride levels. In patients with a triglyceride level of 500 mg/dL or higher, triglyceride lowering should be a priority as these levels are associated with pancreatitis. In these patients, a very-low fat diet, weight loss, exercise, and often a fibrate, nicotinic acid, and/or omega-3 fatty acids in the form of Lovaza® are indicated.

Similarly, in patients with low HDL levels, treatment should primarily be directed at achieving goal LDL levels, and secondarily non-HDL goals if the triglycerides are elevated. In patients with isolated low HDL and normal triglycerides, treatment with nicotinic acid or a fibrate should be considered if there is a CAD risk equivalent.

Summary

Dyslipidemias are extremely common disorders of lipid metabolism and composition which can result from familial or environmental causes. The most important complication from dyslipidemia in most individuals is the development of atherosclerosis and, in particular, CAD. Throughout the past 40 years significant developments have been made in the treatments of dyslipidemias in order to prevent and treat

CAD. The NCEP has developed a set of guidelines which address lifestyle and pharmacologic treatment of hyperlipidemia which are currently being updated. With the appropriate screening, selection, and treatment of patients with dyslipidemia, a large burden of disease can be treated in a safe and efficient manner.

References

1. Third Report of the National Cholesterol Education Program (NCEP) Expert Panel on Detection, Evaluation, and Treatment of High Blood Cholesterol in Adults (Adult Treatment Panel III) final report. Circulation. 2002;106:3143–421.
2. The multiple risk factor intervention trial (MRFIT). A national study of primary prevention of coronary heart disease. JAMA. 1976;235:825–7.
3. Pekkanen J, Linn S, Heiss G, et al. Ten-year mortality from cardiovascular disease in relation to cholesterol level among men with and without preexisting cardiovascular disease. N Engl J Med. 1990; 322:1700–7.
4. Rifkind B, Levy RI. Hyperlipidemia: diagnosis and therapy. New York: Grune & Stratton; 1977.
5. Ross R. Atherosclerosis – an inflammatory disease. N Engl J Med. 1999;340:115–26.
6. Kavey RE, Allada V, Daniels SR, et al. Cardiovascular risk reduction in high-risk pediatric patients: a scientific statement from the American Heart Association Expert Panel on Population and Prevention Science; the Councils on Cardiovascular Disease in the Young, Epidemiology and Prevention, Nutrition, Physical Activity and Metabolism, High Blood Pressure Research, Cardiovascular Nursing, and the Kidney in Heart Disease; and the Interdisciplinary Working Group on Quality of Care and Outcomes Research: endorsed by the American Academy of Pediatrics. Circulation. 2006; 114:2710–38.
7. Fredrickson DS, Lees RS. A system for phenotyping hyperlipoproteinemia. Circulation. 1965;31:321–7.
8. Fredrickson DS. An international classification of hyperlipidemias and hyperlipoproteinemias. Ann Intern Med. 1971;75:471–2.
9. Ridker PM, Rifai N, Cook NR, Bradwin G, Buring JE. Non–HDL cholesterol, apolipoproteins A-I and B100, standard lipid measures, lipid ratios, and CRP as risk factors for cardiovascular disease in women. JAMA. 2005;294:326–33.

10. Austin MA, Hokanson JE, Edwards KL. Hypertriglyceridemia as a cardiovascular risk factor. Am J Cardiol. 1998;81:7B–12B.
11. Amarenco P, Lavallee P, Touboul PJ. Statins and stroke prevention. Cerebrovasc Dis. 2004;17 Suppl 1:81–8.
12. Zandi-Nejad K, Brenner BM. Strategies to retard the progression of chronic kidney disease. Med Clin North Am. 2005;89:489–509.
13. Stefanick ML, Mackey S, Sheehan M, Ellsworth N, Haskell WL, Wood PD. Effects of diet and exercise in men and postmenopausal women with low levels of HDL cholesterol and high levels of LDL cholesterol. N Engl J Med. 1998;339:12–20.
14. Vaughan CJ, Gotto Jr AM. Update on statins: 2003. Circulation. 2004;110:886–92.
15. Downs JR, Clearfield M, Weis S, et al. Primary prevention of acute coronary events with lovastatin in men and women with average cholesterol levels: results of AFCAPS/TexCAPS. Air Force/Texas Coronary Atherosclerosis Prevention Study. JAMA. 1998;279:1615–22.
16. Sever PS, Dahlof B, Poulter NR, et al. Prevention of coronary and stroke events with atorvastatin in hypertensive patients who have average or lower-than-average cholesterol concentrations, in the Anglo-Scandinavian Cardiac Outcomes Trial – Lipid Lowering Arm (ASCOT-LLA): a multicentre randomised controlled trial. Lancet. 2003;361:1149–58.
17. Shepherd J, Cobbe SM, Ford I, et al. Prevention of coronary heart disease with pravastatin in men with hypercholesterolemia. West of Scotland Coronary Prevention Study Group. N Engl J Med. 1995;333:1301–7.
18. Jones P, Kafonek S, Laurora I, Hunninghake D. Comparative dose efficacy study of atorvastatin versus simvastatin, pravastatin, lovastatin, and fluvastatin in patients with hypercholesterolemia (the CURVES study). Am J Cardiol. 1998;81:582–7.
19. Brown AS, Bakker-Arkema RG, Yellen L, et al. Treating patients with documented atherosclerosis to National Cholesterol Education Program-recommended low-density-lipoprotein cholesterol goals with atorvastatin, fluvastatin, lovastatin and simvastatin. J Am Coll Cardiol. 1998;32:665–72.
20. Jones PH, Davidson MH, Stein EA, et al. Comparison of the efficacy and safety of rosuvastatin versus atorvastatin, simvastatin, and pravastatin across doses (STELLAR* Trial). Am J Cardiol. 2003;92:152–60.
21. Randomised trial of cholesterol lowering in 4444 patients with coronary heart disease: the Scandinavian Simvastatin Survival Study (4S). Lancet 1994;344:1383–9.
22. Prevention of cardiovascular events and death with pravastatin in patients with coronary heart disease and a broad range of initial cholesterol levels. The Long-Term Intervention with Pravastatin in Ischaemic Disease (LIPID) Study Group. N Engl J Med. 1998;339:1349–57.

23. MRC/BHF Heart Protection Study of cholesterol lowering with simvastatin in 20,536 high-risk individuals: a randomised placebo-controlled trial. Lancet. 2002;360:7–22.
24. Pfeffer MA, Sacks FM, Moye LA, et al. Cholesterol and recurrent events: a secondary prevention trial for normolipidemic patients. CARE Investigators. Am J Cardiol. 1995;76:98C–106C.
25. Pedersen TR, Faergeman O, Kastelein JJ, et al. High-dose atorvastatin vs. usual-dose simvastatin for secondary prevention after myocardial infarction: the IDEAL study: a randomized controlled trial. JAMA. 2005;294:2437–45.
26. LaRosa JC, Grundy SM, Waters DD, et al. Intensive lipid lowering with atorvastatin in patients with stable coronary disease. N Engl J Med. 2005;352:1425–35.
27. Grundy SM, Cleeman JI, Merz CN, et al. Implications of recent clinical trials for the National Cholesterol Education Program Adult Treatment Panel III guidelines. Circulation. 2004;110:227–39.
28. Jacobson TA. Toward "pain-free" statin prescribing: clinical algorithm for diagnosis and management of myalgia. Mayo Clin Proc. 2008;83:687–700.
29. Paoletti R, Holmes WL. Drugs affecting lipid metabolism. Berlin/New York: Springer; 1987.
30. Keech A, Simes RJ, Barter P, et al. Effects of long-term fenofibrate therapy on cardiovascular events in 9795 people with type 2 diabetes mellitus (the FIELD study): randomised controlled trial. Lancet. 2005;366:1849–61.
31. Rubins HB, Robins SJ, Collins D, et al. Gemfibrozil for the secondary prevention of coronary heart disease in men with low levels of high-density lipoprotein cholesterol. Veterans Affairs High-Density Lipoprotein Cholesterol Intervention Trial Study Group. N Engl J Med. 1999;341:410–8.
32. The Lipid Research Clinics Coronary Primary Prevention Trial results. I. Reduction in incidence of coronary heart disease. JAMA. 1984;251:351–64.
33. Pearson TA, Denke MA, McBride PE, Battisti WP, Brady WE, Palmisano J. A community-based, randomized trial of ezetimibe added to statin therapy to attain NCEP ATP III goals for LDL cholesterol in hypercholesterolemic patients: the ezetimibe add-on to statin for effectiveness (EASE) trial. Mayo Clin Proc. 2005;80:587–95.
34. Kastelein JJ, Akdim F, Stroes ES, et al. Simvastatin with or without ezetimibe in familial hypercholesterolemia. N Engl J Med. 2008;358:1431–43.
35. Taylor AJ, Villines TC, Stanek EJ, et al. Extended-release niacin or ezetimibe and carotid intima-media thickness. N Engl J Med. 2009;361:2113–22.
36. Cannon CP, Giugliano RP, Blazing MA, et al. Rationale and design of IMPROVE-IT (IMProved Reduction of Outcomes: Vytorin

Efficacy International Trial): comparison of ezetimbe/simvastatin versus simvastatin monotherapy on cardiovascular outcomes in patients with acute coronary syndromes. Am Heart J. 2008;156:826–32.

37. Canner PL, Berge KG, Wenger NK, et al. Fifteen year mortality in Coronary Drug Project patients: long-term benefit with niacin. J Am Coll Cardiol. 1986;8:1245–55.

38. Gould AL, Rossouw JE, Santanello NC, Heyse JF, Furberg CD. Cholesterol reduction yields clinical benefit: impact of statin trials. Circulation. 1998;97:946–52.

Chapter 8
Coronary Artery Disease

Benjamin G. Plank, M. James Doling, and Peter A. Knight

Introduction

Coronary artery disease is the leading cause of death for men and women in the USA. A report by the American Heart Association estimates that one out of every six deaths in this country is a consequence of coronary artery disease [1]. An American suffers a heart attack every 25 seconds, and the disease takes a life every minute. As alarming as these statistics may be, improvements in management and prevention have led to a steady decline in the global death rate attributable to coronary artery disease over the past few decades [2, 3].

The prevalence of coronary artery disease in our population is striking. In the USA approximately 17.6 million adults 20 years of age and older have coronary artery disease,

B.G. Plank (✉)
Department of Medicine, Division of Cardiology,
University of Rochester Medical Center, Rochester, NY, USA
e-mail: benjamin_plank@urmc.rochester.edu

M.J. Doling
Division of Cardiology, University of Rochester Medical Center,
Rochester, NY, USA

P.A. Knight
Surgery, Division of Cardiac Surgery,
University of Rochester Medical Center,
Rochester, NY, USA

J.D. Bisognano et al. (eds.), *Manual of Outpatient Cardiology*,   179
DOI 10.1007/978-0-85729-944-4_8,
© Springer-Verlag London Limited 2012

accounting for nearly 8% of the population [1]. Of those, approximately 8.5 million have had a prior myocardial infarction, while 10.2 million suffer from chronic angina pectoris.

Men continue to be affected by coronary artery disease slightly more often than women, but the difference is small. Approximately 9% of US men and 7% of women have coronary artery disease [1]. Among males, the disease is more prevalent in whites (9.4%) than in African Americans (7.8%). The opposite is true for women, with a higher prevalence in African Americans (8.8%) than in whites (6.9%). Latino and Asian adults have a slightly lower prevalence of CAD than whites and African Americans.

The likelihood that an individual will develop coronary artery disease in his or her lifetime is impressive. According to data from the Framingham Heart Study, the lifetime risk of developing coronary artery disease for a previously disease-free 40-year-old individual is 49% for men and 32% for women [4]. Those who live to age 70 without prior disease continue to face a 24–35% risk of developing coronary disease in their lifetime.

Indeed, the burden this disorder places on our society and economy is profound. As our population ages, and as the number of coronary artery disease survivors increases, the core of cardiovascular care will continue to shift from the hospital setting to the clinic. Now more than ever it is imperative that our outpatient medical professionals are skilled in the management of coronary artery disease.

Pathophysiology

The vast majority of coronary artery disease can be attributed to atherosclerosis, a chronic disorder involving lipid accumulation within the walls of arteries. In order to better appreciate the natural history of this disease, the normal arterial anatomy and physiology will be reviewed, and a brief discussion of the pathophysiology of atherosclerosis and coronary artery disease will follow.

Layers of an Arterial Wall

All arteries, including coronary arteries, are composed of three layers – the intima, tunica media, and adventitia, all surrounding the central lumen through which blood flows (Fig. 8.1). Each layer serves a number of essential purposes and plays a central role in vascular homeostasis.

Intima

The intima is the innermost layer of an arterial wall. A single layer of endothelial cells, called the endothelium, lines its luminal aspect. This endothelial monolayer is anchored to a tough matrix called the basal lamina, a collagenous layer that confers structural support to the intima, while maintaining constant contact with blood as it flows through the lumen. Endothelial cells interact with blood through various mechanisms and play a critical role in maintaining continuous flow through the artery.

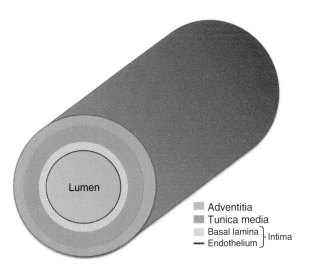

FIGURE 8.1 Cross sectional schematic of an artery and its major layers

As part of the body's natural defense system, blood is primed to clot whenever it is exposed to foreign (non-blood) material. This function is in place to help avert exsanguination and maintain hemostasis in the event of a vascular injury. When triggered, a complex cascade of coagulation protein activation is unleashed. The net result is thrombus formation. The endothelium is not blood and is therefore perceived as foreign by blood, thus generating the potential for coagulation. To prevent intravascular clot from forming, endothelial cells must prevent thrombus formation as blood comes into contact with the intimal wall. They accomplish this through numerous inhibitory mechanisms that are built into endothelial cell membranes.

The luminal surface of endothelial cells exhibits anticoagulant and pro-fibrinolytic proteins. Heparin sulfate proteoglycan molecules, for example, are present on the surface of endothelial cell membranes. As blood comes into contact with the monolayer, the heparin sulfate proteoglycan molecules potentiate antithrombin III production in blood, inhibiting thrombin formation and coagulation. Thrombomodulin is another anticoagulant protein found on the endothelial cell surface. This protein enhances the activation of proteins S and C, which act to inhibit thrombin activation and thrombus formation. In addition to anticoagulant elements, endothelial cell membranes contain fibrinolytic proteins such as tissue plasminogen activator. Tissue plasminogen activator potentiates production of plasmin, a potent fibrinolytic protein that will break down clot if it is generated. These mechanisms work together with various others to prevent blood from clotting as it travels through vessels.

Tunica Media and Adventitia

The intermediate layer of an arterial wall, called the tunica media, consists of concentrically layered smooth muscle cells and a supportive elastic matrix that act to provide the vascular tone and flexibility that are essential for arterial function.

Smooth muscle cells contract and relax in response to various stimuli including adrenergic tone (contraction) and nitric oxide (relaxation). This contraction and relaxation enable small arteries and arterioles to regulate blood flow through vascular beds. In larger arteries, aberrant smooth muscle contraction may lead to vasospasm that can occasionally inhibit blood flow and precipitate tissue ischemia. In addition to maintaining vascular tone, smooth muscle cells produce much of the extracellular matrix that provides the structural support and strength necessary to maintain arterial homeostasis.

The outer layer of an artery, called the adventitia, contains elements necessary to sustain the artery, including the vaso vasorum (tiny blood vessels that supply nutrients to the wall) and nerve endings that deliver stimuli from the autonomic nervous system. In addition, mast cells and fibroblasts reside in small numbers in this layer, providing innate immunologic support when needed.

Atherosclerosis

Atherosclerosis is a condition in which fatty material accumulates within arterial wall and forms an atheroma, or plaque. This process can take decades to evolve, during which time most individuals remain largely asymptomatic. Clinical manifestations of the disease are recognized only after a plaque becomes sizeable enough to hinder blood flow through the vessel lumen, or unstable enough to precipitate an acute and obstructing thrombus (see Fig. 8.2).

The initial step in plaque development involves the buildup of low-density lipoproteins (LDL) within the intimal layer. LDL, often referred to as "bad cholesterol," is a type of lipoprotein that functions to transport fats and cholesterol through the bloodstream. Buildup of LDL in an arterial wall occurs when LDL concentrations are elevated, as may be the case after eating a meal rich in cholesterol and saturated fat or in individuals with a genetic predisposition to hyperlipidemia.

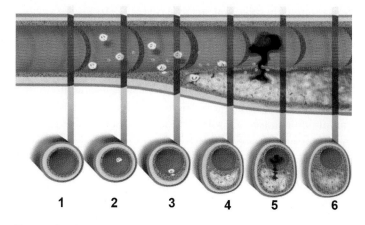

FIGURE 8.2 Stages of coronary atherosclerotic plaque development [5]. The upper drawing is a longitudinal section depicting evolving atheroma at different stages of development. The bottom is the corresponding cross-sectional representation of the vessel. (1) Normal coronary artery. (2) Monocytes are recruited by endothelial cells that were activated by oxidized LDL particles accumulating in the intima. (3–4) Activated monocytes differentiate into macrophages, cross the endothelium, and phagocytize LDL particles to become lipid-laden foam cells. Foam cells recruit smooth muscle cells to the intima, which begin to build a fibrous capsule around the lipid-rich core. (4) Inflammatory mediators stimulate foam cells to produce tissue factor and proteinases. The proteinases begin to degrade the fibrous capsule. (5) Weakened fibrous cap may rupture, exposing lipid-rich core and tissue factor to blood. Coagulation is activated, thrombus is generated. This may cause an acute coronary syndrome. (6) Thrombus is resorbed, atheroma heals, but scar is more collagenous and calcific than before

The LDL particles travel across the endothelial monolayer and bind to intimal matrix proteins. Once bound, the particles are essentially fixed within the vessel wall (Fig. 8.2, stages 1–2).

Over time, enzymes expressed by intimal cells oxidize the LDL particles. The resulting oxidized lipids are pro-inflammatory and induce cytokine production by neighboring smooth muscle cells residing in the tunica media. Inflammatory cytokines such as IL-1 stimulate local endothelial cells to express cell adhesion molecules (VCAM-1, ICAM-1, and selectins) on their luminal surfaces. Circulating mononuclear cells from blood are captured by these adhesion molecules, activated, and make their way across the endothelium and into the intima (Fig. 8.2, stage 3). The activated monocytes differentiate into macrophages, migrate towards the oxidized LDL particles, and bind to and internalize them. These lipid-laden macrophages remain in place and are referred to as "foam cells" due to their foamy appearance under light microscopy. The foams cells accumulate within the intima, eventually forming a "fatty streak," the precursor to an atheroma.

Foam cells release pro-inflammatory cytokines as they gather within the fatty streak. The cytokines stimulate smooth muscle cell migration from the tunica media. Once in the intima, the smooth muscle cells actively proliferate and deposit a fibrous matrix around the lipid rich foam cells. The fatty streak has now become an atheroma (Fig. 8.2, stage 4). Smooth muscle cells and foam cells eventually die, leaving a largely acellular fibrous capsule surrounding a central core filled with necrotic foam cells. The luminal aspect of this fibrous capsule is often referred to as the "fibrous cap," and plays an important role in the pathophysiology of acute coronary syndromes.

As a plaque develops and expands, it slowly pushes the vessel wall outward until it can no longer physically accommodate this movement. After a critical point in advancement is reached the plaque begins to expand inward, infringing upon and narrowing the vessel lumen. Symptoms of coronary artery disease are manifested as the severity of luminal narrowing progresses, usually beyond 60%. Affected individuals may begin to experience exertional chest pain or pressure, often associated with shortness of breath, nausea, or diaphoresis that is relieved by rest or nitroglycerin. This predictable pattern of symptoms is referred to as "stable" angina pectoris, and is often a sign of clinically significant coronary stenosis.

While the chronic narrowing of a coronary artery's lumen may cause stable anginal symptoms, it is acute intracoronary thrombosis that is most commonly responsible for an acute coronary syndrome such as unstable angina or myocardial infarction (Fig. 8.2, stage 5). A coronary plaque is vulnerable to the relentless mechanical stress of blood flow. As smooth muscle cells residing in the plaque's fibrous capsule die, the combination of a weakened fibrous cap and continuous exposure to the mechanical shearing effect of blood can lead to fibrous cap fracturing (plaque rupture) or superficial erosion. Both mechanisms expose the sub-endothelial matrix and the pro-coagulant materials within the necrotic core to blood. Coagulation is activated and an acute intracoronary thrombus is formed. If significant, the thrombus may severely limit or completely obstruct blood flow through the artery resulting in acute myocardial ischemia or infarction.

Risk Factors

As mentioned, most cases of coronary artery disease can be attributed to atherosclerotic involvement of the heart's vascular tree. This same atherosclerotic process is responsible for all cardiovascular disorders including cerebrovascular, peripheral arterial, and aortic diseases. An individual with cardiovascular disease will most likely have atherosclerotic involvement of multiple vascular beds. For this reason, noncoronary vascular disease is regarded as carrying an equivalent risk for future cardiac events as the presence of coronary disease itself [6].

In addition to established cardiovascular disease, observational studies have identified multiple independent risk factors that are linked to the development of coronary artery disease. These factors include advanced age, male sex, a family history of coronary artery disease, hypertension, dyslipidemia, diabetes mellitus, and tobacco abuse. One analysis examined data from three major observational cohorts in an attempt to link patient characteristics to coronary risk [7]. Clinical characteristics from over 380,000 individuals were analyzed, and it was found that nearly all of the approximately 21,000 people who died of a coronary event had at least one of the aforementioned risk factors.

While factors such as advanced age, male sex, and family history are inescapable, others are clearly modifiable. INTERHEART was a large case–control study that sought to quantitate the global impact of potentially modifiable risk factors believed to be associated with coronary disease [8]. More than 15,000 individuals from six continents who presented with an acute myocardial infarction were included along with a similar number of age-matched controls that were free of pre-existing heart disease. A number of modifiable factors were identified that were highly associated with the majority of cases. Hypertension, dyslipidemia, diabetes, smoking, lack of exercise, abdominal obesity, and a diet lacking of fruits and vegetables carried the strongest associations. Of those, INTERHEART found that tobacco use accounted for 36% of the global population-attributable risk (PAR) for a first myocardial infarction (odds ratio 2.87 compared to non-smokers). This was topped only by dyslipidemia, which carried a PAR of 49% (OR 3.25). Diabetes and hypertension were also found to be important predictors of future events (OR 2.37 and 1.91, respectively), while the daily consumption of fruits and vegetables and regular exercise were found to be protective (OR 0.70 and 0.86, respectively).

INTERHEART and similar epidemiologic studies have demonstrated that there is a tremendous potential for disease prevention if risk factors are identified and modified. As medical practitioners, we must carefully screen our patients in order to identify high-risk patients, and then work with them to modify their habits and clinical characteristics that put them in danger of developing cardiovascular disease. If successful, we have the potential to prevent a great deal of heart disease before it has a chance to manifest.

Clinical Consequence of Coronary Artery Disease

The hallmark symptom of obstructive coronary artery disease is chest discomfort, or angina. Often described as a "pressure" or "tightness" located in the left chest region, it may radiate to the neck and jaw or down the left arm and may be associated with other symptoms such as shortness of breath, diaphoresis, nausea, and vomiting. Angina may be characterized as either stable or unstable based on specific aspects of the history and clinical presentation. Unstable angina, together with non-ST-elevation myocardial infarction and ST-elevation myocardial infarction, make up the clinical spectrum known as Acute Coronary Syndrome. All patients presenting with anginal symptoms must be carefully evaluated by a health care professional and triaged appropriately.

Acute Coronary Syndrome

Acute coronary syndrome (ACS) comprises a spectrum of disorders that are most commonly associated with sudden plaque disruption and thrombus formation leading to partial or complete coronary artery obstruction. This spectrum is made up of three clinical conditions: unstable angina, non-ST-elevation myocardial infarction (NSTEMI), and ST-elevation myocardial infarction (STEMI). While a detailed discussion of ACS is outside of the spectrum of this book, a brief overview will be provided here.

Unstable angina is a clinical diagnosis. It differs from stable angina in that it is angina that possesses at least one of the following qualities: (a) occurs at rest; (b) is new in onset, often severe in intensity; (c) occurs in a crescendo pattern (more severe, longer lasting, or more frequent than a patient's chronic stable angina); or (d) is not relieved by rest or nitroglycerin. Unstable angina is an urgent cardiac condition, and patients should be referred to an emergency department for rapid evaluation and treatment.

Individuals with angina who test positive for myocardial cell death with elevated cardiac biomarkers (CK, CK-MB, or Troponin) levels are further classified as having a NSTEMI. Patients with UA/NSTEMI require inpatient treatment and telemetry monitoring, serial cardiac biomarkers, intensive medical management, and noninvasive testing (for lower-risk patients with UA) or angiography and revascularization.

Those who present with chest discomfort and have ST elevations on their ECG are having an STEMI and require emergent cardiac care including immediate angiography and revascularization, which is best accomplished with PCI if available or thrombolytics if transfer to a cardiac catheterization laboratory is more than 60 min away. The goal is to open the occluded coronary artery within 90 min after the patient presents to the emergency department.

It is important to note that while most cases of acute coronary syndrome are the result of atherosclerotic plaque rupture and thrombus formation, other etiologies are possible. Coronary vasoconstriction may occur due to a number of mechanisms including excessive adrenergic stimulation, cocaine, cold immersion, and endothelial dysfunction. Prinzmetal angina (also called Variant angina), is a form of intermittent coronary vasoconstriction, the mechanism of which is still not completely understood. Other etiologies for acute coronary syndrome include progressive luminal narrowing (as seen in stent restonosis following PCI and transplant graft arteriopathy), coronary arteritis, and coronary embolism.

Stable Angina

Angina that occurs predictably with certain levels of exertion or emotional stress and is relieved within 5–15 min by rest or nitroglycerin is referred to as stable angina. As discussed above, stable angina is the result of myocardial ischemia caused by a coronary plaque that has grown large enough to impinge upon the vessel lumen. Stable symptoms may range from mild to severe, and may significantly impair an individual's quality of life.

All patients with stable angina should be referred to a Cardiologist for non-invasive stress testing to determine the extent of the ischemia and to decide whether coronary revascularization would be beneficial. For many individuals, symptom management can be adequately achieved with an anti-ischemic medication regimen. The most common classes of anti-ischemic drugs used to treat stable angina include nitrates, beta-blockers, and calcium-channel blockers. Therapy should be initiated with a single agent, with the addition of a second drug only if necessary to reduce symptoms.

Beta-blockers are first-line drugs for stable angina. They inhibit myocardial beta-adrenergic receptors, resulting in a reduction of both heart rate and contractility. The net result is lower myocardial work during exertion. In addition to symptom relief, beta-blockers have been shown to reduce mortality and prevent future heart attacks in patients with angina who have previously suffered a myocardial infarction [9]. According to the guidelines set forth by the American College of Cardiology (ACC) and the American Heart Association (AHA), beta-blockers are recommended for all patients with stable angina who have a history of a prior MI or for those who have left ventricular dysfunction [10]. Cardio-selective beta-blockers (those that act on beta-1 receptors specifically) such as metoprolol and atenolol are recommended for stable angina, as they tend to have fewer extra-cardiac side effects than non-selective beta-blockers.

Nitrates promote vascular dilation by inducing smooth muscle relaxation within the vessel wall. Their anti-ischemic effects are largely the result of the decreased myocardial workload brought about by systemic vasodilation and cardiac afterload reduction. When afterload is reduced, the heart muscle contracts and pumps blood forward against a lower resistance, requiring less work and thus less oxygen. Nitrates are available in long-acting and short-acting preparations. Short-acting nitrates, such as sublingual nitroglycerin, are used as needed to treat acute anginal symptoms. Long-acting preparations such as isosorbide mononitrate are used daily for maintenance therapy. Tolerance is a common problem encountered with chronic nitrate therapy. Care must be given to dose long-acting nitrates properly to assure adequate nitrate-free periods within each 24-h period, in order to prevent tolerance from developing. In general, this can be accomplished by prescribing nitrates according to their dosing instructions provided by the manufacturer.

Calcium channel blockers inhibit voltage-gated calcium channels in cardiac muscle and blood vessels, which results in a decrease in intracellular calcium in myocytes and vascular smooth muscle cells. When these cells are prompted to contract, a process dependent upon intracellular calcium, they are only able to do so to a lesser extent. The net result is a decrease in cardiac contractility and peripheral arterial vasodilatation and afterload reduction, which decreases myocardial oxygen demand. Long-acting calcium channel blockers are recommended for stable angina, such as diltiazem, amlodipine, or felodipine. Short-acting dihydropyridine calcium channel blockers such as nifedipine should be avoided, as they may increase the risk of mortality and myocardial infarction in select patients [11, 12].

Ranolazine, a late sodium channel blocker, is a newer antianginal medication that has been shown to reduce symptoms of chronic stable angina [13, 14]. Approved by the FDA in 2006 for management of stable angina, this drug is recommended for patients who have anginal symptoms that are refractory to other anti-anginal medications. An important side-effect of Ranolazine is prolongation of the QT interval, a factor which precludes its recommendation as a first-line agent for angina.

All patients with stable angina should take measures to improve their overall aerobic capacity and to reduce their cardiovascular risk. A regular, low-impact aerobic exercise program should be recommended for patients who do not have contraindications. Aerobic conditioning lowers cardiac oxygen requirements and increases exercise tolerance. In addition, daily aspirin therapy (81 mg daily) should be initiated, unless contraindicated. If aspirin is contraindicated, clopidogrel should be considered. Modification of other cardiovascular risk factors including smoking, weight loss, hypertension, dyslipidemia, and glycemic control is imperative for the management of patients with stable angina.

The current ACC/AHA guidelines recommend that patients with stable angina be referred for noninvasive stress testing [15]. A detailed discussion of the indications for stress testing and the types of stress tests available is found in Chap. 4. Individuals with intermediate- or high-risk findings on stress testing, or those with severe anginal symptoms that are refractory to optimal medical therapy, may be referred for coronary angiography. Based on those findings, coronary revascularization will be offered to those with disease patterns that have been shown to benefit from the procedure.

Coronary Revascularization

Coronary revascularization is the restoration of blood flow to regions of myocardium that are poorly perfused due to a coronary obstruction. Revascularization may be accomplished percutaneously using a series of catheters, balloons, and stents (percutaneous coronary intervention, or PCI) or surgically (coronary artery bypass grafting, or CABG). The decision to proceed with revascularization and the approach chosen is dependent upon the patient's clinical presentation, risk profile, and coronary anatomy.

Patients presenting with an acute coronary syndrome may require urgent or emergent coronary angiography and revascularization in order to salvage myocardium that is at risk of death. As discussed, a care provider should refer any patient expected of having an acute coronary syndrome to a medical center for urgent evaluation and treatment by a specialist. A detailed discussion concerning the indications for and methods of coronary revascularization in patients with an acute coronary syndrome is outside the scope of this text.

Coronary artery disease manifesting as stable angina is commonly encountered in the outpatient setting. If left untreated, the disorder will lead to worsening symptoms and an increased risk of myocardial infarction, heart failure, and death. Patients presenting with stable coronary artery disease require aggressive medical optimization to slow or prevent the progression of coronary artery disease and to lower their cardiovascular risk. As discussed previously, all patients with stable angina should be risk-stratified with a non-invasive stress test prior to making a decision to proceed with angiography. Those who have severe disease identified on angiography or with persistent lifestyle-altering symptoms despite maximal medical therapy may be candidates for coronary revascularization. The options for revascularization include CABG or PCI.

Coronary Artery Bypass Grafting

Coronary artery bypass grafting is a surgical procedure in which a Cardiothoracic Surgeon restores blood flow to a region of myocardium supplied by an obstructed coronary artery. To accomplish this, blood vessels harvested from other parts of the body, called grafts, are reattached to the coronary circuit downstream from the obstruction. The vessels used for grafting include arteries (most commonly one or more internal thoracic arteries or a radial artery) and veins (typically saphenous veins harvested from the patient's leg). Developed in 1964, the procedure has been refined and is now one of the most commonly performed operations in the USA.

For patients with chronic refractory angina, early and intermediate post-operative outcomes are excellent when compared to medications alone. The Coronary Artery Surgery Study (CASS) demonstrated a marked reduction in anginal symptoms in those who underwent surgery, with over 60% of CABG patients remaining symptom-free at 5 years compared to fewer than 40% of those on medical therapy alone [16]. This symptom benefit disappeared at 10 years however, with statistically similar rates of angina seen in both groups.

The long-term symptomatic benefits of bypass surgery are most likely limited by the development of graft failure. Arterial grafts are known to have excellent long-term patency [17, 18]. Left internal thoracic arterial grafts have a patency rate of greater than 95% at 10 years. Vein grafts, on the other hand, carry a 10–15 year patency rate of only 60%. This difference in graft durability is reflected in long-term survival outcomes following bypass surgery. Patients with severe three-vessel disease undergoing CABG who received an arterial graft to the left anterior descending coronary artery, alone or in combination with other vein grafts, had an 83% survival rate at 10 years compared to 71% of those who received vein grafts alone [19]. A subsequent analysis found that this survival benefit was still present at 15 years [20].

While a primary goal of surgical revascularization in patients with stable coronary artery disease is symptom management, it has been proven that some patients gain a mortality benefit from CABG over medical therapy alone. Those with high-risk anatomy identified by angiography including severe left main coronary artery disease, three-vessel disease, and two-vessel disease including severe proximal LAD stenosis were found in a number of studies to have a significantly lower risk of mortality when treated with bypass surgery [21–23]. In addition, patients who received bilateral internal thoracic arterial grafting gained an added benefit over a single internal thoracic graft, with 50% survival at 20 years in the dual-ITA group versus 37% in the single-ITA group [24].

Percutaneous Coronary Intervention

Percutaneous coronary intervention is an invasive procedure performed by an Interventional Cardiologist. Using fluoroscopic guidance, a catheter is advanced to the heart through an arterial access point in the wrist (radial artery) or groin (femoral artery). The coronary arteries are selectively engaged with the catheter and injected with contrast dye, allowing visualization of coronary blood-flow within the arteries. Narrowing or blockages within the coronary vascular tree are identified in this way. If a severe lesion is identified, revascularization may be possible by balloon angioplasty or, more commonly now, stent placement.

Balloon angioplasty dates back to the 1970s. Originally developed to offer an alternative to coronary artery bypass grafting, the procedure involves a small, deflated balloon that is passed through a coronary lesion and then inflated, stretching the blockage and breaking its fibrous and calcific skeleton. After deflating and removing the balloon, blood is able to pass freely through the dilated vessel. Revascularization has been accomplished. The biggest problem with balloon angioplasty is its relatively high restenosis rate, with approximately 40% of treated lesions narrowing within 6 months of the procedure [25]. This restenosis is associated with recurrence of anginal symptoms in up to 75% of patients, and leads to repeat revascularization in around 30%[26]. The introduction of coronary artery stents in the 1990s has brought about a dramatic decline in PCI restenosis rates.

A coronary artery stent is a small metallic meshwork tube that is used to open a blocked segment of a coronary artery. There are two basic categories of stents: bare metal stents (BMS) and drug-eluting stents (DES). Both are made of a strong, expandable metal alloy. Drug-eluting stents differ from BMS in that they are impregnated with a chemo-inhibitory medication (most often paclitaxel or sirolimus) that acts to prevent stent "restenosis." Restenosis is the overgrowth of cellular and fibrotic tissue that can infringe upon the vessel lumen and inhibit blood flow. The decision regarding which type of stent to use is based on multiple clinical factors.

The first intra-coronary stents developed were bare metal. Since their introduction into clinic practice in the late 1980s they have been shown to provide a definite benefit over balloon angioplasty, cutting the overall restenosis rate down by approximately 30% and the target lesion revascularization rate (the rate at which patients must undergo an additional PCI procedure to revascularize their previously-opened lesion) by 15% compared to balloon angioplasty alone [27, 28].

Drug-eluting stents were developed to further reduce the restenosis and target lesion revascularization rates. These stents work by chemically inhibiting neo-intimal hyperplasia within the stent lumen. The benefit of DES was illustrated in a large meta-analysis published in 2007 that evaluated data from 38 randomized trials (including more than 18,000 patients) comparing DES to BMS. The study identified a marked reduction in the target lesion revascularization rate in patients who received a drug-eluting stent, with similar rates of death and myocardial infarction [29].

While restenosis is an important complication of percutaneous interventions using stents, stent thrombosis is a potentially devastating problem that practitioners must be wary of. Stents are essentially foreign bodies implanted directly into the bloodstream. As blood comes into contact with metal, platelets and other clotting factors are triggered, increasing the risk of thrombus formation within the stent. Stent thrombosis may result in complete obstruction of flow through the artery, leading to an acute myocardial infarction. A dual antiplatelet regimen including aspirin and a thienopyridine (clopidogrel, ticlopidine, or prasugrel) has been shown to reduce the risk of stent thrombosis and is therefore a critical part of post-PCI management.

Over time, endothelial cells overgrow, or "endothelialize," the stent, effectively eliminating direct contact between blood and metal. This process significantly reduces the risk of stent thrombosis. Due to the inhibitory medication secreted by a DES, neointimal growth takes longer to mature compared to bare metal stents. This point has important clinical implications and lengthens the recommended duration of dual antiplatelet therapy for those patients receiving a drug-eluting stent.

Most cases of stent thrombosis occur within the first month after placement, although the overall thrombosis rate is very low (less than 1%) when patients are treated with an appropriate dual-antiplatelet regimen, regardless of whether a DES or BMS was used [30, 31]. Similarly, the rates of stent thrombosis in drug-eluting and bare metal stents are both less than 1% up to a year after placement [32]. The risk of very late stent thrombosis (more than a year after implantation) is low, but has been shown to be slightly higher in those who received a DES versus BMS [33]. Despite this increased risk of very late stent thrombosis, patients receiving a DES had a markedly reduced risk of target lesion revascularization due to restenosis and had no significant difference in death or myocardial infarction compared to those who received a BMS [34].

The benefits and limitations of percutaneous intervention in the management of patients with stable coronary artery disease was demonstrated in COURAGE, published in 2007. COURAGE was a large randomized clinical trial comparing outcomes in patients with stable angina and high-risk coronary anatomy who were randomized to treatment with PCI plus optimal medical management or medical management alone [35]. The majority of patients in the intervention group received bare-metal stents, as drug-eluting stents were not yet approved for use during the majority of the enrollment period. After a mean follow-up of almost 5 years, there was no difference in death or myocardial infarction between the two groups. Further review found that anginal symptoms were better controlled in the PCI group at 6 month compared to the medical group, but this benefit was gone at 3 years, likely reflecting progression of underlying chronic coronary disease [36].

PCI Versus CABG

As discussed, the goals of medical therapy and revascularization are to improve symptoms and prevent the complications of coronary artery disease including myocardial infarction, heart failure, and death. When a decision has been made to pursue coronary revascularization, multiple factors must be considered in order to determine the best method to accomplish a successful result.

Several early studies compared outcomes in patients who were revascularized with balloon angioplasty versus coronary artery bypass grafting (CABG). Some of the more prominent trials included BARI, RITA, GABI, and CABRI [37–40]. In general, these studies found that overall survival was similar in the angioplasty and CABG groups. However, patients undergoing angioplasty were more likely to have recurrent angina that required an additional revascularization procedure. While the results are telling, these studies do not accurately reflect modern practice as most percutaneous interventions now involve stent placement.

Bare metal stents were compared to CABG in patients with stable CAD in the Arterial Revascularization Therapies Study Part I (ARTS I) and Stent or Surgery (SoS) trials. In ARTS I, over 1,200 patients with multi-vessel disease were randomized to undergo bypass surgery or bare-metal stent placement [41]. At 5 years there was no mortality difference between the two groups, but there was a significantly higher risk of repeat revascularization in the BMS group (30% vs. 9%). Similarly, the SoS trial randomized nearly 1,000 patients to BMS or CABG and found a significantly higher risk of repeat revascularization in the stent group (21% vs. 6%) at 6 years [42]. In addition, this analysis found that mortality was significantly higher in the PCI group (11% vs. 7%). The reason for increased mortality in the PCI group was unclear and was not seen in similar studies. A meta-analysis comparing BMS to CABG was published soon after SoS and included data from ARTS I, SoS, and two other large randomized trials [43]. This report found no difference in mortality at 5 years between the two groups, but again noted a significantly higher rate of repeat revascularization in the BMS group (29% vs. 8%).

Drug-eluting stents were designed to decrease the risk of restenosis and have been shown to carry a lower rate of restenosis compared to BMS while maintaining a similar risk of myocardial infarction and death. The SYNTAX trial compared long-term outcomes in patients with stable coronary artery disease who received PCI with DES to those who underwent CABG [44]. The study randomized 1,800 patients with severe coronary artery disease (three-vessel disease or left main coronary artery stenosis) to either PCI with DES or surgical intervention with CABG. At 12 months, the composite risk of death, stroke, and MI was similar between the PCI and CABG groups (7.6% vs. 7.7%, respectively). However, as seen in prior studies, the risk of repeat revascularization due to recurrent anginal symptoms was significantly higher in the PCI group (13.5% vs. 5.9%). The stroke risk at 1 year was higher in the CABG group (2.2% vs. 0.6%), a finding which may be a due to the fact that PCI patients were more likely than CABG patients to be treated with a dual-antiplatelet regimen following revascularization.

Of the outcome measures considered following revascularization, quality of life (QOL) is among the most important. The original SYNTAX trial assessed major adverse cardiovascular events in patients with stable CAD receiving PCI with DES compared to CABG. The SYNTAX authors went on to publish an additional report comparing QOL between the two groups [45]. Using standardized questionnaires to assess health-related QOL, the group found that while patients who received PCI reported better QOL compared to CABG in all categories immediately following revascularization, the CABG patients were more likely to be angina-free at 12 months compared to PCI (71.6% vs. 76.3% $P=0.05$).

The question of which revascularization approach is best is difficult to answer, and the risks and benefits of PCI and CABG must be carefully weighed for each individual patient. Those with chronic stable angina who fail medical management and who are considering revascularization should be referred to a Cardiologist for further assessment, risk stratification, and discussion of the different treatment options.

Risk Reduction in Patients with Coronary Artery Disease

Patients with a history of coronary artery disease, including those with stable angina or a prior myocardial infarction, are at an increased risk of developing further cardiovascular complications such as myocardial infarction, stroke, and death. For these high-risk individuals, aggressive risk factor reduction is imperative, and a balanced approach should be pursued consisting of lifestyle modification, medical therapy, and regular medical follow-up.

Smoking Cessation

As discussed earlier in this chapter, tobacco abuse is a powerful independent risk factor for a first myocardial infarction. Smoking cessation is an integral part of cardiovascular risk reduction in patients who have had a coronary event.

There is powerful data illustrating the importance of smoking cessation. One study found that for smokers who survived their first heart attack, the relative risk of a second attack within the next 3 years was 1.17 in those who quit compared to 1.51 in those who continued to smoke, when compared to nonsmokers [46]. Another study found that smokers with coronary artery disease who quit have a significant mortality benefit over those who continue to smoke [47]. The long-term relative risk of death in the cessation group was 0.64 (95% CI 0.58–0.71) when compared to the smoking group.

While smoking cessation has been proven to be an effective way to reduce cardiovascular risk, it is among the most difficult steps for any smoker to take. It is the duty of the medical practitioner to ask patients about smoking at every visit and to encourage and educate smokers about the benefits of quitting. When a patient is ready to quit smoking the medical professional should discuss options that may assist in achieving cessation, including medical therapy and community support groups.

Lipid Lowering

Aggressive lipid management is a vital element of risk reduction in patients with established coronary artery disease. Patients with underlying heart disease and elevated plasma cholesterol are at a significantly increased risk of death compared to similar patients without CAD [48]. A number of management techniques have been tested over the years, including lifestyle modification and medical therapy.

Lifestyle modifications including regular exercise, a diet low in cholesterol and saturated fat, and smoking cessation have long been an integral part of cardiovascular risk reduction, and the potential benefits have been demonstrated in multiple studies. The STARS trial, for one, demonstrated that after 3 years the progression of vessel narrowing in patients with coronary artery disease significantly decreased, regression of lesions increased, and angina severity decreased in individuals treated with a low-fat, low-cholesterol diet compared to standard care alone [49]. Similarly, the Lifestyle Heart Trial demonstrated that patients with CAD who were assigned to an aggressive life-style modification regimen including a vegetarian diet, smoking cessation, moderate exercise, and stress management experienced a significant regression in coronary atherosclerotic lesions at 1 year as well as a decrease in coronary symptoms compared to conservative management [50]. In both studies, LDL levels were found to decrease in the intervention groups compared to the controls.

While lifestyle modification has been proven to play a central role in cardiovascular risk management, studies have shown that pharmacologic lipid reduction significantly improves coronary atherosclerosis and clinical outcomes over lifestyle modification alone [51–53]. Of the lipid-lowering drugs on the market today, statins are the only ones that have been proven to improve overall mortality in patients with established coronary disease. Multiple randomized trials have been published in the past two decades demonstrating that lowering LDL cholesterol with statin medications reduces the incidence of cardiovascular complications such as myocardial infarction and death [54–57]. More recently, several trials have tested the notion that intense lipid control is beneficial compared to more relaxed control.

The IDEAL trial, published in 2003, investigated whether intensive lipid management was beneficial in patients with stable coronary artery disease [58]. Nearly 9,000 patients with stable disease were evaluated and randomized to 20 mg of simvastatin (conservative therapy) or 80 mg of atorvastatin (intensive therapy) per day. They were followed for 5 years, and the primary outcome was a composite of coronary death, nonfatal MI, and cardiac arrest. The intensive therapy group achieved a lower mean LDL level than the conservative group (81 mg/dL vs. 104 mg/dL). The primary endpoint occurred in 10.4% of patients in the simvastatin group and 9.3% in the atorvastatin group, a difference that was not found to be statistically significant (HR 0.89, CI 0.78–1.01, $P = 0.07$).

The question of what the optimal LDL goal should be in patients who have had an acute coronary event was addressed in the PROVE IT-TIMI 22 trial, published in 2004 [59]. More than 4,000 patients hospitalized for an acute coronary syndrome within the past 10 days were enrolled and were randomized to 40 mg of pravastatin (standard therapy) or 80 mg of atorvastatin (intensive therapy). The primary endpoint was a composite of all cause mortality, MI, unstable angina, revascularization, and stroke, and mean follow-up was 2 years. As expected, a more robust reduction in LDL cholesterol was achieved in the atorvastatin group (62 mg/dL) compared to the pravastatin group (95 mg/dL). The primary endpoint occurred in 26.3% of patients in the pravastatin group compared to 22.4% in the atorvastatin group, reflecting a 16% reduction in the hazard ratio in favor of atorvastatin ($P = 0.005$, CI 5–26%). These results indicate that patients with a history of an acute coronary syndrome benefit from more intensive LDL reduction.

The Treating New Targets (TNT) trial, published in 2005, was another major study that examined the effects of intensive lipid management in patients with established CAD [60]. Ten thousand patients with a history of CAD and LDL cholesterol of less than 130 mg/dL were randomized to receive 10 mg vs. 80 mg of atorvastatin daily. Patients were followed for an average of almost 5 years, and the primary endpoint was death from a complication of CAD, nonfatal MI, cardiac arrest, or stroke. The high-dose atorvastatin group achieved a mean LDL of 77 mg/dL compared to 101 mg/dL in the low-dose group. The primary outcome occurred in 8.7% of patients in the high-dose group compared to 10.9% in the low-dose group, reflecting a 22% relative risk reduction in those treated with high-dose atorvastatin (HR 0.78; CI 0.69–0.89).

While statin medications clearly improve outcomes in patients with coronary disease, the benefits of other lipid-lowering medications have not been as strongly supported in the literature. Fibrate drugs such as gemfibrozil and fenofibrate, for example, have not been shown to improve overall mortality in patients with coronary artery disease [61]. This was illustrated in the ACCORD Lipid Trial, in which 5,500 patients with type 2 diabetes and cardiovascular disease or multiple risk factors were randomized to fenofibrate or placebo in addition to simvastatin therapy [62]. The patients were followed for approximately 5 years. LDL was found to be similar in the two groups, HDL was slightly higher in the fenofibrate group, and triglycerides were lower in the fenofibrate group. Despite these differences, there was no significant difference in heart attack, stroke, or death between the two groups.

The results of these and other trials illustrate the importance of good lipid management in patients with coronary artery disease, and are echoed in the most recent guidelines for lipid management. Both the 2004 ATPIII and the 2006 AHA/ACC guidelines for secondary prevention recommend an LDL cholesterol goal of less than 100 mg/dL for all patients with coronary artery disease or a risk equivalent including atherosclerosis, diabetes, and chronic kidney disease, with an optional goal of <70 mg/dL in particularly high-risk patients. These goals should be met with a combination of lifestyle modification plus medical therapy, preferably a statin [63, 64].

Antiplatelet Therapy

Antiplatelet therapies including aspirin and thienopyridine analogs such as clopidogrel (Plavix) have been shown to improve outcomes in patients with coronary artery disease. Over the past two decades, there have been numerous studies and two major meta-analyses examining the effects of antiplatelet therapy on clinical outcomes in high-risk patients.

The Antithrombotic Trialists' Collaboration included data from nearly 300 randomized trials that investigated antiplatelet regimens in patients with underlying cardiovascular disease [65]. The main outcome measure was a composite of non-fatal MI, non-fatal stroke, or fatal vascular event (MI or stroke). The majority of patients in the study group were on aspirin, while a small portion were on a thienopyridine drug such as clopidogrel. In these high-risk patients, antiplatelet therapy was found to significantly reduce the relative risk of vascular events by 22% when compared to individuals who were not on antiplatelet medications.

Another large meta-analysis examined the protective effects of low-dose (75–150 mg per day) aspirin versus no aspirin in patients with stable cardiovascular disease (prior MI, stable angina, or stroke/TIA) [66]. Data from six randomized trials for a total of almost 10,000 patients were included. Aspirin use was found to be associated with a 21% reduction in all cardiovascular events and a 26% reduction in risk of nonfatal MI, as well as a 25% reduction in stroke and a 13% reduction in all-cause mortality.

In high-risk patients who are unable to tolerate aspirin therapy, clopidogrel is a reasonable alternative. The CAPRIE trial, published in 1996, was a major randomized trial designed to determine the comparative efficacy of clopidogrel (75 mg daily) versus aspirin (325 mg daily) in reducing the risk of cardiovascular events (stroke, MI, or vascular death) in patients with underlying cardiovascular disease [67]. Nearly 20,000 patients were randomized and followed for 2 years. The analysis showed a small but significant reduction in the average annual risk of a cardiovascular event in the clopidogrel group compared to the aspirin group (5.32% vs. 5.83%, $p = 0.043$, CI 0.3–16.5). The risk of a severe complication, including major bleeding, was statistically similar in the two groups. Given the very small absolute risk reduction with clopidogrel compared to aspirin (0.51%) and the significantly higher cost of clopidogrel, it is reasonable to reserve this therapy for individuals with stable disease who cannot tolerate aspirin.

The CHARISMA trial was published in 2006 to address the question of whether the addition of clopidogrel (75 mg daily) to low-dose aspirin (75–162 mg daily) therapy offers any outcome benefit in patients with stable cardiovascular disease or with multiple risk factors for cardiovascular disease [68]. The study randomized over 15,000 patients to clopidogrel plus aspirin or placebo plus aspirin, and the primary endpoint was a composite of non-fatal MI, stroke or cardiovascular death. After a median 28 months of follow-up, no significant difference was identified between the clopidogrel and placebo groups (6.8% vs. 7.3%, respectively; RR 0.93; CI 0.83–1.05; $P=0.22$). In addition, there was a small trend towards an increase in severe bleeding in the clopidogrel group (1.7% vs. 1.3%, CI 0.97–1.61, $P=0.09$), suggesting that the potential risks of adding clopidogrel to aspirin may outweigh the benefits in this stable population.

It is important to note that the CAPRIE and CHARISMA trials examined the efficacy of clopidogrel in patients with stable cardiovascular disease. Patients who required clopidogrel for other specific reasons, such as those with an acute coronary syndrome or with a prior coronary stent, were excluded from the analysis. Multiple studies that have demonstrated that dual antiplatelet therapy with aspirin and a thienopyridine analog improves outcomes in patients who have received a coronary stent. The PCI-CURE and CREDO trials showed that prolonged therapy with clopidogrel in addition to aspirin after PCI with a bare metal stent significantly prevented major cardiac events at 9 months and 1 year, respectively, compared to aspirin alone [69, 70]. In patients who have received drug-eluting stents, studies have demonstrated an increase in stent thrombosis in patients who discontinue thienopyridine therapy within the first year after implantation [71, 72].

Recent evidence has demonstrated that the thienopyridine drug prasugrel offers a benefit over clopidogrel in patients with acute coronary syndrome undergoing PCI. The TRITON-TIMI 38 trial randomized close to 14,000 patients with an acute coronary syndrome who received a stent to receive prasugrel versus clopidogrel [73]. All patients were placed on aspirin indefinitely. The patients were followed for 6–15 months, and the primary endpoint was cardiovascular death, nonfatal MI, or nonfatal stroke. In the end, 12.1% of patients receiving clopidogrel reached the primary endpoint, versus 9.9% receiving prasugrel (HR 0.81; CI 0.73–0.90; $P<0.001$). Despite the apparent benefit of prasugrel compared to clopidogrel, there was a greater risk of major bleeding in the prasugrel group (2.4% vs. 1.8%; HR 1.32; 95% CI 1.03–1.68; $P=0.03$). Overall, mortality was not significantly different between the two groups.

The updated 2009 ACC/AHA/SCAI Guidelines on Percutaneous Coronary Intervention recommend a minimum of 12 months of therapy with a thienopyridine such as clopidogrel or prasugrel, along with a lifetime of aspirin therapy, in all patients with acute coronary syndrome receiving a stent [74]. If the risk of mortality due to bleeding outweighs the benefit given by the thienopyridine, early discontinuation should be carefully considered.

Blood Pressure Control

Hypertension management is an important part of risk reduction in patients with underlying cardiovascular disease. Blood pressure goals have been studied in a number of clinical trials including INVEST and ACCORD BP [75, 76]. Both trials found that there was no significant difference in nonfatal MI, stroke, or cardiovascular death between standard and intensive blood pressure treatment groups. The current AHA/ACC Guidelines recommend maintaining a blood pressure goal of <140/90 mmHg in patients with coronary artery disease [77]. Patients with diabetes or chronic kidney disease should be maintained below 130/80 mmHg.

Beta-Blockers

Beta-blockers reduce myocardial oxygen demand by reducing heart rate, contractility, and left-ventricular wall stress. In patients with stable angina, beta-blockers have been proven to significantly reduce chest pain and increase exercise tolerance [78, 79]. In addition, beta-blockers have been shown to improve survival in high-risk patients with angina who have a history of myocardial infarction or heart failure. The current AHA/ACC Guidelines recommend that a beta-blocker be initiated as first-line therapy for all patients with stable coronary disease, unless contraindicated [80].

Despite the proven benefits of beta-blocker therapy in patients with coronary artery disease, the drug is frequently not prescribed to eligible patients [81, 82]. Historically, many practitioners have been uncomfortable prescribing beta-blockers to patients with various co-morbid conditions including chronic obstructive pulmonary disease (COPD), asthma, and left ventricular dysfunction or heart failure. Despite well-intentioned concerns, studies have demonstrated that these high-risk individuals gain a definite survival benefit when treated long-term with a beta-blocker compared to those who are not [83–85]. Individuals for whom beta-blockers should be used with caution or temporarily avoided include patients with active bronchospasm, profound hypotension or shock, severe bradycardia, or high-degree heart block. When these conditions have improved, these individuals should be re-evaluated for beta-blocker therapy.

Angiotensin Converting Enzyme Inhibitors and Angiotensin Receptor Blockers

Angiotensin converting enzyme inhibitors (ACE-inhibitors) and angiotensin receptor blockers (ARB's) are proven to benefit patients following an acute myocardial infarction. When an individual suffers a myocardial infarction, the infarcted region undergoes remodeling and scar formation. ACE-inhibitors and ARB's reduce ventricular remodeling in the days and weeks following an acute MI.

The ISIS-4 and GISSI-3 trials demonstrated a significant early and late mortality benefit in patients who received an ACE-inhibitor within the first 24 h following an acute MI. In ISIS-4, nearly 60,000 patients with an acute MI were randomized to receive captopril or placebo for 1 month [86]. The captopril group experienced a 7% proportional reduction in mortality at 5 weeks compared to the placebo group, with a persistent benefit noted at 1 year. In GISSI-3, over 19,000 patients with an acute MI were randomized to lisinopril or placebo for 6 weeks [87]. A 10% relative reduction in mortality was identified in the lisinopril group, with benefit extending up to 4 years. Similarly, a large meta-analysis that included nearly 100,000 patients demonstrated an early mortality benefit in patients who were started on an ACE-inhibitor within the first 36 h following an acute MI [88]. At 30 days, mortality was 7.6% in the control group and 7.1% in the ACE-inhibitor group (RR 0.93, 95% CI 0.89–0.98).

A greater benefit has been seen in patients with left ventricular dysfunction following a myocardial infarction. The SAVE trial randomized over 2,000 patients with an LVEF of 40% or less to captopril or placebo within 16 days following an MI [89]. After three and a half years of follow-up, there was a 19% decrease in mortality, a 37% reduction in the occurrence of heart failure, and a significant reduction in heart failure hospitalizations in the captopril group compared to placebo. The HOPE trial demonstrated that this mortality benefit extends to all high-risk patients, regardless of prior MI or LV dysfunction [90].

The current ACC/AHA Guidelines recommend ACE-inhibitor therapy in all post-MI patients with either an EF≤40%, hypertension, diabetes, or chronic kidney disease. They are considered optional in patients with a normal LVEF and well-controlled cardiovascular risk factors (class IIa). ARB's should be used in similar patients who are unable to tolerate ACE-inhibitors.

Aldosterone Antagonists

Aldosterone antagonists such as spironolactone and eplerenone have been shown to improve outcomes in patients with systolic heart failure. The benefit of spironolactone was demonstrated in the RALES trial. Over 1600 patients with NYHA Class III or IV heart failure symptoms and an LVEF of≤35% were randomized to receive spironolactone or placebo in addition to a standard heart failure regimen [91].

The study was discontinued early at 24 months, as a significant 30% relative risk reduction in mortality was demonstrated in the spironolactone group.

The recent EMPHASIS-HF trial examined the role of epleronone in patients with mild heart failure symptoms [92]. Almost 3,000 patients with NYHA Class II heart failure symptoms and an LVEF ≤30% or an LVEF >30% and ≤35% with a prolonged QRS duration (>130 ms) were randomized to eplerenone plus standard therapy versus standard therapy alone. This study was also terminated early (at 21 months) due to a significantly lower rate of cardiovascular death or heart failure hospitalizations in the treatment group (18.3% vs. 25.9%, HR 0.63; 95% CI 0.54–0.74). Patients in the eplerenone group were also found to have a significant decrease in all-cause mortality compared to placebo (12.5% vs. 15.5%; HR 0.76; 95% CI 0.62–0.94).

The current ACC/AHA Guidelines recommend aldosterone inhibitors such as spironolactone and eplerenone be used in patients who have had a myocardial infarction who are already on a beta-blocker and ACE-inhibitor and who have an LVEF of ≤40%.

References

1. Lloyd-Jones D, Adams RJ, Brown TM, et al. Executive summary: heart disease and stroke statistics – 2010 update: a report from the American Heart Association. Circulation. 2010;121(7):948–54.
2. Cooper R, Cutler J, Desvigne-Nickens P, Fortmann SP, et al. Trends and disparities in coronary heart disease, stroke, and other cardiovascular diseases in the United States: findings of the national conference on cardiovascular disease prevention. Circulation. 2000; 102(25):3137–47.
3. Levi F, Chatenoud L, Bertuccio P, et al. Mortality from cardiovascular and cerebrovascular diseases in Europe and other areas of the world: an update. Eur J Cardiovasc Prev Rehabil. 2009;16(3):333–50.
4. Lloyd-Jones DM, Larson MG, Beiser A, Levy D. Lifetime risk of developing coronary heart disease. Lancet. 1999;353(9147):89–92.
5. Libby P. Current concepts of the pathogenesis of the acute coronary syndromes. Circulation. 2001;104:365–72.

6. National Cholesterol Education Program (NCEP) Expert panel on detection, evaluation, and treatment of high blood cholesterol in adults (Adult Treatment Panel, III). Circulation. 2002; 106:3143.

7. Greenland P, Knoll MD, Stamler J, et al. Major risk factors as antecedents of fatal and nonfatal coronary heart disease events. JAMA. 2003;290(7):891–7.

8. Yusuf S, Hawken S, Ounpuu S, et al. Effect of potentially modifiable risk factors associated with myocardial infarction in 52 countries (the INTERHEART study): case-control study. Lancet. 2004; 364(9438):937–52.

9. Teo KK, Yusuf S, Furberg CD. Effects of prophylactic antiarrhythmic drug therapy in acute myocardial infarction. An overview of results from randomized controlled trials. JAMA. 1993;270(13): 1589–95.

10. Fraker T, Fihn S, Yancy C, et al. 2007 chronic angina focused update of the ACC/AHA 2002 guidelines for the management of patients with chronic stable angina: a report of the American College of Cardiology/American Heart Association Task Force on Practice Guidelines Writing Group to develop the focused update of the 2002 guidelines for the management of patients with chronic stable angina. J Am Coll Cardiol. 2007;50(23):2264–74.

11. Furberg CD, Psaty BM, Meyer JV. Nifedipine. Dose-related increase in mortality in patients with coronary heart disease. Circulation. 1995;92(5):1326–31.

12. Psaty BM, Heckbert SR, Koepsell TD, et al. The risk of myocardial infarction associated with antihypertensive drug therapies. JAMA. 1995;274(8):620–5.

13. Chaitman B. Ranolazine for the treatment of chronic angina and potential use in other cardiovascular conditions. Circulation. 2006;113(20):2462–72.

14. Chaitman B, Skettino S, Parker J, et al. Anti-ischemic effects and long-term survival during ranolazine monotherapy in patients with chronic severe angina. J Am Coll Cardiol. 2004;43(8):1375–82.

15. Kushner FG, Hand M, Smith SC, et al. 2009 focused updates: ACC/AHA guidelines for the management of patients with ST-elevation myocardial infarction (updating the 2004 guideline and 2007 focused update) and ACC/AHA/SCAI guidelines on percutaneous coronary intervention (updating the 2005 guideline and 2007 focused update) a report of the American College of Cardiology Foundation/American Heart Association Task Force on Practice Guidelines. J Am Coll Cardiol. 2009;54(23):2205–41.

16. Rogers WJ, Coggin CJ, Gersh BJ, et al. Ten-year follow-up of quality of life in patients randomized to receive medical therapy or coronary artery bypass graft surgery. The Coronary Artery Surgery Study (CASS). Circulation. 1990;82(5):1647–58.

17. Tatoulis J, Buxton BF, Fuller JA. Patencies of 2127 arterial to coronary conduits over 15 years. Ann Thorac Surg. 2004;77(1):93–101.
18. Sabik JF 3rd, Lytle BW, Blackstone EH, Houghtaling PL, Cosgrove DM. Comparison of saphenous vein and internal thoracic artery graft patency by coronary system. Ann Thorac Surg. 2005;79(2): 544–51.
19. Loop FD, Lytle BW, Cosgrove DM, et al. Influence of the internal-mammary-artery graft on 10-year survival and other cardiac events. N Engl J Med. 1986;314(1):1–6.
20. Cameron A, Davis KB, Green G, Schaff HV. Coronary bypass surgery with internal-thoracic-artery grafts – effects on survival over a 15-year period. N Engl J Med. 1996;334(4):216–9.
21. The Veterans Administration Coronary Artery Bypass Surgery Cooperative Study Group. Eleven-year survival in the Veterans Administration randomized trial of coronary bypass surgery for stable angina. N Engl J Med. 1984;311:1333–9.
22. Yusuf S, Zucker D, Peduzzi P, et al. Effect of coronary artery bypass graft surgery on survival: overview of 10-year results from randomised trials by the Coronary Artery Bypass Graft Surgery Trialists Collaboration. Lancet. 1994;344(8922):563–70.
23. Myers WO, Schaff HV, Gersh BJ, et al. Improved survival of surgically treated patients with triple vessel coronary artery disease and severe angina pectoris. A report from the Coronary Artery Surgery Study (CASS) registry. J Thorac Cardiovasc Surg. 1989;97(4):487–95.
24. Lytle B, Blackstone E, Sabik J, et al. The effect of bilateral internal thoracic artery grafting on survival during 20 postoperative years. Ann Thorac Surg. 2004;78:2005–14.
25. Guiteras-Val P, Varas-Lorenzo C, Garcia-Picart J, et al. Clinical and sequential angiographic follow-up six months and 10 years after successful percutaneous transluminal coronary angioplasty. Am J Cardiol. 1999;83(6):868–74.
26. Cannan CR, Yeh W, Kelsey SF, Cohen HA, Detre K, Williams DO. Incidence and predictors of target vessel revascularization following percutaneous transluminal coronary angioplasty: a report from the National Heart, Lung, and Blood Institute Percutaneous Transluminal Coronary Angioplasty Registry. Am J Cardiol. 1999;84(2):170–5.
27. Serruys PW, de Jaegere P, Kiemeneij F, et al. A comparison of balloon-expandable-stent implantation with balloon angioplasty in patients with coronary artery disease. Benestent Study Group. N Engl J Med. 1994;331(8):489–95.
28. Fischman DL, Leon MB, Baim DS, et al. A randomized comparison of coronary-stent placement and balloon angioplasty in the treatment of coronary artery disease. Stent Restenosis Study Investigators. N Engl J Med. 1994;31(8):496–501.

29. Stettler C, Wandel S, Allemann S, et al. Outcomes associated with drug-eluting and bare-metal stents: a collaborative network meta-analysis. Lancet. 2007;370(9591):937–48.

30. Moreno R, Fernandez C, Hernandez R, et al. Drug-eluting stent thrombosis: results from a pooled analysis including 10 randomized studies. J Am Coll Cardiol. 2005;45(6):954–9.

31. Leon M, Baim D, Popma J, et al. A clinical trial comparing three antithrombotic-drug regimens after coronary-artery stenting. Stent Anticoagulation Restenosis Study Investigators. N Engl J Med. 1998;339(23):1665–71.

32. Roiron C, Sanchez P, Bouzamondo A, Lechat P, Montalescot G. Drug eluting stents: an updated meta-analysis of randomised controlled trials. Heart. 2006;92(5):641–9.

33. Bavry AA, Kumbhani DJ, Helton TJ, Borek PP, Mood GR, Bhatt DL. Late thrombosis of drug-eluting stents: a meta-analysis of randomized clinical trials. Am J Med. 2006;119(12):1056–61.

34. Stone GW, Moses JW, Ellis SG, et al. Safety and efficacy of sirolimus- and paclitaxel-eluting coronary stents. N Engl J Med. 2007;356(10): 998–1008.

35. Boden WE, O'Rourke RA, Teo KK, et al. Optimal medical therapy with or without PCI for stable coronary disease. N Engl J Med. 2007; 356(15):1503–16.

36. Weintraub W, Spertus J, Kolm P, et al. Effect of PCI on quality of life in patients with stable coronary disease. N Engl J Med. 2008;358:677.

37. Chaitman BR, Rosen AD, Williams DO, et al. Myocardial infarction and cardiac mortality in the Bypass Angioplasty Revascularization Investigation (BARI) randomized trial. Circulation. 1997;96(7):2162–70.

38. RITA Trial Participants. Coronary angioplasty versus coronary artery bypass surgery: the Randomized Intervention Treatment of Angina (RITA) trial. Lancet. 1993;341(8845):573–80.

39. Hamm CW, Reimers J, Ischinger T, Rupprecht HJ, Berger J, Bleifeld W. A randomized study of coronary angioplasty compared with bypass surgery in patients with symptomatic multivessel coronary disease. German Angioplasty Bypass Surgery Investigation (GABI). N Engl J Med. 1994;331(16):1037–43.

40. Kurbaan AS, Bowker TJ, Ilsley CD, Rickards AF. Impact of postangioplasty restenosis on comparisons of outcome between angioplasty and bypass grafting. Coronary Angioplasty versus Bypass Revascularisation Investigation (CABRI) Investigators. Am J Cardiol. 1998;82(3):272–6.

41. Serruys PW, Unger F, Sousa JE, et al. Comparison of coronary-artery bypass surgery and stenting for the treatment of multivessel disease. N Engl J Med. 2001;344(15):1117–24.

42. Booth J, Clayton T, Pepper J, et al. Randomized, controlled trial of coronary artery bypass surgery versus percutaneous coronary intervention in patients with multivessel coronary artery disease: six-year follow-up from the Stent or Surgery Trial (SoS). Circulation. 2008;118(4):381–8.

43. Daemen J, Boersma E, Flather M, et al. Long-term safety and efficacy of percutaneous coronary intervention with stenting and coronary artery bypass surgery for multivessel coronary artery disease: a meta-analysis with 5-year patient-level data from the ARTS, ERACI-II, MASS-II, and SoS trials. Circulation. 2008;118(11):1146–54.

44. Serruys PW, Morice MC, Kappetein AP, et al. Percutaneous coronary intervention versus coronary-artery bypass grafting for severe coronary artery disease. N Engl J Med. 2009;360(10):961–72.

45. Cohen D, Van Hout B, Serruys P, et al. Quality of life after PCI with drug-eluting stents or coronary-artery bypass surgery. N Engl J Med. 2011;364:1016–26.

46. Rea TD, Heckbert SR, Kaplan RC, Smith NL, Lemaitre RN, Psaty BM. Smoking status and risk for recurrent coronary events after myocardial infarction. Ann Intern Med. 2002;137(6):494–500.

47. Critchley JA, Capewell S. Mortality risk reduction associated with smoking cessation in patients with coronary heart disease: a systematic review. JAMA. 2003;290(1):86–97.

48. Pekkanen J, Linn S, Heiss G, Suchindran CM, Leon A, Rifkind BM, et al. Ten-year mortality from cardiovascular disease in relation to cholesterol level among men with and without preexisting cardiovascular disease. N Engl J Med. 1990;322(24):1700–7.

49. Watts GF, Lewis B, Brunt JN, et al. Effects on coronary artery disease of lipid-lowering diet, or diet plus cholestyramine, in the St Thomas' Atherosclerosis Regression Study (STARS). Lancet. 1992;339(8793):563–9.

50. Ornish D, Brown SE, Scherwitz LW, et al. Can lifestyle changes reverse coronary heart disease? The Lifestyle Heart Trial. Lancet. 1990;336(8708):129–33.

51. Cashin-Hemphill L, Mack WJ, Pogoda JM, et al. Beneficial effects of colestipol-niacin on coronary atherosclerosis. A 4-year follow-up. JAMA. 1990;264(23):3013–7.

52. Brown G, Albers JJ, Fisher LD, et al. Regression of coronary artery disease as a result of intensive lipid-lowering therapy in men with high levels of apolipoprotein B. N Engl J Med. 1990;323(19):1289–98.

53. Blankenhorn D, Azen S, Kramsch D, et al. Coronary angiographic changes with lovastatin therapy. The Monitored Atherosclerosis Regression Study (MARS). Ann Intern Med. 1993;119:969–76.

54. Scandinavian Simvastatin Survival Study Group. Randomized trial of cholesterol lowering in 4444 patients with coronary heart disease: the Scandinavian Simvastatin Survival Study (4 S). Lancet. 1994;344(8934):1383–9.

55. Sacks F, Pfeffer M, Moye L, et al. The effect of pravastatin on coronary events after myocardial infarction in patients with average cholesterol levels. N Engl J Med. 1996;335:1001–9.

56. Tonkin AM, Colquhoun D, Emberson J, et al. Effects of pravastatin in 3260 patients with unstable angina: results from the LIPID study. Lancet. 2000;356(9245):1871–5.

57. Heart Protection Study Collaborative Group. MRC/BHF Heart Protection Study of cholesterol lowering with simvastatin in 20,536 high-risk individuals: a randomised placebo-controlled trial. Lancet. 2002;360(9326):7–22.

58. Pedersen TR, Faergeman O, Kastelein JJ, et al. High-dose atorvastatin vs. usual-dose simvastatin for secondary prevention after myocardial infarction: the IDEAL study: a randomized controlled trial. JAMA. 2005;294(19):2437–45.

59. Cannon CP, Braunwald E, McCabe CH, et al. Intensive versus moderate lipid lowering with statins after acute coronary syndromes. N Engl J Med. 2004;350(15):1495–504.

60. LaRosa JC, Grundy SM, Waters DD, et al. Intensive lipid lowering with atorvastatin in patients with stable coronary disease. N Engl J Med. 2005;352(14):1425–35.

61. Rubins HB, Robins SJ, Collins D, et al. Gemfibrozil for the secondary prevention of coronary heart disease in men with low levels of high-density lipoprotein cholesterol. Veterans Affairs High-Density Lipoprotein Cholesterol Intervention Trial Study Group. N Engl J Med. 1999;341(6):410–8.

62. ACCORD Study Group, Ginsberg HN, Elam MB, Lovato LC, et al. Effects of combination lipid therapy in type 2 diabetes mellitus. N Engl J Med. 2010;362(17):1563–74.

63. Grundy SM, Cleeman JI, Merz CN, et al. Implications of recent clinical trials for the National Cholesterol Education Program Adult Treatment Panel III guidelines. Circulation. 2004;110(2):227–39.

64. AHA; ACC; National Heart, Lung, and Blood Institute, Smith Jr SC, Blair SN, Bonow RO, et al. AHA/ACC guidelines for secondary prevention for patients with coronary and other atherosclerotic vascular disease: 2006 update endorsed by the National Heart, Lung, and Blood Institute. J Am Coll Cardiol. 2006;47(10):2130–9.

65. Antithrombotic Trialists' Collaboration. Collaborative meta-analysis of randomised trials of antiplatelet therapy for prevention of death, myocardial infarction, and stroke in high risk patients. BMJ. 2002; 324(7329):71–86.

66. Berger JS, Brown DL, Becker RC. Low-dose aspirin in patients with stable cardiovascular disease: a meta-analysis. Am J Med. 2008; 121(1):43–9.

67. CAPRIE Steering Committee. A randomised, blinded, trial of clopidogrel versus aspirin in patients at risk of ischaemic events (CAPRIE). Lancet. 1996;348(9038):1329–39.

68. Bhatt DL, Fox KAA, Hacke W, et al. Clopidogrel and aspirin versus aspirin alone for the prevention of atherothrombotic events. N Engl J Med. 2006;354:1706–17.

69. Mehta SR, Yusuf S, Peters RJ, et al. Effects of pretreatment with clopidogrel and aspirin followed by long-term therapy in patients undergoing percutaneous coronary intervention: the PCI-CURE study. Lancet. 2001;358(9281):527–33.

70. Steinhubl SR, Berger PB, Mann JT 3rd, Fry ET, DeLago A, Wilmer C, et al. CREDO Investigators: Early and sustained dual oral anti-platelet therapy following percutaneous coronary intervention: a randomized controlled trial. JAMA. 2002;288(19):2411–20.

71. Airoldi F, Colombo A, Morici N, Latib A, et al. Incidence and predictors of drug-eluting stent thrombosis during and after discontinuation of thienopyridine treatment. Circulation. 2007;116(7):745–54.

72. Spertus JA, Kettelkamp R, Vance C, et al. Prevalence, predictors, and outcomes of premature discontinuation of thienopyridine therapy after drug-eluting stent placement: results from the PREMIER registry. Circulation. 2006;113(24):2803–9.

73. Wiviott SD, Braunwald E, McCabe CH, Montalescot G, et al. Prasugrel versus clopidogrel in patients with acute coronary syndromes. N Engl J Med. 2007;357(20):2001–15.

74. Kushner FG, Hand M, Smith Jr SC, King SB, et al. 2009 Focused Updates: ACC/AHA Guidelines for the Management of Patients with ST-Elevation Myocardial Infarction and ACC/AHA/SCAI Guidelines on Percutaneous Coronary Intervention: A report of the ACC Foundation/AHA Task Force on practice guidelines. Circulation. 2009;120:2271–306.

75. Pepine CJ, Handberg EM, Cooper-DeHoff RM, et al. A calcium antagonist vs. a non-calcium antagonist hypertension treatment strategy for patients with coronary artery disease. The International Verapamil-Trandolapril Study (INVEST): a randomized controlled trial. JAMA. 2003;290(21):2805–16.

76. ACCORD Study Group, Cushman WC, Evans GW, Byington RP, et al. Effects of intensive blood-pressure control in type 2 diabetes mellitus. N Engl J Med. 2010;362(17):1575–85.

77. Smith SC, Allen J, Blair S, et al. AHA/ACC guidelines for secondary prevention for patients with coronary and other atherosclerotic vascular disease: 2006 update: endorsed by the National Heart, Lung, and Blood Institute. Circulation. 2006;113:2363–72.

78. Warren SG, Brewer DL, Orgain ES. Long-term propranolol therapy for angina pectoris. Am J Cardiol. 1976;37(3):420–6.

79. Jackson G, Harry JD, Robinson C, Kitson D, Jewitt DE. Comparison of atenolol with propranolol in the treatment of angina pectoris with special reference to once daily administration of atenolol. Br Heart J. 1978;40(9):998–1004.

80. Fraker TD, Fihn SD, Gibbons RJ, et al. 2007 Chronic angina focused update of the ACC/AHA 2002 guidelines for the management of patients with chronic stable angina. A report of the American College of Cardiology/American Heart Association Task Force on Practice Guidelines Writing Group to develop the focused update of the 2002 guidelines for the management of patients with chronic stable angina. Circulation. 2007;116:2762–72.

81. Soumerai SB, McLaughlin TJ, Spiegelman D, Hertzmark E, Thibault G, Goldman L. Adverse outcomes of underuse of beta-blockers in elderly survivors of acute myocardial infarction. JAMA. 1997;277(2):115–21.

82. Brand DA, Newcomer LN, Freiburger A, Tian H. Cardiologists' practices compared with practice guidelines: use of beta-blockade after acute myocardial infarction. J Am Coll Cardiol. 1995;26(6):1432–6.

83. Chen J, Radford MJ, Wang Y, Marciniak TA, Krumholz HM. Effectiveness of beta-blocker therapy after acute myocardial infarction in elderly patients with chronic obstructive pulmonary disease or asthma. J Am Coll Cardiol. 2001;37(7):1950–6.

84. Gottlieb SS, McCarter RJ, Vogel RA. Effect of beta-blockade on mortality among high-risk and low-risk patients after myocardial infarction. N Engl J Med. 1998;339(8):489–97.

85. Dargie HJ. Effect of carvedilol on outcome after myocardial infarction in patients with left-ventricular dysfunction: the CAPRICORN randomised trial. Lancet. 2001;357(9266):1385–90.

86. ISIS-4 (Fourth International Study of Infarct Survival) Collaborative Group. ISIS-4: a randomised factorial trial assessing early oral captopril, oral mononitrate, and intravenous magnesium sulphate in 58,050 patients with suspected acute myocardial infarction. Lancet. 1995;345(8951):669–85.

87. Gruppo Italiano per lo Studio della Sopravvivenza nell'infarto Miocardico: GISSI-3: effects of lisinopril and transdermal glyceryl trinitrate singly and together on 6-week mortality and ventricular function after acute myocardial infarction. Lancet. 1994;343(8906):1115–22.

88. ACE Inhibitor Myocardial Infarction Collaborative Group. Indications for ACE inhibitors in the early treatment of acute myocardial infarction: systematic overview of individual data from 100,000 patients in randomized trials. Circulation. 1998;97(22):2202–12.

89. Pfeffer MA, Braunwald E, Moyé LA, Basta L, et al. Effect of captopril on mortality and morbidity in patients with left ventricular dysfunction after myocardial infarction. Results of the survival and ventricular enlargement trial. The SAVE Investigators. N Engl J Med. 1992;327(10):669–77.

90. Yusuf S, Sleight P, Pogue J, Bosch J, Davies R, Dagenais G. Effects of an angiotensin-converting-enzyme inhibitor, ramipril, on cardiovascular events in high-risk patients. The Heart Outcomes Prevention Evaluation Study Investigators. N Engl J Med. 2000;342(3):145–53.

91. Pitt B, Zannad F, Remme WJ, Cody R, Castaigne A, Perez A, et al. The effect of spironolactone on morbidity and mortality in patients with severe heart failure. Randomized Aldactone Evaluation Study Investigators. N Engl J Med. 1999;341(10):709–17.

92. Zannad F, McMurray JJ, Krum H, van Veldhuisen DJ, Swedberg K, Shi H, et al. Eplerenone in patients with systolic heart failure and mild symptoms. N Engl J Med. 2011;364:11–21.

Chapter 9
Valvular Heart Disease

Ryan J. Hoefen and Eugene Storozynsky

Variations in the acuity and severity of a few distinct valve lesions yield a wide variety of presentations among patients with valvular heart disease. While this can make valve disease seem confusing, a basic knowledge of the underlying physiology can actually make these conditions, including the presenting symptomatology, natural course, and treatment, more understandable. Such an understanding is essential since patients with severe valve disease may be critically ill, but are very treatable when the etiology is promptly recognized. Early recognition of mild or moderate disease is also essential since early treatment may allay complications and the need for risky mechanical intervention. In this chapter, we will systematically review the common etiologies, pathophysiology, natural course, diagnosis, and treatment for the most common valve lesions.

R.J. Hoefen (✉)
Department of Medicine, Division of Cardiology,
University of Rochester Medical Center, Rochester, NY, USA
e-mail: Ryan_Hoefen@urmc.rohester.edu

E. Storozynsky
Division of Cardiology, University of Rochester Medical Center,
Rochester, NY, USA

J.D. Bisognano et al. (eds.), *Manual of Outpatient Cardiology*,   217
DOI 10.1007/978-0-85729-944-4_9,
© Springer-Verlag London Limited 2012

Aortic Stenosis

Etiology

Aortic outflow obstruction is classified by the level at which the obstruction occurs as either valvular aortic stenosis (AS), subvalvular AS, or supravalvular AS. Valvular AS is by far the most common of the three and will be discussed in detail. Subvalvular AS can be the result of either a fixed obstruction from abnormal tissue in the aortic outflow tract, which usually presents in children with other associated cardiac malformations, or a dynamic obstruction due pronounced hypertrophy of the septal myocardium in patients with hypertrophic cardiomyopathy, which will be discussed briefly elsewhere. Supravalvular AS, the least common of the three, primarily presents during childhood in patients with a mutation of the gene encoding elastin and may be associated with stenosis of other vessels including the coronary arteries, descending aorta, and pulmonary artery.

Valvular AS is generally the result of inflammation with slowly progressive calcification and fibrosis of the aortic leaflets, fusing them together, and thus preventing them from fully opening and permitting free flow into the aorta. The most common cause is *age-related degenerative calcific AS* in elderly patients, which is thought to be mediated by chronic inflammation similar to that of atherosclerosis within vessel walls. However, AS may occur in younger patients if they are predisposed to valvular inflammation by congenital abnormality (i.e. bicuspid aortic valve) or rheumatic disease. The presence of a bicuspid aortic valve often signifies an underlying aortic abnormality, so coexistence of aortic dissection, aneurysm, and/or coarctation should be considered.

Pathophysiology

As aortic valve area decreases, there is increasing resistance to ventricular outflow and a growing pressure gradient between the left ventricle and the aorta. Initially, left ventricular systolic pressures increase to maintain a normal stroke volume. Over time, this pressure overload results in concentric hypertrophy (see Figure 9.1b). Patients are usually asymptomatic in the early stages and are not aware of the increasing transvalvular gradient or ventricular hypertrophy.

As stenosis progresses, a point is reached where the compensatory increase in contractility by hypertrophy becomes maximally extended and can even become detrimental. At this point, the patient will begin to experience one or more of the classic triad of symptoms: angina, syncope, and dyspnea. Angina is the result of the increased oxygen demand of the thickened ventricle wall combined with decreased perfusion due to high transmural pressures as the ventricle strains against the obstructed outlet. While many patients suffer from concomitant coronary artery disease, some patients may have classic angina despite an absence of coronary lesions. Syncope occurs due to inability of the maximally extended heart to further increase cardiac output and meet systemic demand during exertion. Dyspnea is caused by pulmonary edema secondary to the increased left ventricular diastolic pressures needed to fill the stiff ventricle, which are transmitted to the left atrium and pulmonary vasculature. The impaired filling is exacerbated by tachycardia (i.e. during exertion) since there is decreased diastolic filling time, which results in even higher filling pressures. Prior to the wide availability of surgical valve replacement, the mean amount of time between the first symptoms of AS and death was about 3 years, often occurring as a result of sudden cardiac death.

Physical Exam

Characteristic physical exam findings of AS include *pulsus parvus et tardus* (slowly rising pulse with a sustained peak), delayed aortic closure (aortic closure may occur simultaneous with or even after pulmonic closure, the latter of which is termed paradoxic splitting of the S2), and a low-pitched, raspy crescendo/decrescendo systolic murmur heard best at the heart base with transmission to the carotid arteries. As the valve area narrows, the murmur peaks later in systole and may become softer. Other findings of AS are those typical of LV hypertrophy, including lateral displacement of the apical impulse, S4 heart sound, and accentuation of the venous *a* wave on inspection of the jugular veins.

Diagnostic Testing

Transthoracic echocardiography is a very sensitive and specific method for detecting AS. With the use of Doppler imaging, the trans-valvular gradient and valve area can be estimated with good accuracy. However, in some cases, it is difficult to align the echo probe with the aortic outflow, in which case Doppler ultrasound will underestimate the severity of the stenosis. This is also true of transesophageal echocardiography, where proper alignment of the probe parallel to aortic outflow can be very difficult. Therefore, when patients have symptoms that are out of proportion to the echo findings, invasive measurement of the cardiac output and transvalvular gradient should be performed in the catheterization laboratory.

Patients with a low cardiac output of any cause may be found to have a low calculated aortic valve area and a low transvalvular pressure gradient on diagnostic testing – so-called "low-gradient AS" – whether or not there is true AS because the severely depressed cardiac output may not be sufficient to fully open the aortic valve. To distinguish whether there is fixed valve disease or its appearance as a result of poor cardiac performance, a dobutamine echo should be performed to assess the valve with augmented cardiac output. If there is fixed aortic stenosis, this will increase the transvalvular gradient but the calculated aortic valve area will remain low. On the other hand, the gradient will remain low and the calculated valve area will increase if the appearance of a low valve area was due to cardiomyopathy of another cause.

Treatment

No medical treatment has been shown to be of benefit in the treatment of asymptomatic AS. Statins have been hypothesized to slow the progression of AS by decreasing inflammatory destruction of the valve, but clinical trials have failed to demonstrate any benefit thus far.

The primary treatment for symptomatic AS is aortic valve replacement (AVR). Severe AS with symptoms and/or LV systolic dysfunction (ejection fraction less than 50%) is a Class I indications to perform AVR, as is the presence of severe AS in a patient who is undergoing CABG or surgery of the aorta or other heart valves. Patients with asymptomatic critical AS should be monitored with annual echocardiograms and undergo surgery if symptoms or LV systolic dysfunction develop. Balloon valvuloplasty is an alternative that is primarily used in children with congenital, non-calcific AS. In adults, there is a high rate of restenosis, so it is usually reserved for palliation or as a "bridge" to surgery in patients who are too ill to undergo surgery. Transcatheter aortic valve implantation (TAVI), a method of percutaneous valve replacement, is currently under investigation and has shown promising results in patients who are not candidates for surgical valve replacement in initial studies.

Aortic Regurgitation

Etiology

Aortic regurgitation (AR) is due to a primary disorder of the aortic valve or the aortic root. Aortic root disease, which has become more common than primary valvular etiologies, may be due to connective tissue disorders (Marfans or Ehlers-Danlos), severe hypertension, or aortic dissection. Primary valvular causes include rheumatic disease, rheumatoid spondylitis, and congenital abnormalities. Acute AR may occur as a result of infective endocarditis or trauma. AR can also occur with mixed AS, which is almost always due to rheumatic or congenital disease.

Pathophysiology

In AR, regurgitation of a portion of the total stroke volume with each heartbeat compromises the effective forward stroke volume. In chronic AR, the effective forward stroke volume is maintained by increasing the total stroke volume, which is primarily achieved by LV dilation. As the LV dilates, the aortic root may enlarge and further separate the aortic cusps, thus exacerbating the aortic regurgitation (see Figure 9.1d). At this early stage, the dynamic blood flow may produce palpitations in the chest or head, particularly with exertion, which may be quite uncomfortable for some patients.

As LV dilation progresses, the myocardium must generate increasing wall tension in order to maintain sufficient cardiac output. Eventually, the LV cannot maintain a sufficient effective forward stroke volume, particularly during exertion. As this occurs, cardiac output may be normal at rest, but fails to rise normally with exertion, producing exertional dyspnea. Regurgitant flow also increases LV diastolic filling pressure, causing secondary elevation in left atrial and pulmonary pressures, leading to patient complaints of orthopnea and paroxysmal nocturnal dyspnea. Ischemia may also occur in these patients with longstanding AR even in the absence of coronary artery disease because oxygen demand is increased by LV dilatation and wall tension while coronary blood flow is reduced by decreased diastolic pressure.

While patients with chronic AR may tolerate significant amounts of regurgitation because of compensatory mechanisms, patients with acute AR experience a rapidly increased LV diastolic pressure, secondarily elevating left atrial and pulmonary pressures. Pulmonary edema and cardiogenic shock may occur rapidly in these patients.

Physical Examination

Many of the characteristic findings of aortic regurgitation are a result of the hyperdynamic blood flow and widened pulse pressure in the major arteries, although they may not be present in advanced or acute AI where there is elevated LV diastolic pressure and poor LV systolic function. These findings may include bobbing of the head with systole or even jarring of the entire body, a "water-hammer" pulse (abrupt distention and collapse of the large arteries), a loud "pistol-shot" sound (Traube's sign) or a "to-and-fro" murmur (Duroziez's sign) when slight compression is applied to the femoral artery with a stethoscope, and alternate flushing and blanching at the root of the fingernails when pressure is applied at the tip (Quincke's pulse). There may also be a heaving LV impulse that is displaced laterally and inferiorly and a diastolic thrill at the left sternal border as well as a systolic thrill transmitted along the carotid arteries.

Cardiac auscultation may reveal an absence of aortic closure, S3 and S4 sounds, and a high-pitched, blowing, decrescendo diastolic murmur along the left sternal border that becomes louder and longer as the disease progresses. The murmur is accentuated by sitting, leaning forward, with breath held in forced expiration. There may also be a loud systolic ejection murmur at the base of the heart transmitted to the carotids that is higher pitched and shorter than the murmur of AS. There may also be a soft, low-pitched, rumbling mid-diastolic bruit thought to be due to displacement of the anterior mitral valve leaflet by the AR jet (Austin Flint murmur). The features of AR are accentuated by handgrip due to increased systemic vascular resistance.

Diagnostic Testing

Transthoracic echocardiography is very sensitive for detecting AR and helpful in determining severity as well as helping to identify the cause or at least in differentiating primary valve disorders from aortic root disorders. Transesophageal echocardiography provides higher resolution imaging of the aortic valve and may clarify the mechanism of regurgitation. Catheterization, including aortography for further visualization of the dimensions of the ascending aorta and the amount of aortic regurgitation, as well as coronary angiography to identify coexistent coronary disease, can also be helpful, particularly prior to a planned surgical valve replacement.

Treatment

Although surgery is the only definitive treatment, symptoms of heart failure can be improved with digitalis, salt restriction, diuretics, vasodilators, and ACE inhibitors. Long acting nifedipine has been shown to delay the need for surgery. Nitrates are typically not as helpful for angina as they are in ischemic cardiomyopathy, but may still provide some relief.

The key issue regarding surgery is that of timing. Since chronic AR progresses slowly, not all patients will require surgery. Rather, they should be monitored closely and generally followed by echocardiogram every 6 months. Surgery is generally indicated when there are either severe symptoms or LV dysfunction (EF<55% or LV end-systolic volume >55 mL/m^2). If surgery is delayed too long, LV fibrosis may prevent significant functional recovery.

Mitral Stenosis

Etiology

Mitral stenosis (MS) is the result of the valve leaflets being thickened and fused by fibrous tissue and/or calcium deposits. The disease progresses over time as the thickened leaflets become further calcified due to immobilization. This is nearly always caused by rheumatic fever. Thus its incidence appears to be decreasing in developed countries. It often coexists with mitral regurgitation, which is discussed below. Less common causes of mitral stenosis include congenital defects, malignant carcinoid, systemic lupus erythematosis, and rheumatoid arthritis.

Pathophysiology

A normal mitral valve has an area of approximately 6 cm^2 and allows unimpeded flow from the left atrium to the left ventricle with essentially no pressure gradient between the two chambers. As the valve narrows to less than 2 cm^2, left atrial pressure increases as resistance to flow across the valve increases (see Figure 9.1c). The increased pressure gradient is exacerbated when heart rate increases since shortened diastole requires higher flow rates across the valve to achieve appropriate LV filling. As a result, patients may experience shortness of breath with exertion at this stage. Cardiac output may also fail to rise normally with exertion. Other causes of increased heart rate including emotional stress, thyrotoxicosis, and pregnancy can also produce symptoms. Similarly, as elevated left atrial pressure produces progressive left atrial enlargement, there is a propensity to develop atrial fibrillation, which often hastens or exacerbates symptoms since the uncontrolled heart rate and loss of atrial contraction further reduce ventricular filling.

Critical stenosis of the mitral valve (generally considered a valve area less than 1 cm^2) is associated with a high transvalvular pressure gradient (approximately 20 mmHg or more), resulting in significant pulmonary hypertension and, if left untreated, eventual right ventricular failure and systemic venous congestion. This may be accompanied by orthopnea, paroxysmal nocturnal dyspnea, hemoptysis, abdominal bloating, ascites, and lower extremity edema. Cardiac output may become suboptimal at rest and may not rise (in fact, it may even worsen) with activity.

Physical Examination

Physical exam may reveal an apical diastolic thrill with the patient in left lateral decubitus position. Characteristic auscultatory findings include a mitral opening snap most audible during expiration medial to the cardiac apex followed by a low rumbling murmur at the apex with the patient in the left lateral decubitus position, then an accentuated, snapping, and slightly delayed S1 sound. Pulmonary hypertension may be apparent as a closely split or fixed S2 with an accentuated P2, and pulmonary systolic ejection click.

Diagnostic Testing

Transthoracic echocardiography is highly sensitive and specific for detecting MS since satisfactory alignment of the echo probe with the mitral flow for determination of transvalvular gradient and valve area can generally be achieved by an experienced sonographer. Transesophageal echocardiography can also be helpful in many cases for detailed analysis of the valve structure and the subvalvular apparatus, which may determine the most appropriate treatment, as will be discussed below.

Left and right heart catheterization may also be performed to determine cardiac output, transvalvular gradient, and calculated valve area, but is more prone to error than Doppler-derived measurements. Coronary angiography is also helpful to evaluate for coronary artery disease when surgical repair is being considered.

Treatment

Medical treatment of mitral stenosis is quite limited and is primarily aimed at treating complications of the disease. Sodium restriction and diuresis may improve symptoms of pulmonary congestion. Since atrial fibrillation exacerbates symptoms, cardioversion or rate control may provide relief. All patients with atrial fibrillation due to mitral stenosis should be placed on long-term anticoagulation due to a high risk of thromboembolic complications.

Balloon valvotomy, the inflation of a balloon placed across the mitral valve via percutaneous right heart catheterization with septal puncture, is the preferred method of valve repair in appropriate candidates because of lower morbidity and mortality compared to surgical repair. This procedure is most successful if leaflets are thin and not significantly calcified. It is contraindicated if there is moderate to severe mitral regurgitation or left atrial thrombus. It is primarily indicated in patients who are symptomatic or have moderate to severe valve stenosis with pulmonary hypertension (PA systolic pressure >50 mmHg or >60 mmHg during exercise). Surgical valve repair may be required if balloon valvotomy is not possible, unsuccessful, or results in restenosis. Mitral valve replacement is also necessary if there is co-existent mitral regurgitation, the valve is damaged from a previous repair, or if the valve cannot be sufficiently repaired.

Mitral Regurgitation

Etiology

The cause of mitral regurgitation (MR) may be mitral valve prolapse, rheumatic heart disease, congenital defects of the endocardial cushion, ischemia (either ischemic cardiomyopathy resulting in chronic MR or ischemia at the base of the papillary muscle causing acute or even intermittent MR), or left ventricular dilation of any cause resulting in enlargement of the mitral annulus. Acute causes of MR include ischemia, infectious endocarditis, and trauma. MR may complicate a myocardial infarction and should be suspected in patients recovering from MI who are found to have a new systolic murmur.

Pathophysiology

The major hemodynamic effects of MR are: (1) decreased forward cardiac output through the aortic valve due to ejection of a significant portion of the stroke volume through the dysfunctional mitral valve, and (2) increased pressure in the left atrium as it receives the regurgitant flow.

As in aortic regurgitation, the compensatory mechanism for reduced forward cardiac output in chronic MR is left ventricular dilation and increased ejection fraction. Ventricular dilation may further exacerbate MR since enlargement of the mitral annulus further prevents closure of the mitral leaflets (see Figure 9.1e). Continued dilation of the ventricle requires increased wall stress generation to maintain the hyperdynamic ejection fraction necessary for a normal forward cardiac output, which eventually cannot be sustained and the left ventricular ejection fraction and cardiac output begin to decline, producing symptoms of fatigue.

Elevated left atrial pressure is transmitted to the pulmonary vasculature, where it causes dyspnea and eventually right ventricular failure and systemic venous congestion. However, the degree to which the left atrial pressure is transmitted to the pulmonary vasculature is tempered by the left atrial compliance. In chronic MR, the left atrial compliance increases, so patients may tolerate high left atrial pressures without significant symptoms. Patients who develop high compliance of the left atrium may have predominant symptoms of decreased cardiac output from left ventricular dysfunction (primarily fatigue, as discussed above) rather than symptoms of pulmonary congestion. On the other hand, patients with acute MR generally have low atrial compliance and quickly develop severely elevated pulmonary pressures and pulmonary edema. Elevated left atrial pressures also cause enlargement of the left atrium over time. As a result, patients with chronic, severe MR nearly always develop atrial fibrillation.

Physical Examination

In patients with MR, S1 is usually absent, soft, or buried in the murmur. The murmur is typically a loud holosystolic or decrescendo apical murmur radiating to the axilla. The location of the murmur may vary depending on the direction of the regurgitant jet. It has been said to have a "cooing" quality if there is a flail leaflet. The murmur is exacerbated by isometric strain, such as Valsalva. The aortic valve may close prematurely, causing wide splitting of S2. There may also be an audible S3 and/or S4. Associated findings may include a palpable systolic thrill at the cardiac apex, which is often laterally displaced.

Diagnostic Testing

Transthoracic echocardiography is very sensitive and specific for identification of MR. Good alignment of the probe with mitral flow is possible, allowing good visualization of the degree of regurgitation. However, the rapid development of high left atrial pressure in acute, severe MR reduces the regurgitant velocity, potentially making the diagnosis less apparent on Doppler echocardiography. Echocardiography is also important for determining left ventricular function in patients with MR. Transesophageal echocardiography is not usually necessary to make the diagnosis of mitral regurgitation however its superior resolution of the valve and the subvalvular apparatus can be helpful in determining the underlying mechanism for the MR, such as by visualizing vegetations associated with endocarditis or a ruptured chordae tendonae. If the severity is unclear by transthoracic echocardiography, assessment of flow reversal within the pulmonary veins by transesophageal echocardiographic Doppler analysis will further ascertain the severity of MR.

Cardiac catheterization may also be helpful. Left ventriculography allows direct visualization of the regurgitant flow and can help determine its severity if echocardiography imaging is too limited. Coronary angiography should also be performed in patients with planned surgical treatment to determine if coronary bypass is indicated.

Treatment

Conservative treatment of chronic MR includes restricting physical activities that produce dyspnea/fatigue, reducing sodium intake and enhancing sodium excretion with diuretics. Vasodilators may help increase forward cardiac output. ACE inhibitors are an excellent choice for chronic MR. Intravenous nitroprusside or nitroglycerin may be helpful in acute or severe MR. Anticoagulation and/or leg binders may help to prevent thromboembolic disease in late stages.

The only definitive treatment for mitral regurgitation is surgery. Asymptomatic or minimally symptomatic patients with normal LV function (EF>60%) may remain stable for years and should not undergo surgery. However, if symptoms have a significant impact on the patient's lifestyle or there is LV dysfunction, surgical treatment should be offered, which may yield significant LV functional improvement. In many cases, the mitral valve can be reconstructed or an annuloplasty ring can be placed, but valve replacement is often necessary. The valve may be replaced with a bioprosthetic or a mechanical bileaflet valve. Bioprosthetic valves are prone to late mechanical dysfunction while mechanical valves require lifelong anticoagulation therapy and thus are associated with risks of bleeding or thromboembolism. Therefore, careful consideration must be made in deciding which type of valve is most appropriate at the time of surgery.

Tricuspid Stenosis

Tricuspid stenosis (TS) is generally caused by rheumatic fever and only occurs in association with other valve lesions (generally MS). As the pressure gradient across the valve increases, so does the right atrial pressure, resulting in right atrial enlargement and systemic venous congestion. The decreased right heart output may decrease pulmonary pressures despite the presence of MS, thus improving symptoms of (or even masking) MS. Patients will typically complain of discomfort due to ascites and edema, as well as fatigue secondary to low CO. The diastolic murmur of TS is best heard along the left sternal border and is accentuated during inspiration due to increased flow across the valve and decreased during expiration and Valsalva maneuver. Intensive salt restriction and diuresis may improve symptoms of systemic venous congestion and improve surgical risk. Valve repair or replacement is typically carried out at the time of mitral valve surgery.

Tricuspid Regurgitation

Tricuspid regurgitation (TR) is generally secondary to RV dilatation of any other cause, but can also be due to rheumatic fever, infarction of RV papillary muscles, tricuspid prolapse, infective endocarditis, trauma, or congenital defects. Its primary effects are systemic venous congestion and reduced cardiac output. Like TS, it can reduce the signs and symptoms of pulmonary hypertension. It produces a holosystolic murmur along the lower left sternal border that intensifies during inspiration and diminishes during expiration or Valsalva maneuver. Atrial fibrillation is often present due to atrial enlargement. Isolated TR in the absence of pulmonary hypertension (such as in infectious endocarditis or trauma) may be well-tolerated and not require further treatment. In many cases, TR may resolve if the underlying cause of RV enlargement is treated, such as surgical repair of a mitral valve when pulmonary hypertension causes RV enlargement. However, recovery may be speeded with tricuspid valvuloplasty. In cases of TR with severe valve deformity due to rheumatic disease, surgical valve repair or replacement should be carried out, particularly if there is no pulmonary hypertension (and hence little chance of improvement with correction of the underlying cause for pulmonary hypertension).

Pulmonic Valve Dysfunction

Pulmonic valve dysfunction is far less common than the other forms of valvular disease described above. Regurgitation may result from infective endocarditis or dilatation of the pulmonic valve ring by severe pulmonary hypertension, but these are unlikely to be of hemodynamic consequence. Pulmonic stenosis is an uncommon congenital defect and may be progressive if the obstruction is moderate or severe leading to presentation in adulthood. The obstruction may limit flow sufficiently to prevent cardiac output from meeting metabolic demand during exertion, producing exertional dyspnea, fatigue, and syncope. The RV undergoes hypertrophy and a forceful atrial contraction is required for RV filling. If RV systolic pressures exceed that of the LV, right-to-left shunt may occur through a patent foramen ovale or atrial septal defect, resulting in cyanosis. On physical exam, the murmur of pulmonic stenosis is a harsh systolic crescendo-decrescendo sound at the upper left sternal border. The strong atrial contraction may be manifested by prominent *a* waves in the jugular venous pulse or even pre-systolic pulsation of the liver. The ECG may show right axis deviation, RV hypertrophy, and RA enlargement. Treatment is usually performed by balloon valvuloplasty, but may sometimes require surgical valve repair.

Endocarditis Prophylaxis

Infectious endocarditis (IE) is a rare, but serious condition occurring when bacteremia leads to colonization of the cardiac valves or other cardiac structures. The great majority of occurrences of bacteremia do not lead to endocarditis since the normal endothelium is resistant to bacterial adhesion and colonization. Disruption of the normal endothelial lining by either erosive exposure of the underlying matrix (such as by exposure to high-velocity, turbulent flow from regurgitant valve lesions) or placement of prosthetic materials may increase the risk of bacterial adhesion and colonization in some patients. Since some dental, respiratory, gastrointestinal, and genitourinary procedures can cause transient bacteremia, it has been common practice for many years to give prophylactic antibiotics to patients thought to have elevated risk of IE due to disruption of the normal endothelium, although this practice has been driven largely by small, observational studies and expert opinion rather than large, randomized trials.

The American Heart Association and The American College of Cardiology have issued joint guidelines on appropriate use of antibiotics for IE prevention for over 50 years with nine major revisions to date. While past iterations of the guidelines have recommended prophylaxis for patients with a wide variety of valvular and congenital heart defects undergoing any of a large number of procedures, the most recent revision, published in 2007, significantly narrows both the patients and procedures that are thought to be appropriate for antibiotic pretreatment. This reflects currently-held beliefs that endocarditis is much more likely to result from frequent bacteremia associated with daily activities (eating, brushing, flossing, etc.) than it is from a medical or dental procedure, so the number of cases of IE prevented by antibiotic prophylaxis is exceedingly small – to the point that antibiotic-associated adverse events outweigh the benefit of prophylaxis. Therefore, the role of proper oral hygiene is emphasized and antibiotic prophylaxis prior to procedures is limited to only the patients who are at highest risk of developing IE, which includes patients with the following:

- Prosthetic cardiac valves or prosthetic materials used for valve repair
- Previous IE
- Unrepaired cyanotic CHD (including palliative shunts and conduits)
- CHD repaired with prosthetic materials within the prior 6 months (since complete endothelialization typically occurs within 6 months of implantation)
- Repaired CHD with residual defect at or near the site of a prosthetic patch or device (which inhibits endothelialization)
- Cardiac transplant patients who develop valvular disease

The scope of procedures for which antibiotic pretreatment is thought to be appropriate for high-risk patients has also been narrowed to only those that produce significant bacteremia, including dental procedures that involve manipulation of the gingival tissue or periapical region of the teeth or perforation of the oral mucosa and procedures of the respiratory tract that involve incision or biopsy of the respiratory mucosa (this does not include routine brochoscopy). In contrast to prior versions of the guidelines, use of antibiotics prior to diagnostic EGD and colonoscopy is no longer recommended. It is also not recommended to give prophylactic antibiotics prior to cystoscopy unless the patient has an enterococcal urinary tract infection or colonization.

Since the current guidelines recommend antibiotic prophylaxis in a small subset of patients and procedures compared to previous iterations of the guidelines, there are many patients with valve dysfunction, such as mitral prolapse, who have previously been advised to take antibiotics prior to procedures who should now be counseled that this is no longer recommended.

The appropriate antibiotic regimen given to high risk patients undergoing an appropriate procedure should be one that is active against causative pathogens of IE that are present in the region where the procedure is being performed. For dental procedures, the first choice, according to the 2007 AHA/ACC guidelines, is oral amoxicillin (2 g) in a single dose 30–60 min prior to the procedure. For patients who are allergic to penecillins, cephalexin (2 g; unless there is a history of anaphylaxis, angioedema, or urticarial to penecillins), clindamycin (600 mg), azithromycin (500 mg), or clarithromycin (500 mg) may be given. For patients unable to take an oral antibiotic, ampicillin (2 g), cefazolin (1 g), ceftriaxone (1 g), or clindamycin (600 mg) may be given intramuscularly or intravenously.

→

FIGURE 9.1 Ventricular response to valve dysfunction. (**a**) Normal valvular and cardiac function with unrestricted flow across the mitral and aortic valves. (**b**) Severe aortic stenosis with a high pressure gradient across the aortic valve causing concentric hypertrophy of the left ventricle. As the ventricle thickens, it becomes stiff and filling pressures increases, which causes left atrial enlargement. (**c**) Severe mitral stenosis with a high pressure gradient across the mitral valve causing left atrial enlargement. The left ventricle is not significantly affected. Later, increased pulmonary pressures may result in right ventricular enlargement. (**d**) Severe aortic regurgitation is compensated by enlargement of the left ventricular cavity. The regurgitant flow also causes elevates diastolic filling pressures, which results in left atrial enlargement. (**e**) Severe mitral regurgitation is also compensated by left ventricular cavity enlargement. The regurgitant flow directly increases left atrial pressure, which causes left atrial enlargement

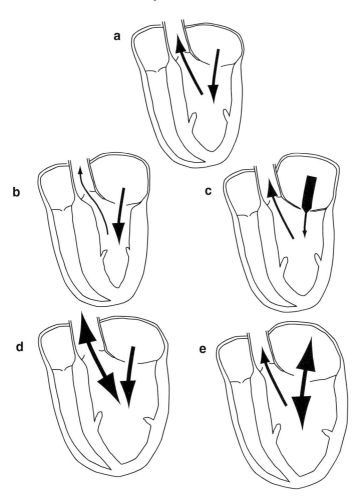

Chapter 10
Ambulatory Arrhythmias

Andrew J. Brenyo and Mehmet K. Aktas

Normal cardiac function relies on the exquisitely coordinated flow of electrical impulses through the heart. Abnormalities of this electrical flow are known as arrhythmias and are amongst the most common clinical problems encountered in both the inpatient and outpatient setting. The presentation of arrhythmia can range from a benign sensation of palpitations to cardiovascular collapse and death. Therefore, a thorough basic understanding of the mechanisms, basic evaluation and treatment of arrhythmia is important to the daily practice of outpatient clinical medicine.

This chapter describes the anatomy of the conduction system followed by a description of the mechanisms of arrhythmia and initial steps in their diagnostic evaluation and therapeutic management. Arrhythmias will initially be divided and discussed en masse in rapid (tachyarrhythmia) or slow (bradyarrhythmia) conduction sections with individual arrhythmias (fast and slow) and ECG examples

A.J. Brenyo
Division of Cardiology, University of Rochester Medical Center,
Rochester, NY, USA
e-mail: andrew_brenyo@urmc.rochester.edu

M.K. Aktas
Division of Cardiology–Electrophysiology,
University of Rochester Medical Center,
Rochester, NY, USA

J.D. Bisognano et al. (eds.), *Manual of Outpatient Cardiology*,   237
DOI 10.1007/978-0-85729-944-4_10,
© Springer-Verlag London Limited 2012

following the respective general discussion section. The chapter structure should mirror the bedside outpatient evaluation and diagnostic evaluation of arrhythmias with the initial dichotomizing value being the presenting heart rate and symptoms followed by electrocardiographic assessment finally diagnostic and therapeutic maneuvers that are particular to each arrhythmia. Tachyarrhythmia and bradyarrhythmia sections will include a bedside consultant section with practical rules regarding when to be concerned and refer the patient from the outpatient setting to an acute care facility or consider acute cardiology consultation.

Conduction System Anatomy and Basic Physiology

The specialized conduction system responsible for coordinated electrical impulse flow includes the sinoatrial (SA) node, the atrioventricular (AV) nodal region and the ventricular conduction system composed of the bundle of His, right and left bundle branches, and the Purkinje fibers (Fig. 10.1). Electrical impulse formation arises from the intrinsic automaticity present within each of these specialized structures. The tissue with the fastest impulse formation (typically the SA node) determines the heart rate. As noted in Fig. 10.1 all of the structures that compose the conduction system have a natural impulse formation rate: SA node 60–80/min, AV node 40–50/min, left and right bundle branches and purkinje fibers 30–40/min.

With the SA node generally having the fastest impulse formation, each normal electrical impulse flows through the atrial tissue to the AV node where it is slowed, thereby giving the atria time to empty and fill the ventricles. Following its slowing at the AV node, electricity moves through the bundle of His and into the right and left bundle branch resulting in ventricular systole and generation of ventricular systole felt peripherally as a pulse. Although very simplified, this description provides the basic framework for understanding basic cardiac conduction system anatomy and function allowing a more detailed discussion of arrhythmia mechanisms.

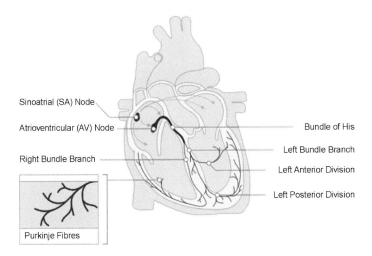

Sinoatrial (SA) Node

Atrioventricular (AV) Node

Right Bundle Branch

Bundle of His

Left Bundle Branch

Left Anterior Division

Left Posterior Division

Purkinje Fibres

FIGURE 10.1 Illustration of the cardiac conduction system. Pertinent anatomic structures are identified

Tachyarrhythmias

Any abnormality in electrical conduction that results in a heart rate and peripheral pulse of greater than 100 bpm is what defines a tachyarrhythmia. There are three potential mechanisms behind electrical impulse formation at a higher than normal rate: (1) reentry, (2) enhanced automaticity, (3) triggered activity. Each mechanism will be discussed in depth in the following paragraphs with the underlying process, electrocardiographic appearance of the resulting arrhythmia, and treatment individual to each mechanism.

Reentry

Reentry is a very common mechanism by which electrical stimuli are altered leading to tachyarrhythmia. A reentrant rhythm represents a self-sustaining electrical circuit that repeatedly depolarizes a section of myocardial tissue. Examples of reentry include atrial flutter, atrial fibrillation, AV nodal reentrant tachycardia (AVNRT), ventricular tachycardia, etc.

The requirements for a reentrant rhythm to form include the presence of the "short circuit" along with some form of ectopic beat such as premature atrial contractions (PACs) for atrial flutter or AVNRT, premature ventricular contractions (PVCs) for VT and pulmonary vein extra electrical stimulation for atrial fibrillation. Reentry is a very complex phenomenon involving more than one pathway with different conduction and repolarization properties to form the short circuit that will not be discussed in full here.

In short, a reentrant rhythm is the result of a short circuit within the cardiac tissue that, when an electrical impulse enters it at just the right time, can start a self perpetuating electrical racetrack that with each lap acts to depolarize the surrounding myocardium and takeover as the dominant pacemaker of the heart. Thus if the rate of the circuit is 300/min, the surrounding myocardium will depolarize at 300/min. Therefore, the location of the reentrant circuit determines its effect. For instance, a supraventricular (above the ventricle) location may result in a variable heart rate due to the action of the AV node as a gate keeper to ventricular activation while a ventricular reentrant circuit location will have a direct effect on heart rate only dependent on the speed of the reentrant circuit.

The nice thing about reentrant tachyarrhythmias is that interruption of the circuit utilizing physical and pharmacologic maneuvers (of which there are numerous) will result in termination of the arrhythmia and are often diagnostic.

Enhanced Automaticity

Cardiac tissue injury, typically as the result of systemic illness, can result in areas outside of the normal conduction system developing automaticity and, if faster than the SA node automaticity rate, take over as the dominant pacemaker within the heart. Enhanced automaticity is not always a pathologic process as in sinus tachycardia where increased sympathetic tone results in a faster sinus rate to meet higher metabolic demands due to systemic illness. However, arrhythmias due to enhanced automaticity are almost always secondary to another primary process and are more a marker of illness than a primary arrhythmic process. Examples of enhanced automaticity include sinus tachycardia, atrial tachycardia "atach" (automaticity from an area within the atria that is not the SA node), multifocal atrial tachycardia "MAT", wandering atrial pacemaker "WAP" (similar to MAT but with a HR < 100), some forms of ventricular tachycardia (VT), and automated idiopathic ventricular rhythm "AIVR" (similar to VT but with HR < 100).

The mainstay of therapy for these arrhythmias is diagnosis and aggressive treatment of the underlying process resulting in the abnormal rhythm. Pharmacologic therapies (typically beta and calcium channel blockers) to stabilize the cellular membranes and decrease the rate of these arrhythmias can also be considered with the caveat that the abnormal rhythm may be physiologic and acting to provide hemodynamic support to the patient. Therefore, they are not usually first line therapies and only used once the primary process has been identified and treated.

Triggered Activity

Under certain conditions an electrical stimulus can result in the onset of a rapid ventricular rhythm with variable electrical axis and morphology typically called "Torsades de pointes" or twisting of the points. Generally the inciting electrical stimulus needs to come within the vulnerable period when repolarization of the myocardium has begun but not completed. The reason why this period is vulnerable stems from the fact that repolarization during this time is heterogeneous and an electrical impulse of sufficient strength occurring at this time can begin to wander through the partially depolarized myocardium and become self perpetuating as in torsades de pointes.

A rough estimation of the time that repolarization is taking is the interval from the onset of the QRS complex to the end of the T wave on surface 12 lead ECG. The longer this interval is the longer the vulnerable period is going to be and the greater the risk is that an early or ectopic beat will find it. This is why patients with congenitally long QT intervals are at higher risk for ventricular arrhythmias and sudden cardiac death and also why the QT interval is closely monitored in patients receiving drugs that are known to prolong it. There is a large role for prevention of triggered arrhythmias as there are a number of medications that are known to prolong the QT interval including many commonly prescribed outpatient medications (Fig. 10.2) and assessment of the QT interval in patients presenting with syncope may result in the identification of congenital long QT syndrome and an opportunity to prevent ventricular arrhythmia and death. Acute treatment of arrhythmias resulting from triggered activity, mostly torsades de pointes, usually centers around acute emergency department referral, defibrillation and reversal of the inciting cause followed by implantable defibrillator therapy dependent on the situation.

FIGURE 10.2 Algorithm for the electrocardiographic diagnosis of tachyarrhythmia's [1]. *Cardiology Consultant Comment:* As can be seen schematically below, the thought process for the ECG diagnosis of a tachyarrhythmia centers around three questions: (1) wide or narrow QRS complex, (2) regular or irregular QRS-QRS interval and (3) are there p waves visualized. Having an answer to these three questions will best allow a cardiology provider to assist via telephone with the diagnosis and therapy for the tachyarrhythmia in question. In the setting where the diagnosis remains unclear even after adequately addressing these questions, additional maneuvers (vagal/adenosine) as outlined in the bedside tachyarrhythmia diagnostic section are often fruitful. Performance of such is not necessary prior to contacting cardiology although they are likely to be recommended

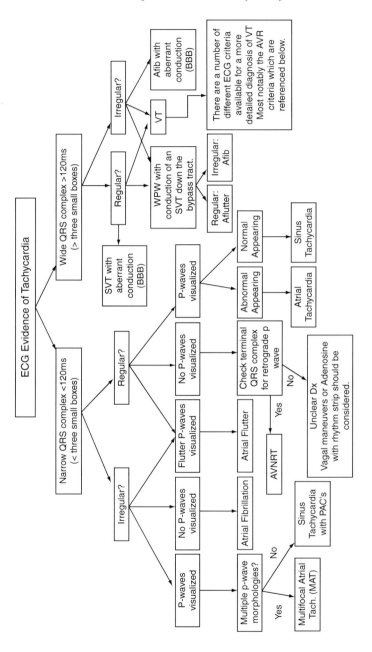

Evaluation of Tachyarrhythmias

Similar to the evaluation of any other cardiovascular process, the evaluation of a tachyarrhythmia starts with a thorough history and physical exam followed by ECG performance and interpretation. Patients tend to present in one of three ways: (1) ongoing symptoms and tachycardia on presentation, (2) no symptoms but incidental finding of tachycardia on presentation, and (3) prior symptoms of tachycardia but absent tachycardia on presentation. Each situation is approached differently although the diagnostic foundation in all three situations remains the history, physical and ECG.

An algorithmic discussion regarding the electrocardiographic diagnosis and therapeutic approaches for tachyarrhythmia's are presented in Figs. 10.2 and 10.3 respectively.

Ongoing Symptoms and Tachycardia on Presentation

By far the most straightforward and potentially serious situation is the patient presenting with symptoms and correlating tachyarrhythmia on ECG. In this setting evaluation of the patient is dependent on the vital signs and ECG interpretation. Hemodynamic instability, regardless of the electrocardiographic findings, warrants emergency department referral with an accompanying ECG and, dependent on the arrhythmia, inpatient cardiology consultation. Many outpatient clinics have an AED on site and its use in this setting should be considered.

The outpatient evaluation of patients that are hemodynamically stable is more extensive and with the use of simple bedside maneuvers can also prove to be therapeutic. Once the patient is deemed stable with ongoing tachycardia the focus shifts to assessment of the electrocardiogram and definitive identification of the arrhythmia. If available, an old ECG should always be utilized for comparison to the tachyarrhythmia. Two relatively broad brush dichotomizing ECG variables at the start of the ECG diagnostic tree are whether the QRS complex narrow (<120 ms) or wide (>120 ms) and

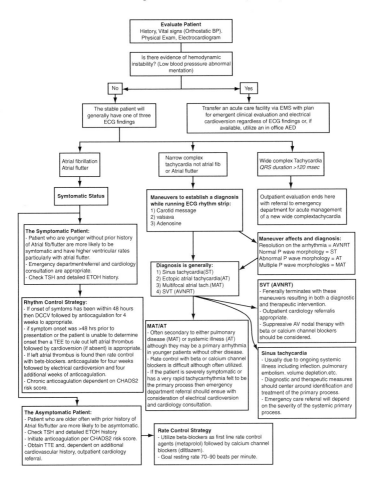

FIGURE 10.3 Bedside tachyarrhythmia evaluation and therapeutic strategy algorithm

whether it is regular or irregular. Irregularity to the QRS complex generally points toward a diagnosis of atrial fibrillation which is by far the most common tachyarrhythmia seen in the outpatient setting. Even in the setting of a wide complex tachycardia, irregular r-r intervals (irregular QRS complex) make ventricular tachycardia unlikely as it would need to be torsades de pointes (polymorphic VT) and would likely be accompanied by hemodynamic instability. An old ECG is particularly helpful to determine if the irregular wide complex tachycardia is atrial fibrillation in the setting of a bundle branch block that may have been present on the previous ECG.

Further definitive diagnosis rests on whether p waves are visualized or not. If p waves are absent, then a diagnosis of atrial fibrillation can be made; please see the section discussing specific outpatient therapeutic strategies for atrial fibrillation. If p waves are visualized there are two remaining possibilities: atrial flutter and multifocal atrial tachycardia (MAT). MAT is characterized by multiple different p wave morphologies and a ratio of p waves to QRS complexes of 1:1. If multiple p wave morphologies (3 on a standard 12 lead ECG) are visualized then proceed to the section dealing specifically with the diagnostic evaluation and therapeutic options for MAT. Atrial flutter characteristically has a "saw tooth pattern" in the inferior limb leads and a p wave to QRS ratio greater than 1:1, often 2:1 or 3:1. Therapy for atrial flutter will be further discussed in the section dealing with atrial fibrillation given their similarities.

Wide complex tachycardias that are hemodynamically stable come in two flavors: monomorphic ventricular tachycardia and pre-excited tachycardia as the result of a bypass tract. The outpatient management of wide complex tachyarrhythmias centers on rapid emergency department referral with an accompanying ECG displaying the wide complex rhythm. Once there, urgent cardiology consultation is generally sought for advanced ECG interpretation and management of the rhythm typically followed by admission and further inpatient evaluation.

Regular narrow complex tachycardias are often more difficult to definitively diagnose than atrial fibrillation or MAT given that the QRS complex and t wave often act to obscure any atrial activity necessary to make the diagnosis. If p-waves are visualized and appear to have a normal morphology (upright in the limb leads I, II, III) with a heart rate of

100–130 a diagnosis of sinus tachycardia can be made. With abnormal p-wave morphology in the limb leads, particularly after double checking for correct placement, along with a heart rate that is usually 120–150, a diagnosis of ectopic atrial tachycardia is evident. If there are not any p-waves and the rhythm is regular, it is most likely AV nodal reentrant tachycardia (AVNRT).

To definitively arrive at a diagnosis there are a number of maneuvers that can be performed bedside that will likely prove diagnostic and potentially therapeutic. The first and most important maneuver is getting a continuous rhythm strip from the available ECG machine to record the change in the rhythm. Following adequate patient positioning and with a rhythm strip running one of three maneuvers are generally used: (1) carotid massage, (2) valsalva, and (3) IV adenosine administration. Of the three the most invasive and anxiety provoking for the patient is adenosine administration as it requires an IV and, if successful, results in transient complete AV block that will be felt by the patient. As a result, the first line of diagnostic maneuvers is generally carotid massage and valsalva.

Carotid massage is performed on one carotid artery generally just superior to the sternocleidomastoid muscle where the carotid pulse can be palpated. Pressure is applied in a constant fashion for 5–7 s. A relative contraindication to its performance is known carotid disease as theoretically it can dislodge plaque that could act as a source of embolus. Valsalva is performed by asking the patient to strain against a closed glottis producing a similar feeling to having a bowel movement and hold for 5–10 s. Both of these maneuvers increase vagal tone resulting in a decrease in conduction through the AV node acting to lengthen the r-r interval and allow visualization of atrial activity or termination of the arrhythmia in the case of AVNRT. Similarly, 6 mg of adenosine pushed IV through an antecubital IV induces transient complete AV block allowing visualization of persistent p waves (sinus tach, ectopic atrial tach, multifocal atrial tach), flutter waves (atrial flutter), no p-waves (atrial fibrillation) or termination of the arrhythmia and return of normal sinus rhythm (AVNRT). Once a diagnosis is definitively made, specific therapy for the identified arrhythmia should be initiated as detailed in the following section along with cardiology consultation dependent on the final arrhythmia diagnosis.

Asymptomatic Patient with Incidental Finding of Tachycardia on Presentation

The patient that presents with an incidental finding of tachycardia on entry physical exam or ECG is managed much the same as the symptomatic patient in situation one. Asymptomatic patients are increasingly likely to have been in the arrhythmia chronically and to tolerate it better, thus decreasing the urgency of the evaluation. Elderly patients with atrial fibrillation are probably the most likely to present in such a fashion and as a result represent the most common presentation scenario. That said the same approach should be utilized toward definitive diagnosis of the arrhythmia as detailed in situation 1, followed by the therapeutic strategies listed under the individual arrhythmias in the following section.

Prior Symptoms of Tachycardia but Absent Tachycardia on Presentation

Probably the most difficult of the three situations is the patient who presents with symptoms of tachyarrhythmia including palpitations, syncope, and irregular pulse but without these symptoms or electrocardiographic abnormalities on initial office evaluation. Generally these patients are very stable upon initial evaluation with a lingering concern for arrhythmic death post office evaluation. Patient populations presenting in this way that are at increased risk for serious arrhythmic events include those with a prior history of coronary disease, known abnormal ejection fraction, and a family history of sudden cardiac death in an otherwise young patient; all pointing toward a more serious ventricular arrhythmia or ventricular arrhythmic syndrome (e.g. Long QT/Brugada syndrome).

Symptoms that are particularly concerning include syncope without prodrome followed by rapid asymptomatic recovery, palpitations associated with chest pain or exercise induced symptoms up to and including syncope. Again all of these symptoms are indicative of a more serious ventricular arrhythmia and merit a combination of ECG assessment for sings of prior myocardial infarction, left bundle branch block, electrolyte abnormalities (hyperkalemia) and prolongation of the QT interval, followed by outpatient telemetric monitoring (48 h holter or event monitor), trans-thoracic echocardiography and urgent outpatient cardiology evaluation. Certainly if the electrocardiogram is markedly abnormal with what appears to be an acute process such as hyperkalemia then emergency department referral is appropriate. In the absence of concerning historical elements, patient characteristics or symptom complex it is reasonable to initiate the evaluation with outpatient holter monitor placement, trans-thoracic echocardiography and non-urgent outpatient cardiology referral.

Bedside Cardiology Consultant

The acuity of the situation generally dictates my level of concern. In the unstable patient acute therapies need to be initiated often specific to the arrhythmia and, dependent on the clinical scenario, often towards other ongoing clinical processes that are acting to drive the arrhythmia. As a cardiologist the focus is really: Is the arrhythmia causing the patients instability or is the arrhythmia the result of the instability? Often ongoing processes such as infection, volume depletion, etc. can throw gas on the arrhythmic fire through an increase in adrenergic tone and with only a slight propensity to develop an arrhythmia, result in the onset of an arrhythmia to maintain the cardiac output. Generally the arrhythmia is atrial fibrillation that is very similar to sinus tachycardia in this situation due to its secondary relationship to another ongoing primary process that requires therapy more urgently than the atrial fibrillation. Moreover, treating the arrhythmia with chronotropic agents or cardioversion may actually do harm in this setting as the arrhythmia is almost physiologic as it is the patients compensatory mechanism to maintain cardiac output in the setting of the ongoing systemic illness. Although concern is generally focused on the telemetry or ECG, my concern is often focused on making sure that any occult primary process inciting the arrhythmia is identified. Certainly in the unstable patient, cardiology consultation is appropriate, generally during emergency department or inpatient stay along with a thorough basic evaluation for possible driving processes including basic blood work, cardiac biomarkers, urinanalysis, blood cultures and chest xray.

Wide complex tachycardias are almost uniformly concerning to a cardiologist and often require extensive evaluation for precipitating factors such as myocardial ischemia, infiltrative ventricular disease such as sarcoidosis or more rare forms of arrhythmic syndromes such as idiopathic ventricular tachycardia. The details surrounding these individual disease processes are not as important as the acute patient management designed to bring the patient to the attention of a cardiologist, often in the inpatient setting.

The most important thing to perform prior to cardiology consultation is electrocardiographic recording of the arrhythmia and collecting an old ECG for comparison. If possible, performance of the diagnostic bedside maneuvers in the case where definitive diagnosis is not present on the initial ECG is also helpful, but not necessary. Without an ECG displaying the arrhythmia we will generally recommend the evaluation detailed in situation 3 in the previous section or a period of inpatient observation to hopefully catch the arrhythmia on telemetry.

Diagnostic and Therapeutic Strategies for Individual Tachyarrhythmias

Sinus Tachycardia

Characterized by a regular rhythm and rate of 100–125 with normal p wave morphology and one p wave for every QRS complex. Arises as the result of enhanced automaticity usually due to systemic illness increasing adrenergic tone causing faster depolarization of the SA node. Often mentioned as the "most dangerous arrhythmia on the ward" due to its association with an occult primary process that may initially elude identification and subsequently appropriate therapy. The most important therapeutic measure is to assess thoroughly for a primary process that will explain the presence of sinus tachycardia such as pneumonia, urinary tract infection, pulmonary embolism, etc. and while that evaluation is ongoing to provide resuscitative IV fluids. Concerning findings center around hemodynamic instability and the severity of the primary process. Emergency department referral in the setting of hemodynamic instability or dependent on the acute primary process is appropriate. Generally cardiology consultation is not appropriate.

Sinus tachycardia ECG example:

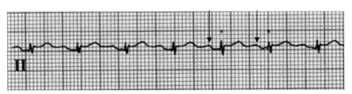

Characteristic of sinus tachycardia is a regular tachycardia with one p wave (*arrow*) for every QRS complex (*star*).

Atrial Fibrillation/Flutter

Although very different at the level of the reentrant circuit responsible for the arrhythmia, atrial fibrillation and atrial flutter are often discussed together due to the similarities in their management surrounding rate vs. rhythm control and the necessary consideration of systemic anticoagulation.

The hallmark of atrial fibrillation is irregularity of the QRS complexes and the absence of p waves on ECG. Atrial fibrillation pulse rates can vary with the health of the AV node; younger patients with robust AV node conduction tend to be more symptomatic and tachycardic than elderly patients with an age associated decline in AV node conductivity. Afib is a reentrant tachycardia that originates from electrical activity of the pulmonary veins that when it spreads to the left atrium can provide the nidus for the onset of the innumerable disorganized small reentrant circuits that are responsible for the irregularity of the QRS complex and the absence of p waves on the surface 12 lead ECG. Afib is a common secondary arrhythmia in patients with ongoing systemic illness although it is the most common primary arrhythmia encountered in medicine today.

Atrial flutter is often described as having a "saw tooth" pattern in the inferior leads on surface 12 lead ECG. The single reentrant circuit present in the right atrium is responsible for this appearance. As the reentrant circuit is organized, regular and has a rate of 300 bpm, atrial flutter is often a regular tachycardia with a rate of 150 bpm and stable two (atrial impulse) to one (QRS complex) conduction. Often conduction through the AV node is variable resulting in inconsistent conduction ratios of 2:1, 3:1, 4:1 etc. Therefore atrial flutter may be regular or irregular but is always characterized by flutter waves usually visualized best in the inferior leads or V1. If you are faced with an ambiguous regular tachycardia on ECG that has a rate of 150 bpm, a guess of atrial flutter will probably put you in the right 85% of the time. However, this is the situation where the bedside maneuvers detailed in the general tachycardia evaluation section above should be utilized.

The management of atrial fibrillation and atrial flutter are very similar. After ECG diagnosis is made the next step is determined by the hemodynamics of the patient, any concurrent primary process that may be responsible for the development of Afib/flutter as a secondary arrhythmia and their symptomatic status. If the patient is hemodynamically unstable, referral to an acute care facility for initiation of resuscitative efforts followed by cardiology consultation and possibly cardioversion is appropriate.

When faced with a hemodynamically stable patient the evaluation should then shift to the evaluation of possible inciting or exacerbating factors responsible for the development of the arrhythmia. Hyperthyroidism, recent ETOH abuse, infection (pneumonia, uti, etc.), volume depletion (gastroenteritis, decreased intake), electrolyte disturbances (renal failure), obstructive sleep apnea are all common primary processes that need either historic or basic laboratory attention for appropriate therapy to be delivered and to minimize risk of recurrence of the arrhythmia. If the afib/flutter is felt to be secondary (usually due to ongoing infection or volume depletion) the first step is administration of intravenous fluids followed by the initiation of rate control agents (metoprolol or diltiazem) once the patient is resuscitated and treatment for the primary process has begun.

In the instance where the afib/flutter is felt to be primary, management is dictated by the age, symptomatic status of the patient. Generally, younger patients are more likely to be symptomatic with atrial fibrillation and require inpatient cardiology input for rhythm control strategies. When confronted by a young symptomatic patient with new onset atrial fibrillation cardioversion is often pursued dependent on the duration of symptoms; if symptomatic for less than 72 h then cardioversion can be performed followed by anticoagulation with coumadin and bridging with lovenox/fragmin for 4 weeks due to the loss of atrial systole after cardioversion and the risk of atrial embolus formation as a result.

With symptoms ongoing for greater than 3 days then transesophageal echocardiography to assess for left atrial appendage thrombus is typically recommended and in the absence of an appendage thrombus, cardioversion is generally performed during the same procedure. If an appendage thrombus is identified then rate control agents (oral metoprolol/diltiazem) and anticoagulation are started with bridging for 4 weeks followed by cardioversion and another 4 weeks of anticoagulation. This rhythm control strategy is colored by the high rate of spontaneous conversion of atrial fibrillation in the young symptomatic population that will usually make anticoagulation and cardioversion unnecessary. Obviously the plan surrounding rhythm control will be determined in close consultation with a cardiologist and likely follow up post cardioversion.

Atrial fibrillation ECG example:

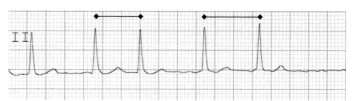

Atrial fibrillation is most characterized by two findings displayed within the figure: (1) irregularity of the QRS-QRS (RR) interval as shown by the different length brackets displayed in the figure and (2) absence of p waves.

Atrial flutter ECG example:

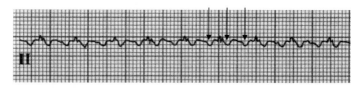

Atrial flutter is best distinguished by the "saw tooth" pattern to the tracing in the inferior leads, particularly lead II. As shown above there are multiple atrial flutter p waves (*arrows*) to every QRS complex in a 2:1 ratio.

AVNRT

Regular tachyarrhythmia generally with a rate of 130–150 bpm characterized by the absence of p waves with the major difference from atrial fibrillation being the regularity of the tachycardia. AVNRT is an AV node localized reentrant arrhythmia requiring variable conductive properties within the AV node along with an episode of ectopic atrial activity such as a premature atrial contraction to set off the self sustaining reentrant rhythm. Once established, the reentrant circuit sends electrical impulses down to the ventricles and retrograde back through the atrium from the AV node, typically causing an abnormality of the terminal QRS complex termed a pseudo s or r wave. Often it is difficult to tell the difference between AVNRT and atrial flutter on surface 12 lead ECG. Having an old ECG in this setting is imperative as the difference in the terminal portion of the QRS complex, where the retrograde p wave is buried, is key in the electrocardiographic differentiation of AVNRT from aflutter.

In the setting of probable AVNRT vs. atrial flutter the evaluation detailed in the tachyarrhythmia section above should be utilized. Classically the arrhythmia will break with vagal maneuvers or adenosine administration differing from atrial flutter that will generally not terminate, displaying persistent atrial flutter waves without QRS complexes when complete AV block via vagal or pharmacologic means is achieved. With this finding in hand the patient can be instructed as to the use of vagal maneuvers to break the arrhythmia if and when it returns. For the patient with multiple recurrences or inability to self terminate the arrhythmia with vagal maneuvers either chronic suppressive or as needed at the onset of symptoms "pill in the pocket" therapy with calcium channel blockers is reasonable. Outpatient electrophysiology referral for ablation therapy in this patient population is appropriate with ablation proving curative in over 90% of patients. Counseling regarding avoidance of exacerbating factors such as caffeine or sleep deprivation should also be provided.

If the tachyarrhythmia is persistent or does not terminate with vagal maneuvers the patient should be referred to an acute care setting for definitive diagnosis and cardiology evaluation preferentially with documentation of diagnostic efforts as noted in the tachyarrhythmia evaluation section. Generally AVNRT is tolerated well hemodynamically, but in the rare instance that the patient presents with hemodynamic instability, emergency department referral is appropriate.

AVNRT ECG example:

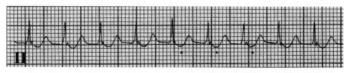

The above strip displays the classic findings of AVNRT with a regular tachycardia that typically has a rate of 150 bpm (two large boxes between each QRS) and evidence of retrograde conduction of p waves (*star*). Retrograde atrial activity is not always seen but with careful inspection of a baseline ECG can often be seen.

Ectopic Atrial Tachycardia

Is a regular tachycardia with one p wave for every QRS complex very similar to sinus tachycardia except the tachycardia generating foci is not the sinus node, rather it is another area within the atrium. Often it has a visually abnormal p wave morphology or axis noted as inverted p waves in the limb leads in the absence of limb lead reversal. EAT arises as the result of enhanced automaticity usually due to systemic illness increasing adrenergic tone causing the regular depolarization of tissue outside of the SA node. Particularly in younger female patients without structural heart disease or ongoing acute illness it can present as a primary arrhythmia that is very amenable to ablation therapy after consultation with an electrophysiologist. The most important first step (beyond ECG diagnosis) in evaluating atrial tachycardia is a thorough evaluation for exacerbating or inciting factors that are potentially correctable. Typically chronotropic agents are not very successful in controlling the rate but given the limited options otherwise they are generally employed. Generally if a patient presents with atrial tachycardia, acute care referral is appropriate due to the likelihood of occult illness and the need for advance electrophysiologic input regarding both medical and ablative therapy.

EAT ECG example:

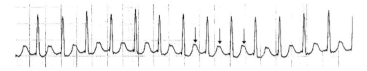

After adenosine 6 mg IV:

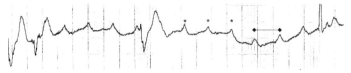

Atrial tachycardia is a regular tachyarrhythmia character-ized by a p wave rate of slower than 300 bpm (one large box) as displayed by the bracket in the lower tracing. With adenos-ine administration there is often persistence of the p waves as displayed in the bottom row and a return to tachycardia after the adenosine has ceased to act. In the above tracing the atrial tachycardia p waves are hidden in the preceding t wave (*arrows*).

Multifocal Atrial Tachycardia

Characterized by an irregular rhythm with one p wave for every QRS complex but multiple different p wave morpholo-gies (at least 3) on a standard 12 lead ECG. The mechanism is felt to be enhanced automaticity resulting in multiple atrial foci depolarizing often increasing the rate 130–140 bpm. Commonly associated with chronic pulmonary disease although may present as a primary arrhythmia. Therapeutic options are limited as they focus on treatment of the underlying pulmo-nary disease but do include the use of AV node agents such as metoprolol (if acceptable given the often underlying pulmo-nary disease) and diltiazem. Typically chronotropic agents are not very successful in controlling the rate but given the limited options otherwise they are generally employed. Advanced electrophysiologic management (ablation, antiarrhythmic therapy) is not utilized for MAT given the multiple atrial foci responsible for the tachyarrhythmia and due to its nature as a secondary process.

MAT ECG example:

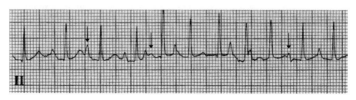

MAT is often irregular, as seen in the above tracing, with three or greater p wave morphologies on standard 12 lead rhythm strip (*arrows*).

Wide Complex Tachycardia/WPW

In the outpatient setting the most common wide complex (>120 ms or three small ECG boxes) tachyarrhythmia encountered is atrial fibrillation/flutter in the setting of a bundle branch block. The main differentiating ECG feature is the subtle irregularity of the QRS complexes supporting the diagnosis of a supraventricular tachyarrhythmia instead of the more concerning ventricular arrhythmia. Numerous ventricular tachycardia ECG diagnostic algorithms have been described and utilized with varying degrees of accuracy. When a wide complex tachyarrhythmia is encountered in the outpatient setting, emergency department referral is appropriate regardless of the final diagnosis of the arrhythmia: VT, atrial fibrillation with a bundle branch block, WPW all are appropriate to evaluate in the inpatient setting.

WPW in particular may come to the outpatient practitioners' attention in the absence of tachycardia as ECG evidence of preexcitation may be visualized on a resting ECG. Often patients will experience symptoms of palpitations, presyncope or syncope but present in normal sinus rhythm. WPW syndrome or preexcitation due to an accessory conduction pathway around the AV node will often display a shortened p-r interval or a slurring of the initiation of the QRS complex commonly termed a delta wave. Such electrocardiographic abnormalities should prompt outpatient cardiology and potentially electrophysiology referral.

There are numerous forms of ventricular tachycardia that may present in the outpatient setting. In the USA the most common form of ventricular tachycardia is ischemia or scar associated VT with electrical reentry around infracted scarred myocardium. Typically this form of VT will be found in patients with a history of coronary disease, acute chest pain and or abnormal left ventricular function. More benign forms of VT also exist in young patients without any known coronary disease, either as the result of increased automaticity or microreentry including ventricular outflow tract VT (LVOT and RVOT VT), bundle branch reentry VT, and idiopathic LV VT (Bellhausen's VT). An in depth discussion of these arrhythmias is not necessary given that the outpatient management of them is the same: emergency department referral with urgent cardiology consultation.

Wide complex (ventricular) tachycardia ECG example:

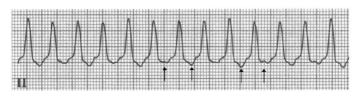

Ventricular tachycardia is characterized by a wide complex (>120 ms or three small boxes) tachycardia that classically displays AV disassociation: more QRS complexes than p waves (*arrows*) without any relationship between the two.

Bradyarrhythmias

Any abnormality in electrical conduction that results in a heart rate and peripheral pulse of less than 60 bpm is what clinically defines a bradyarrhythmia. There are a number of mechanisms for bradyarrhythmia formation including an amazing spectrum of illness at each end of the age spectrum. Benign, congenital, acquired, ischemic, and iatrogenic forms of bradyarrhythmia are commonly encountered in outpatient clinical practice. All forms of bradyarrhythmia involve either slowed or completely blocked electrical impulse propagation within the normal conduction system. Often backup pacemakers provide an "escape rhythm" by which cardiac output is maintained during high grade or complete AV node conduction block.

The basic evaluation of patients presenting with a bradyarrhythmia include a thorough general medical exam, historical assessment for symptoms related to the bradycardia: syncope, presyncope, orthostatic lightheadedness, chest pain, dyspnea on exertion or rest, heart failure, and lower extremity edema followed by ECG diagnosis of the bradyarrhythmia.

Management of bradyarrhythmia centers around two main elements: (1) removal or correction of exacerbating or inciting factors and (2) initiation of temporary followed by permanent pacing in the event that there are not inciting factors to correct or that correcting the inciting elements is unlikely to result in the return of normal conduction. More severe forms of heart block (Mobitz II and complete heart block) do not require associated symptoms for initiation of permanent pacing, whereas Mobitz I and sinus bradycardia require direct correlation of the arrhythmia with patient symptoms to merit device therapy.

Often the majority of the acute evaluation is undertaken in the inpatient setting after referral from an initial outpatient evaluation has been completed. Patients that present with symptoms felt to be directly related to the bradycardia, particularly in the setting of high grade AV block or in the absence of exacerbating medications that could be held pending quick outpatient reevaluation followed by potential inpatient referral, are appropriate to send to the acute care inpatient setting for medical stabilization and electrophysiologic evaluation. Hypotension, extreme bradycardia, syncope, and orthostatic hypotension are all concerning symptoms that should prompt emergency department referral and likely inpatient cardiology evaluation.

As with any other arrhythmic process, the majority of the diagnostic weight is placed upon correct interpretation of the electrocardiogram. The therapeutic approach and diagnostic evaluation of individual bradyarrhythmias will be discussed below.

Bedside Cardiology Consultant

When dealing with a bradyarrhythmia the most important pieces of information are the patient's vital signs particularly the heart rate and blood pressure along with the type of bradyarrhythmia seen on ECG. With profound bradycardia or hypotension, regardless of the ECG, often the patient needs to be referred to the emergency department for acute evaluation, definitive ECG interpretation and hemodynamic stabilization, typically in consultation with a cardiologist. Evidence of AV block beyond and including second degree heart block should be referred to the inpatient setting with an accompanying ECG. Patients with recurrent syncope, hemodynamic instability or complete heart block should be transported via ambulance. Generally any bradycardia that is felt to be causing symptoms will require inpatient evaluation if only for a brief period of observation, medication adjustment and intravenous fluids. Mobitz II and complete heart block are going to receive permanent pacemaker therapy with more benign forms receiving conservative therapy as first line followed by permanent device therapy only in the evidence of severe persistent symptoms.

Often patients will present with onset of symptoms, typically presyncope or syncope with a bradycardic bystander pulse assessment and a normal in office ECG. This situation is difficult as it is unclear whether or not the assessment is correct and even if it is correct, whether or not the bradycardia caused or was a result of the syncope. Inpatient referral for telemetry and basic electrolyte assessment is reasonable when the concern of the clinician is for a cardiogenic cause of syncope. If the level of concern by the provider is low and the patient is receiving therapy with agents that will act to slow the heart rate, it is a reasonable first step to stop them and place an outpatient Holter monitor with short term follow up. Without any evidence of conduction disease on baseline ECG, Holter monitor and no recurrence of symptoms then medications can be slowly restarted with reassurance provided to the patient.

Diagnostic and Therapeutic Strategies for Individual Bradyarrhythmias

Sinus Bradycardia

Characterized by a heart rate of <60 bpm and one p wave for every QRS complex with a constant PR interval. Typically sinus bradycardia is a normal finding in 25–30% of the population over the age of 25, the elderly and the young fit patient. In the asymptomatic patient, sinus bradycardia is not a concerning finding with reassurance and education provided to the patient regarding potential symptoms associated with bradycardia. Patients receiving chronotropic or antihypertensive therapy with digoxin, beta or calcium channel blockers who present with asymptomatic sinus bradycardia should have any possible offending agent decreased or stopped based upon the opinion of the individual clinical practitioner. Other pharmacologic agents such as lithium, antiarrhythmics including amiodarone and sotalol can also cause asymptomatic sinus bradycardia and require dose adjustment as a result. Systemic causes of asymptomatic sinus bradycardia include increased intracranial pressure, vagal stimuli such as nausea and vomiting, obstructive sleep apnea, hypothyroidism and hypothermia.

Symptomatic sinus bradycardia is generally the result of two clinical processes. The first and most common is overdosing of chronotropic or antihypertensive agents, particularly combination therapy with calcium channel and beta blockers for atrial fibrillation in the elderly.

The decision regarding ongoing outpatient management with medication adjustment vs. emergency department referral is subjective with slower heart rates and more profound symptoms leading towards emergency department referral. The majority of the evaluation for symptomatic sinus bradycardia can be performed as an outpatient via short term follow up with inpatient referral also appropriate based upon the comfort level of the involved practitioner. The mainstay of therapy for this form of sinus bradycardia is cessation of the offending agent. Symptoms that persist beyond a washout of the offending agent may require placement of a permanent pacemaker in consultation with an electrophysiologist.

Sinus bradycardia ECG example:

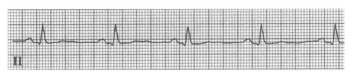

Sinus bradycardia characterized by one p wave for every QRS complex with a rate of less than 60 bpm.

Sick Sinus Syndrome

Sinus node dysfunction is a less common cause of symptomatic sinus bradycardia and is an amalgam of three different clinical presentations: sinus node arrest, sinus node exit block and tachy-brady syndrome. This form of sinus bradycardia is less common but when present is more likely to be symptomatic.

A sinus pause or arrest is defined as the transient absence of sinus P waves on the ECG that may last from 2.0 s to several minutes. This abnormality is an alteration in discharge by the SA pacemaker; as a result, the duration of the pause has no arithmetical relationship to the basic sinus rate (i.e. the cycle length of the pause is not a multiple of the basic sinus cycle length as would occur with 2:1 or 3:1 SA nodal block). The pause or arrest often allows escape beats or rhythms to occur, but lower pacemakers may be sluggish or even absent. A pause that is roughly 2 s does not necessarily indicate disease, since it can occur in the normal heart, but longer pauses (typically 5 s or greater) often result in symptoms of dizziness, presyncope, syncope, and rarely, death. A documented pause of 5 s or greater should receive permanent device therapy regardless of symptoms.

Sinus exit block is similar to a sinus pause on the surface as a pause is visualized on the surface electrocardiogram. The major difference is the timing of the dropped beat being completely in sync with the preceding and following beats. This indicates that the sinus node tried to pace but due to fibrotic electrically non-conducting tissue surrounding it, was not able to get the electrical impulse to the atrium to generate an atrial contraction resulting in a dropped beat. The timing relationship can be visualized in the sinus exit block example below where following the preceding p to p interval through the dropped beat results in landing directly on the p wave of the first beat following the pause. The details surrounding sinus exit block vs. sinus arrest are mainly academic and with evidence of these on surface ECG, inpatient referral for stabilization and cardiology evaluation are appropriate. Generally sinus exit block is not as severely symptomatic as a sinus pause as the interval between QRS complexes is usually shorter in sinus exit block. However, recurrent symptoms regardless of the duration between QRS complexes should receive permanent pacemaker therapy.

Tachy-Brady syndrome is a form of sick sinus syndrome where a tachycardia, typically atrial filbrillation but not limited to such, terminates to a long pause similar to a sinus arrest (see ECG example below). This pause results in the patient experiencing symptoms similar to a sinus arrest: syncope, presyncope, palpitations. Due to the desire to minimize the tachycardia with chronotropic agents and treat the symptomatic pauses, pacemaker placement followed by the initiation of beta or calcium channel blocker therapy is pursued during an inpatient stay. Patients presenting in the outpatient setting with documented tachy-brady syndrome can often be referred to cardiology as an outpatient with inpatient referral and immediate device therapy appropriate for patients with frequent, severe symptoms (frequent syncope with injury).

Therapy for patients with sick sinus syndrome starts with cessation of any possible exacerbating medications. Patients with documented symptomatic bradycardia, including frequent sinus pauses that produce symptoms should receive permanent pacemaker therapy. In some patients, bradycardia is iatrogenic and will occur as a consequence of essential long-term drug therapy of a type and dosage for which there are no acceptable alternatives. For patients with inappropriate heart rate response to exercise (abnormal chronotropic competence) pacemaker placement is also indicated. In cases where it is unclear as to whether sinus node dysfunction is present and accounting for the patients symptoms, invasive assessment of the sinus node via an electrophysiology study is indicated and will provide objective evidence as to abnormal sinus node function requiring permanent pacing.

Sinus arrest/pause ECG example:

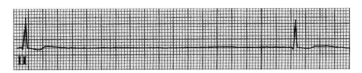

Sinus arrest/pause shown above without any atrial activity during an amazingly long pause, typically resulting in syncope.

Sinus exit block ECG example:

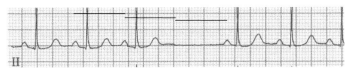

Sinus exit block with what appears to be an absent p wave as the atrial rhythm after the short pause is an exact multiple of the preceding p wave interval (*caliper lines*).

Tachy-Brady ECG example:

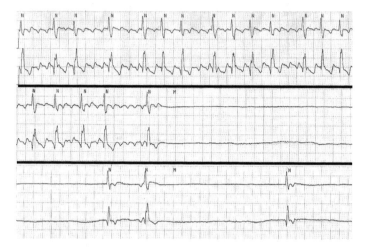

Atrial flutter is displayed in the topmost strip followed by termination of the atrial flutter to a long sinus arrest (*middle strip*) and syncope by the bottom strip. Typically the symptoms of tachy-brady syndrome are associated with the sinus arrest seen above post termination of a supraventricular arrhythmia (typically atrial fibrillation or atrial flutter).

First Degree AV Node Block

Electrocardiographic abnormality characterized by prolongation of the PR interval to greater than 200 ms or one large box on standard 25 mm/s paper speed ECG. Calling this PR prolongation a form of AV block is slightly misleading as it is actually slow electrical conduction through the right atrium and not a delay through the AV node that results in the PR prolongation. There is no therapeutic or diagnostic consideration for this form of AV block although patients that do have first degree AV block are at higher risk for progression to higher grade AV block.

First degree AV block ECG example:

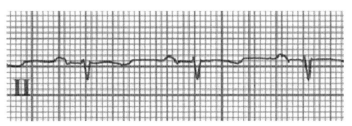

First degree AV block noted for a PR interval (onset of p wave to onset of QRS complex) of greater than one large box in duration.

Second Degree AV Node Block

This is where the threshold for real conduction disease is located with the more benign form of AV block being Wenckebach or Mobitz type I block and Mobitz type II block, a progressive and serious form of AV node disease typically treated with permanent pacemaker placement both included under the umbrella of second degree AV block.

Mobitz I (Wenckebach) AV block is characterized by a progressive prolongation of the PR interval and resulting shortening of the QRS-QRS (aka RR) interval followed by a dropped beat where the p wave is not conducted. It is often due to vagal stimuli (nausea or in a young fit athletic patient), acidosis, electrolyte disturbance, AV nodal chronotropic medications (digoxin, beta and calcium channel blockers) and myocardial ischemia acting to decrease conductivity through the AV node. Less common causes include myo-carditis, post surgical (aortic and mitral valve surgery) and as the result of congenital heart disease.

Mobitz II also includes dropped beats but differs from Mobitz I in that the PR interval does not vary in relation to the non-conducted p wave. In contrast to Mobitz I that involves the AV node and generally has a benign prognosis, Mobitz II is associated with disease of the His bundle below the AV node and has a much higher rate of progression to complete heart block and a resulting increased risk of death.

Therefore determining Mobitz I from Mobitz II with a high degree of certainty is of importance.

From an electrocardiographic perspective the best technique for differentiating the two is a caliper measurement of the PR interval before and after the dropped beat. In Mobitz I the PR interval will be different and Mobitz II it will be the same, coming back to the variable and constant PR intervals that characterizes Mobitz I and II respectively. The RR interval will shorten in the setting of Mobitz I, again due to prolongation of the PR interval, while the RR interval in Mobitz II will remain constant, similarly due to the constant PR interval.

Clinical maneuvers can also be helpful in distinguishing the two types of second degree AV block that are particularly useful in the setting of 2:1 P to QRS block where there is only one PR interval and it is not possible to tell if prolongation is occurring prior to the dropped beat. Generally Mobitz I will improve with exertion or atropine due to the role of vagal tone in inducing the AV block and Mobitz II will worsen as the enhanced conductivity of the AV node (due to the exertion and removal of vagal tone) will be met with no unchanged block distal to the AV node in the His bundle. Increased vagal tone will act to decrease the sinus node rate and may allow more time for excitability to recover in or below the bundle of His, and facilitate conduction. Therefore either getting the patient up to walk around while on telemetry or while the pulse is monitored to record any change in heart rate can provide key information to whether or not the AV block is Mobitz I or II.

Generally, even in the absence of symptoms, Mobitz II AV block is treated with permanent dual chamber pacemaker therapy usually in the inpatient setting with an electrophysiologist's input. Mobitz I is typically treated through removal of the offending agent including treating any nausea or holding chronotropic antihypertensive agents such as beta or calcium channel blockers and antiarryhthmics such as sotalol or amiodarone. If a patient with Mobitz I is symptomatic without exacerbating or correctable factors or after their removal then permanent pacing can be considered, again only with the input of electrophysiology in the inpatient setting.

When it remains unclear whether or not the patient has more severe distal conduction disease (Mobitz II) an invasive electrophysiology study can be performed to document conduction below the AV node. If distal conduction is found to be abnormal it is consistent with Mobitz II, and the patient will receive permanent pacemaker therapy.

Mobitz I ECG example:

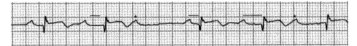

Mobitz I (Wenckebach) AV block with prolongation of the PR interval (*caliper lines*) prior to a non-conducted p wave (*star*). The PR interval before and after the dropped p wave (first and second caliper line are the same length) are not the same a finding that is key to the diagnosis of Mobitz I and removes the more serious Mobitz II as a possible diagnosis.

Mobitz II ECG example:

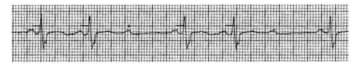

Mobitz II is notable for a constant PR interval (*caliper lines*) prior to a non-conducted p wave (*star*). The sudden loss of AV node conduction often signals more severe distal conduction disease typically requiring permanent pacing or electrophysiology study.

2:1 AV block ECG example:

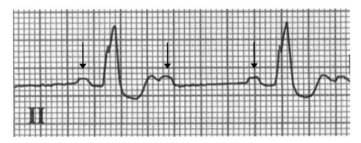

2:1 AV block presents a diagnostic problem as it is not clear if this is Mobitz I or II due to having only one PR interval prior to the dropped beat. Often atropine or exertion (if the patient is able) is utilized to differentiate the two. AV conduction and consequently heart rate in Mobitz I will improve with exertion or atropine and in Mobitz II it will worsen.

Third Degree AV Block

Also termed complete heart block where atrial electrical impulses do not reach the ventricles. The block can exist in the AV node or in the infra-nodal specialized conduction system.

The electrocardiogram is characterized by no relationship between the p waves and the QRS complexes that are typically the result of an escape rhythm where a pacemaker other than the sinus node has sufficient time to depolarize, attain threshold, and produce a depolarization. Multiple non-conducted p waves are seen for every QRS complex resulting in p/QRS ratio of greater than 1.

In complete heart block, the escape rhythm that controls the ventricles can occur at any level below that of the conduction block and the morphology of the QRS complex can help to determine the location at which this is occurring. A narrow QRS complex generally means a junctional escape with a rate of 40–50 bpm and a wide QRS complex is usually the result of a ventricular escape with a rate of less than 40 and often is unreliable, resulting in a very slow rate or asystole. Syncope and death are common presentations in this setting. As a rough rule the slower the escape the more symptomatic the patient and the more urgency to the situation with regard to emergency department referral.

Complete heart block is typically the result of either progressive degenerative conduction disease or the same acute processes resulting in Mobitz II heart block, just further along in the course of illness. Once ischemia and reversible etiologies (medications, acidosis, electrolyte disturbance) have been thoroughly evaluated and eliminated permanent dual chamber pacemaker placement generally ensues. The decision to initiate trans-cutaneous or temporary trans-venous pacing is dictated by inpatient practitioner preference and the clinical stability of the patient. Generally patients presenting with hemodynamic compromise, ventricular escape with slow or inconsistent escape rate or ventricular arrhythmia due to triggered activity secondary to the prolongation of the QT interval seen with a ventricular rhythm are treated with temporary pacing measures.

Complete heart block ECG example:

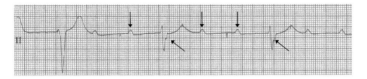

Complete heart block is characterized by two central items: bradycardia and lack of a relationship between the p waves (*arrows*) and QRS complexes. Escape rhythms are typically either wide (QRS > 120 ms) coming from the ventricle with more profound bradycardia as in this case, or narrow (QRS < 120 ms) and coming from the His bundle with rates of 40 bpm or greater.

Basic Device Review

Implanted devices come in two flavors: those with defibrillation capacity (ICDs) and those without (pacemakers). Both of these devices along with indications for their placement will be discussed separately along with clinical and electrocardiographic techniques to differentiate the two in the following paragraphs.

Pacemakers are typically placed for asymptomatic advanced conduction system disease (Mobitz II, complete heart block), symptomatic bradycardia with or without conduction system disease and the tachy-brady syndrome where rate control agents will be used to control the tachycardia while not compromising the patient during bradycardic episodes. For a thorough list of indications the ACC/AHA guidelines provide a complete framework of the indications for permanent pacing (PPM).

Implantable cardioverter defibrillators (ICDs) have revolutionized the treatment of arrhythmic death and have consequently saved countless lives. With the increasing complexity surrounding the computerized analysis of intracardiac electrocardiography utilized by today's ICDs only a limited discussion of their function is possible here. Most ICDs detect the cycle length (rate) of electrical activity primarily from the right ventricular lead with some also obtaining information from the atrial lead in dual chamber configurations. Based upon the rate and other advanced discriminatory settings the device "decides" what the arrhythmia is and treats it as it is programmed. Therefore if the patient has ventricular tachycardia that is not fast enough to cross the programmed ventricular tachycardia rate threshold it will not be treated as VT and in contrast a rapid atrial tachyarrhythmia that is fast enough to cross the VT threshold will be treated as VT even though it is clearly not.

The indications for ICD placement are for primary and secondary prevention of ventricular arrhythmias. Patients with known LV dysfunction (LVEF<35%) either due to ischemic or non-ischemic disease are often considered appropriate for primary prevention ICD therapy based upon data from a number of large clinical trials. After ventricular arrest or presentation with a ventricular arrhythmia, referral of the patient to electrophysiology for secondary prevention of future ventricular arrhythmias and sudden cardiac death is indicated. Although limited in scope, these are the two main indications for ICD placement utilized and for a more thorough discussion please see the ACC/AHA guidelines for ICD therapy.

In the USA two device configurations are commonly used: right ventricular lead only and right atrial and right ventricular lead (dual chamber) pacemaker/defibrillators. The type of system implanted dictates the available modes of pacing and sensing. Although both ICDs and pacemakers are both capable of pacing, generally ICDs implanted for treatment of ventricular arrhythmia have a very low set pacing rate of 40 bpm to minimize unnecessary pacing while pacemakers can have set rates that vary between 50 and 90 bpm. Recently there has been a shift from single chamber pacemaker therapy for bradyarrhythmias as it is not synchronous with atrial activity often resulting in atrial and ventricular contraction at the same time. This stretches the atrium and can initiate atrial fibrillation, something that can easily be avoided with the addition of an atrial lead and dual chamber pacing.

Pacemakers can be described according to the chamber *paced*, the chamber *sensed*, and the *response* of the pacemaker to the sensed impulse. A three-letter code correlating to these categories is used to describe pacemaker types. For example, a VVI pacemaker paces the *ventricles*, senses the *ventricles*, and is *inhibited* when it senses a beat, a VOO pacemaker paces the ventricle and does not sense or respond to native electrical activity. In this descriptive label D stands for both atria and ventricle and A stands for atrial only. Based upon the ECG appearance the type of device and setting can often be determined. A basic diagram showing an implanted device along with the common types of pacemakers are displayed in Fig. 10.4 here.

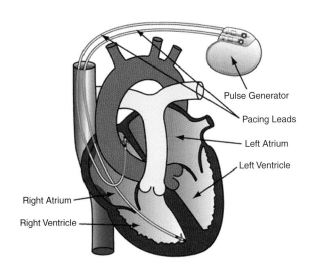

FIGURE 10.4 A basic diagram of a dual chamber device displaying a right atrial and right ventricular lead configuration

Single Lead Ventricular Demand Pacemaker (VVI)

This is by far the most common type of pacemaker. It senses spontaneous ventricular impulses and paces the ventricles only when needed.

VVI PPM ECG example:

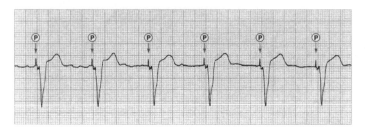

This strip shows ventricular pacemaker capturing every beat. Note absence of mapable P waves, and sharp spikes followed immediately by wide QRS complexes. VVI pacemakers ignore any atrial activity and pace the ventricle where native ventricular activity (PVC or conducted beat from the atria) will inhibit pacing. Dual chamber devices can be set to VVI mode although this is not commonly done. As pacing is initiated in the right ventricle it will propagate via myocardial muscle propagation giving a left bundle branch block conduction pattern on surface 12 lead ECG.

Dual Chamber Demand Pacemaker (DDD)

This pacemaker is also referred to as *fully automatic, universal*, and *physiologic*. It senses both atrial and ventricular activity, and as needed, paces the atria, the ventricles, or both in synchrony. When either atrial pacing or tracking of the patient's native p waves with ventricular paced impulses are seen on surface ECG the device must be a dual chamber pacemaker.

DDD PPM example 1:

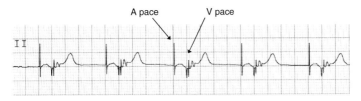

In the above example pacing activity can be seen both in the atrial and ventricular chambers an "AV paced" setting.

DDD PPM example 2:

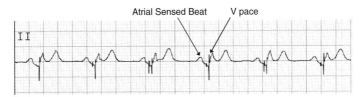

In this example atrial electrical impulses are sensed followed by ventricular pacing after a programmed delay.

Bedside Cardiology Consultant

Common clinical scenarios involving pacemakers and devices in general encountered by the outpatient practitioner include: Is the device a defibrillator or just a pacemaker? When is device interrogation indicated? When should you be concerned regarding device malfunction or lead dislodgement? Can my patient have an MRI with the device?

Is the Device a Defibrillator or Just a Pacemaker?

The simplest way to determine if the device has defibrillator capability is based upon a conversation with the patient and examination of a current or, if available, old chest x-ray. ICDs will generally have coil's evident either in the superior vena cava or within the right ventricle upon the RV lead. The coils are thickened areas of the leads that are required for defibrillation as labeled below on the chest x-ray. Older defibrillators also had larger generators than pacemakers but with improvements in technology and a reduction in the size of both device types, this rule of thumb is less reliable.

Chest x-ray for dual chamber pacemaker

Chest x-ray for dual chamber pacemaker ICD

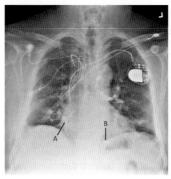 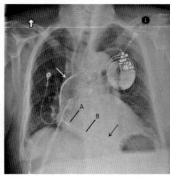

As can be seen above the device that only has pacing ability (on the *left*) does not have the defibrillator coils (*arrows* on *right* image) on its leads. Both devices are dual chamber as atrial leads (**a**) and ventricular leads (**b**) can be seen.

When Is Device Interrogation Indicated?

Device interrogation is reasonable in any situation where device function is in question, the patient has received a shock from the ICD or in the patient presenting with a device and syncope. The device will only have episodes that register as abnormally slow or fast depending on device programming making it of little utility in examining the heart rhythm at a particular point in time unless it was abnormal. Therefore if no abnormalities are found that coincide with the patients episode, it is safe to assume that the episode was not due to either tachy or brady arrhythmias.

Prior to surgical procedure it is reasonable to place a magnet over any device to avoid confusion with electrocautery as either a native heart rhythm or a tachyarrhythmia that would receive inappropriate intraoperative defibrillator therapy. The magnet (large, circular appearing similar to a doughnut) disables sensing and consequently any tachyarrhythmia therapies for an ICD along with initiating asynchronous pacing (VOO) for pacemakers resulting in ventricular pacing at a set backup rhythm without any native sensing. Post magnet application to an ICD non-urgent device interrogation is reasonable to provide reassurance that no changes in tachyarrhythmia therapy occurred with placement of the magnet. Pacemakers do not require routine interrogation after magnet application. For surgical procedures that involve electrocautery within the thoracic cavity or near to the subcutaneously implanted generator the device should be turned off prior to the surgical procedure, essentially accomplishing the same thing as the magnet but without having to keep the magnet in place during surgery. After completion of the surgical procedure the device will require sensing or tachyarrhythmia therapies to be turned back on.

When Should You Be Concerned Regarding Device Malfunction or Lead Dislodgement?

Malfunction of the device or dislodgement of the lead is a rare occurrence that is potentially very serious dependent on the implantation indication. The electrocardiogram and clinical presentation can provide a lot toward determining if the device is not functioning appropriately. A baseline ECG for comparison can prove invaluable in determining if there has been a change in pacing morphology and consequently device function. When pacemaker spikes are not followed by pacing activity or the device is pacing inappropriately due to a failure to sense native activity the device is stated to have "failure to capture" and "failure to sense" respectively, that can signal dislodgement of the pacing lead or device malfunction. Typically accurate determination of either of these scenarios requires the input of either a device specialist or an electrophysiologist. Causes of loss of capture or failure to sense include dislodgement of the lead, progressive heart failure, and electrolyte disturbances with therapeutic measures typically including correcting of the underlying process as well as adjusting device output or sensing thresholds.

In the pacemaker dependent patient (typically placed for complete heart block) loss of device function for any reason can be very serious. Patients unfortunate enough to experience this will often present with profound bradycardia due to suppression of escape rhythms as the result of chronic pacing, syncope and hemodynamic compromise requiring immediate restoration of pacing via either transcutaneous or transvenous modalities.

Migration of the right ventricular lead is thankfully quite uncommon. The typical findings include change from a baseline left bundle branch block pacing pattern to a right bundle branch block and new diaphragmatic stimulation with pacing. If a patient presents with nonstop hiccups or a respiratory rate in the 60s it is reasonable to check a chest x-ray and interrogate the device to determine if the lead has migrated.

Can My Patient Have an MRI with the Device?

This issue is still in flux in cardiology. The concerns with regard to MRI in the setting of a device are both dislodgement and migration of the lead during MRI and the MRI induced induction of arrhythmias. A number of centers have published their experience with MRI in the setting of a device with the following lessons learned: (1) Pacemaker dependent patients should not have an MRI for any reason. (2) Patients with an ICD or those that are not pacemaker dependent should have the device reprogrammed by either a device representative or electrophysiologist prior to the MRI.

The goal with reprogramming is to disable the device's ability to sense thus instructing it to pace independent of any MRI induced artifact. (3) The patient should be monitored during their study often by a cardiologist if available. (4) Post MRI the device should be interrogated and reprogrammed. As device technology evolves and the experience of various academic centers is published these recommendations may be subject to change.

Conclusion

Arrhythmic cardiovascular disease represents some of the most conceptually difficult yet rewarding disease processes within cardiology. As an outpatient care provider the most important pieces of information are the patient's vital signs and electrocardiogram. Based upon the hemodynamic stability of the patient and the electrocardiographic diagnosis, acute emergency department or outpatient cardiology referral may be appropriate. Advanced therapy with antiarrhythmic or device based therapy should be determined during formal inpatient or outpatient cardiology evaluation.

Reference

1. Vereckei A et al. New algorithm using only lead aVR for differential diagnosis of wide QRS complex tachycardia. Heart Rhythm. 2008;5(1):89–98.

Chapter 11
Congestive Heart Failure

Susan F. Lien and Jeffrey D. Alexis

Introduction

Heart failure (HF) is an epidemic disorder that currently affects more than 5 million people in the United States, with an estimated 550,000 new diagnoses each year. Given the increasing age of the population and the improved survival of patients from acute myocardial infarctions and other diseases, the incidence of heart failure will undoubtedly continue to grow. Current data from the NHLBI's Framingham Heart Study suggests that at age 40, the lifetime risk of developing heart failure for both men and women is approximately one in five (or 20%), and 1- and 5-year mortality is about 30% and 50%, respectively. The Framingham study suggests that patients with heart failure have mortality rates four to eight times higher compared to the general population of the same age. Hospital discharges for HF rose from 877,000 in 1996 to 1,106,000 in 2006. Furthermore, the estimated cost of HF in the United States for 2010 is $39.2 billion. However, appropriate recognition and early treatment of heart failure, risk factors, and use of evidence-based therapies in patients already diagnosed with heart failure can help to prevent this expected increase in HF incidence and reduce the mortality,

S.F. Lien (✉) • J. D. Alexis
Department of Internal Medicine, Division of Cardiology,
University of Rochester Medical Center, Rochester, NY, USA
e-mail: susan_lien@urmc.rochester.edu

J.D. Bisognano et al. (eds.), *Manual of Outpatient Cardiology*, 281
DOI 10.1007/978-0-85729-944-4_11,
© Springer-Verlag London Limited 2012

number of hospitalizations, and health care costs associated with this disorder.

Etiology

Although the most common cause of heart failure is ischemic cardiomyopathy (up to two-thirds of all cases), the remaining heart failure conditions do not fit into this category. Appropriate identification of the etiology of heart failure is important to help with therapy.

The causes of heart failure can be further categorized by primary dysfunction (systolic or diastolic). There is considerable overlap with several factors that can independently result in heart failure with systolic dysfunction or heart failure with preserved left ventricular ejection fraction (HFpEF) or a combination of both.

Heart Failure with Systolic Dysfunction

Most simply, heart failure with systolic dysfunction can be defined as a reduction in ejection fraction from impaired contractility of the left ventricle. However, the pathophysiology behind heart failure is complex involving not just impaired myocardial contractility but activation of the neuroendocrine system leading to unfavorable cardiac remodeling that causes chamber enlargement and reduction in ejection fraction.

Chief Complaint/Symptoms

Oftentimes, there is no correlation between the severity of symptoms and the extent of ejection fraction reduction; therefore, a patient with a significantly reduced EF may be asymptomatic. In fact, up to one-half of all patients with left ventricular systolic dysfunction are without symptoms.

However, in patients with symptoms, the most common and earliest presenting symptom is shortness of breath that manifests itself with progressively increasing severity as (1) exertional dyspnea, (2) orthopnea, (3) paroxysmal nocturnal dyspnea, and (4) dyspnea at rest.

1. Exertional dyspnea: As heart failure progresses, the degree of activity needed to induce dyspnea declines. However, as mentioned earlier, there is not always a correlation between exercise capacity and LV function.

2. Orthopnea: This symptom of heart failure presents itself as the heart failure becomes more advanced or in decompensated states. It is defined as shortness of breath that develops when lying down and is relieved with elevation of the head with pillows. Typically, orthopnea is characterized by the number of pillows required for sleeping. The change in the number of pillows needed is important in quantifying the heart failure. In advanced heart failure, orthopnea may be so severe that the patient cannot lie down and must sleep sitting upright in a chair to avoid pulmonary congestion.

3. Paroxysmal nocturnal dyspnea: This symptom occurs as LV failure worsens and is often described as a sudden awakening by the patient after several hours of sleep causing the patient to immediately sit upright, gasping for air, with the associated feelings of severe anxiety/panic and suffocation. Bronchospasm may be present, as well.

4. Dyspnea at rest: This symptom signals failure of compensatory mechanisms and end-stage heart failure. Dyspnea at rest results from decreased pulmonary compliance with increased airway resistance, as well as hypoxemia associated with increased pulmonary capillary wedge pressure, and decreased respiratory muscle function.

Other cardiac symptoms of heart failure include fatigue, weakness, low exercise tolerance, chest pain/pressure, palpitations, dizziness, syncope, anorexia, weight loss, abdominal pain, bloating, cough, insomnia, oliguria, and cerebral symptoms ranging from anxiety to depressed mood to memory impairment and confusion.

Signs/Physical Examination

The physical signs associated with heart failure are dependent upon the degree of compensation, the acuity, and chamber involvement (right-sided versus left-sided heart failure).

1. Volume overload can cause a multitude of physical signs.

   (a) *Pulmonary rales* occur over the lung bases from the accumulation of fluid in the pulmonary interstitium and alveloli caused by elevated pulmonary capillary wedge pressures/left atrial pressures. Acute cardiogenic pulmonary edema is commonly characterized by rales with wheezing and frothy, blood-tinged sputum. However, the presence of pulmonary congestion is not accompanied by rales in 80% of patients with systolic heart failure because of chronic perivascular compensation and increased lymphatic drainage.

   (b) *Dullness* over the lung bases can also be a common sign of volume overload from extravasation of fluid into the pleural space.

   (c) *Jugular venous pulse (JVP)*, measured at a 45° angle, can also be a marker of volume overload. The JVP remains the most accurate and commonly used clinical assessment tool to determine increased left-sided filling pressures with a sensitivity of 70% and specificity of 79%.

   (d) *Third heart sound (S3 gallop)* is an early sign of decompensated heart failure and signifies increased left-sided filling pressures in the setting of diminished LV function.

   (e) *Mitral and tricuspid regurgitation murmurs* often accompany decompensated heart failure with ventricular dilatation. However, there is little correlation between intensity of the murmur to the severity of heart failure as severe mitral regurgitation may have a soft murmur.

   (f) *Edema*, although a hallmark sign of heart failure with volume overload, can also be observed in other conditions, such as nephrotic syndrome, hypoproteine-mia, or chronic venous insufficiency. It should be noted that for peripheral edema to occur requires a gain of at least 5 L of extracellular fluid volume in adults.

(g) *Ascites* occurs in the setting of elevated right-sided filling pressures that causes increased pressures in the portal vein circulation.

(h) *Hepatomegaly* is a common finding in patients with chronic right-sided heart failure; however, with acute heart failure, rapid congestion can cause hepatomegaly with a pulsatile liver that is palpable.

These last three physical findings, edema, ascites, and congestive hepatomegaly, are hallmark signs of right-sided heart failure when elevated right-sided heart pressures are transmitted to the hepatic and gastrointestinal venous circulation that results in previously mentioned symptoms of abdominal pain, bloating, anorexia, and nausea.

2. Pulsus alternans is another sign commonly found with heart failure. It is defined as an alteration of one strong and one weak beat without a change in the cycle length during pulse palpation.

3. Signs of peripheral perfusion (i.e. color, warm or cool extremities, capillary refill) can help gauge the stage of heart failure.

4. Vitals signs can also help monitor the progression of heart failure. Low blood pressure, tachycardia, tachypnea, and narrow pulse pressure often signify an advanced stage of heart failure.

5. Cardiac cachexia is often a sign of chronic heart failure because of anorexia and/or increased total metabolism.

Etiology (Table 11.1)

1. Ischemic cardiomyopathy: As mentioned earlier, it is the most common cause of heart failure caused by coronary artery disease with subsequent wall-motion abnormalities

TABLE 11.1 Common causes of heart failure

Coronary artery disease/ischemic cardiomyopathy

Dilated cardiomyopathy

Infectious cardiomyopathy [Chagas' disease, HIV, CMV, coxsackievirus, influenza, adenovirus, echovirus, enterovirus, bacterial or fungal infections]

Inflammatory cardiomyopathy [lymphocytic, eosinophilic, giant-cell myocarditis]

Hypertensive cardiomyopathy

Valvular Disorders

LV hypertrophy [hypertrophic cardiomyopathy, systemic hypertension, LV outflow obstruction (i.e. aortic valvular stenosis, subvalvular stenosis)]

Restrictive cardiomyopathy [endomyocardial fibrosis, Loeffler's endocarditis, amyloidosis, sarcoidosis, radiation carditis, familial/glycogen storage diseases (i.e. hemochromatosis, Gaucher's disease, Hurler's syndrome, Fabry's disease)]

Constrictive pericarditis

High-Output states [intracardiac left-to-right communications (i.e. VSD, ASD, PDA), extracardiac communications (i.e. dialysis fistula, hereditary hemorrhagic telangiectasias, Osler-Weber-Rendu), anemia]

Arrhythmia [supraventricular or ventricular]

Peripartum cardiomyopathy

Endocrine [thyroid disorders, adrenal insufficiency, pheochromocytoma, acromegaly, diabetes mellitus]

Electrolyte deficiency syndromes [hypokalemia, hypomagnesemia]

Nutritional disorders [kwashiorkor, anemia, beri-beri, selenium]

Toxins [alcohol, catecholamines, cocaine, anthracyclines and other chemotherapeutics, irradiation]

Autoimmune [SLE, polyarteritis nodosa, rheumatoid arthritis, scleroderma, dermatomyositis, polymyositis, Celiac disease]

Congenital/Inherited heart conditions [familial dilated cardiomyopathy, left ventricular noncompaction, muscular dystrophies (i.e. Duchenne's, Becker's, myotonic), neuromuscular (i.e. Friedreich's ataxia, Noonan's disease), inborn errors of fatty acid metabolism, Arrhythmogenic right ventricular cardiomyopathy]

Stress-induced cardiomyopathy (Takotsubo cardiomyopathy)

Idiopathic cardiomyopathy

and left ventricular systolic dysfunction. It is important to stress that stenosis of the coronary arteries does not automatically lead to ischemic cardiomyopathy. However, patients with ischemic cardiomyopathy who have viable myocardium do benefit from percutaneous and surgical revascularization, which can halt or even reverse the progression of heart failure.

2. Dilated cardiomyopathy: Among young people, dilated cardiomyopathy is the most common cardiomyopathy accounting for about 25% of cases. More than 50% of all causes of dilated cardiomyopathy are idiopathic, with the remaining causes being infectious, inflammatory, toxic, high-output states, endocrine, nutritional disorders, autoimmune, congenital/inherited heart conditions, peripartum cardiomyopathy, hypertension, arrhythmia, stress-induced, and electrolyte deficiency. Dilated cardiomyopathy occurs with adverse cardiac remodeling which then leads to cardiac hypertrophy, dilation, and systolic dysfunction. Some nonischemic causes of dilated cardiomyopathy are reversible, and it is important to identify them early to establish appropriate treatment.

3. Infectious cardiomyopathy: Most commonly, viral infections, such as HIV, CMV, coxsackievirus A and B, influenza, adenovirus, herpes viruses, poliovirus, enteroviruses, rubella, rubeola, hepatitis B or C virus, EBV, mumps, parvovirus B19, or echovirus are associated with infectious cardiomyopathy. Other causes can be the tick-borne illness, Rocky Mountain spotted fever, by the bacterial organism, *Rickettsia rickettsii*. In addition, fungi, such as aspergillosis, cryptococosis, coccidioidomycosis, and histoplasmosis, can also lead to a cardiomyopathy. The protozoa, *Trypanosoma cruzi*, leads to Chagas' disease, which causes severe ventricular enlargement, often with apical aneurysm, seen with the cardiomyopathy. It is also associated with arrhythmias, thromboembolic stroke, and sudden death. Chagas disease is most commonly seen in Central and South America. Another protozoa that can cause a cardiomyopathy is Toxoplasmosis gondii.

Helminths, such as trichinosis and schistosomiasis, can also result in a cardiomyopathy. Infectious cardiomyopathies can also be a result of bacterial illnesses by Legionella, Clostridium, streptococci, staphylococci, salmonella, and Shigella. Another reported cause of infectious cardiomyopathies is Lyme disease by the spirochete, *Borelia burgdorferi*.

4. Inflammatory cardiomyopathy: This disease is characterized by the inflammatory infiltration of the myocardium, and therefore, is also known as myocarditis with cardiac dysfunction. Common causes of an inflammatory cardiomyopathy can be from an infectious etiology or from hypereosinophilia, cardiotoxic agents, systemic autoimmune diseases, or collagen vascular diseases. Unfortunately, an inflammatory cardiomyopathy caused by a systemic process has a poor prognosis as it often responds unfavorably to medical therapy and cardiac transplantation. Giant cell myocarditis is a rare, but lethal type of inflammatory cardiomyopathy with a 1-year mortality rate of up to 80%, median survival of 3–5 months from onset of symptoms that are consistent with progressive heart failure.

5. Autoimmune: Systemic lupus erythematosus is one of the common autoimmune disorders that can cause heart failure with systolic dysfunction. It is often associated with myocarditis and an inflammatory cardiomyopathy. Another autoimmune disorder, Celiac disease, can also cause an idiopathic dilated cardiomyopathy. Following a gluten-free diet can reverse the cardiomyopathy and improve cardiac function in these patients.

6. Cardiotoxic agents: Common toxins affecting the heart are chemotherapeutic agents, particularly anthracyclines, alcohol, cocaine, and catecholamines. Chemotherapeutic agents cause myocyte destruction that lead to a dilated cardiomyopathy. It is recommended that prior to chemotherapy, patients have a baseline echocardiogram. Radionuclide ventriculography (MUGA scan) provides very accurate measurements of systolic function. It is often considered the preferred imaging modality in

circumstances where precise measurements of systolic function are needed, such as the case with patients undergoing chemotherapy that undergo periodic cardiac evaluation. Alcohol is another common cause of toxin-mediated cardiomyopathy and accounts for approximately 33% of all cases of dilated cardiomyopathy. In early stages, complete abstinence from alcohol may entirely reverse the cardiomyopathy; however, continued use of alcohol can lead to a 5-year mortality of 50%.

7. Valvular disorders: Valve-related systolic heart failure is associated most commonly with mitral regurgitation, aortic regurgitation, and/or severe aortic stenosis and outflow tract obstruction. Mitral and aortic regurgitation lead to heart failure from a constant state of volume overload, whereas severe aortic stenosis and outflow tract obstruction eventually cause LV dysfunction and heart failure.

8. Endocrine disorders: Because thyroid conditions (i.e. hypo- or hyperthyroidism) can commonly occur, patients with new-onset heart failure should have thyroid function testing as heart failure caused by thyroid disorders is potentially reversible. With hypothyroidism, a decreased cardiac output with bradycardia, and in some cases, a pericardial effusion can occur. In contrast, hyperthyroidism often presents with tachycardia or atrial fibrillation and can be accompanied by fatigue and weight loss. Patients on amiodarone are at an increased risk for developing hyperthyroidism. In Cushing's syndrome, the excess cortisol causes a dilated cardiomyopathy, which can also occur in the presence of excess growth hormone, as seen in patients with acromegaly. In patients with pheochromocytoma, the excess adrenergic stimulants cause direct injury to cardiac myocytes that can lead to systolic dysfunction.

9. Stress-induced cardiomyopathy (Takotsubo cardiomyopathy): Also known as "broken heart syndrome," this cardiomyopathy occurs after an acute stress and is also thought to be a result of the excess sympathomimetic amines following an acutely stressful event. Subsequent echocardiogram shows a reversible apical ballooning.

10. Hypertensive cardiomyopathy: Also known as "burnt-out hypertensive heart," it is the final outcome that initially begins with LV hypertrophy until progression to LV dysfunction thought to be from microvascular ischemia. Hypertensive cardiomyopathy can present in conjunction with ischemic cardiomyopathy as hypertension contributes significantly to coronary artery disease development. With appropriate medical treatment, the negative effects of hypertensive cardiomyopathy can be slowed or reversed.

11. Congenital/inherited cardiomyopathy: Familial dilated cardiomyopathy account for approximately 20–30% of all cases of dilated cardiomyopathy. It carries an unfavorable prognosis and is associated with gene mutations. Arrhythmogenic right ventricular dysplasia (ARVD) is defined by fatty infiltration of the right ventricle that can be difficult to diagnose by endomyocardial biopsy given the patchiness of the disease. However, MRI can be helpful in making the diagnosis. ARVD often occurs in young people, predominantly men, and presents with syncope or ventricular arrhythmias. Although, infrequently, it can occur with right-sided heart failure. Another inherited disorder that affects the right ventricle is Uhl's anomaly. Unlike ARVD, however, Uhl's anomaly is often associated with right-sided heart failure. It is caused by death of cardiac myocytes throughout the right ventricle and is characterized by a paper-thin right ventricular wall. It presents in early childhood and often, the only cure is cardiac transplantation. Left ventricular noncompaction is the abnormal interference of normal ventricular development leading to systolic dysfunction, ventricular arrhythmias, and thromboembolism. Muscular dystrophies, such as Duchenne's and Becker's, arise from genetic mutations and are more commonly associated with a dilated cardiomyopathy. In addition, Fabry's disease, an alpha-galactosidase A deficiency, is a rare occurrence that can lead to LV hypertrophy and dysfunction.

Treatment

The treatment goals for acute decompensated heart failure and chronic heart failure differ. We will discuss the precipitants and management of acute decompensated heart failure later. In chronic heart failure management, the main objectives are to improve symptoms, reduce hospitalizations, and prolong survival. The diagram below illustrates the pathophysiology behind chronic systolic heart failure. Our understanding of this model is the basis behind the main medical therapies used in the treatment of chronic heart failure. These agents target different points of the diagram to interfere with this deleterious cycle to reduce symptoms and adverse effects that ultimately lead to death. Table 11.2 summarizes the main clinical trials for each class of agents critical to the management of chronic heart failure. Table 11.3 summarizes the drug dosing of the primary medical therapies in chronic heart failure treatment.

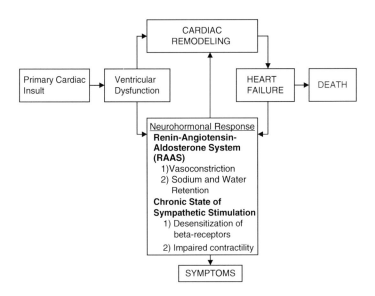

TABLE 11.2 Clinical trials in CHF (grouped by subject)

Trial (year): study design	Purpose	Primary outcome/important points
ACE-I		
CONSENSUS (1987) [8]: Randomized, double-blind, placebo-controlled trial	Study effects of Enalapril on mortality in patients with severe heart failure (NYHA functional class IV)	All cause mortality at 6 months: 26% in Enalapril group vs. 44% in placebo group, $p = 0.002$, RR 0.60. CONSENSUS was the 1st trial to show mortality benefit of ACE-I in CHF. No difference between the two groups in death due to SCD
SOLVD (1991) [41]: Randomized, double-blind, placebo-controlled trial	Evaluate effects of Enalapril on survival in patients with CHF with LVEF ≤35%	All cause mortality: 35.2% in Enalapril group vs. 39.7% in placebo group, $p < 0.0036$, RR 0.82. SOLVD supported results from CONSENSUS and showed mortality benefit of Enalapril in not just NYHA class IV HF but in any class of HF with LVEF <35%
SAVE (1992): Randomized, double-blind, placebo-controlled trial	Study effects of captopril on mortality/ morbidity in patients following an acute MI with LVEF ≤40% without overt heart failure	Mortality from all causes: 20% in captopril group vs. 25% in placebo group, $p = 0.019$, RR 0.81. SAVE was the 1st trial to show a mortality benefit of the addition of an ACE-I to patients following an acute MI with reduced LVEF but no heart failure
ATLAS (2000): Randomized, double-blind trial	Comparison of effects of high-dose lisinopril vs. low-dose lisinopril on mortality and hospitalizations in patients with chronic heart failure NYHA functional class II-IV	Combined endpoint of all-cause mortality and hospitalizations: Risk reduction of 12% seen with the high-dose lis:nopril group vs. low-dose lisinopril, $p = 0.002$

ARBs

Val-HeFT (2001): Randomized, double-blind, placebo-controlled, parallel-group, controlled trial	To evaluate if the addition of valsartan reduces morbidity/mortality in patients with NYHA functional class II-IV heart failure and already on optimal medical therapy (85% on diuretics, 93% on ACE-I, 35% on beta-blockers, 67% on digoxin)	Mortality: 19.7% in valsartan group vs. 19.4% in placebo group, $p = 0.8$, RR 1.02. Combined end point of mortality and morbidity: 28.8% in valsartan group vs. 32.1% in placebo, $p = 0.009$, RR 0.87. Val-HeFT was the first large study to evaluate ARBs in the setting of standard HF therapy. It showed no mortality benefit with the addition of valsartan, and in fact, suggested an increased mortality with the addition of valsartan to beta-blockers and ACE-I. However, Val-HeFT did show a decrease in morbidity with HF
CHARM-Added (2003): Randomized, double-blind, placebo-controlled trial	To evaluate the effects of candesartan added to ACE-I therapy on mortality or heart failure-related hospitalizations in patients with NYHA functional class II-IV HF with LVEF ≤ 40%	Mortality or hospitalization for HF: 37.9% in the candesartan group vs. 42.3% in the placebo group, $p = 0.011$, HR 0.85. CHARM-added also showed a reduction in morbidity with the addition of ARBs to standard therapy. However, unlike Val-HeFT, CHARM-added also demonstrated a reduction in mortality and did not find an increased mortality by adding an ARB to standard therapy of a beta-blocker and ACE-I

(continued)

TABLE 11.2 (Continued)

Trial (year): study design	Purpose	Primary outcome/important points
CHARM-Alternative (2003): Randomized, double-blind, placebo-controlled trial	To evaluate the effects of candesartan on mortality or HF-related hospitalizations in patients with NYHA functional class II-IV HF with LVEF ≤40% and intolerant to ACE-I therapy	Mortality or hospitalization for HF: 33% in candesartan group vs. 40% in placebo group, $p = 0.0004$, HR 0.77. This study demonstrated a 23% relative risk reduction of mortality or hospitalizations with candesartan in patients intolerant to ACE-I
CHARM-Preserved (2003): Randomized, double-blind, placebo-controlled trial	To evaluate the effects of candesartan on mortality or HF-related hospitalizations in patients with NYHA functional class II-IV HF with LVEF >40%	Mortality or hospitalization for HF: 22% in candesartan group vs. 24% in placebo group, $p = 0.118$, HR 0.89. This study was of borderline significance with a possible 11% reduction in the relative risk of mortality or hospitalizations
Aldosterone-antagonists		
RALES (1999): Randomized, double-blind, placebo-controlled trial	To evaluate the effect of spironolactone on morbidity and mortality in patients with severe HF NYHA functional class III-IV and reduced LVEF≤35% already on optimal medical therapy (ACE-I, loop diuretics)	All cause mortality: 35% in spironolactone group vs. 46% in placebo, $p < 0.001$, RR 0.70. RALES was the 1st trial to show a mortality benefit with spironolactone in patients with severe heart failure (NYHA functional class III-IV symptoms) and severely reduced LV systolic function

EPHESUS (2003): Randomized, double-blind, placebo-controlled trial	To evaluate the effect of eplerenone on mortality or cardiovascular-related hospitalizations in patients with reduced LVEF ≤40% with HF symptoms after myocardial infarction and already on optimal medical therapy (87% on ACE-I/ARBs, 75% on beta-blockers)	All cause mortality: 14.4% in eplerenone group vs. 16.7% in placebo group, $p = 0.008$, RR 0.85. Death from cardiovascular causes or first hospitalization for a cardiovascular event: 26.7% in eplerenone group vs. 30% in placebo, $p = 0.002$, RR 0.87
EMPHASIS-HF (2011): Randomized, double-blind, placebo-controlled trial	To evaluate the effects of eplerenone on mortality or CV-related hospitalizations in patients with reduced LVEF ≤35% with NYHA functional class II heart failure and already on optimal medical therapy (95% on ACE-I/ARBs, 86.6% on beta-blockers)	Death from cardiovascular causes or hospitalization for heart failure: 18.3% in eplerenone group vs. 25.9% in placebo group, $p < 0.001$, HR 0.63

(continued)

TABLE 11.2 (Continued)

Trial (year): study design	Purpose	Primary outcome/important points
Beta-blockers		
CIBIS-II (1999): Randomized, double-blind, placebo-controlled trial	To evaluate the effects of bisoprolol on mortality and HF-related hospital admissions in patients with NYHA functional class III-IV symptoms with reduced LVEF≤35% and already on medical treatment (diuretics with ACE-I or vasodilators)	All cause mortality: 11.8% in bisoprolol group vs. 17.3% in placebo group, $p<0.0001$. Estimated annual mortality rate: 8.8% in bisoprolol group vs. 13.2% in placebo, HR 0.66
MERIT-HF (1999) [28]: Randomized, placebo-controlled trial; Blinding during treatment phase not clear	To study effects of metoprolol succinate (CR/XL) on mortality in patients with NYHA functional class II-IV heart failure with reduced LVEF≤40% and already on optimal medical therapy with ACE-I and diuretics	All cause annual mortality rates: 7.2% in metoprolol group and 11% in placebo group, RR 0.66. Yearly risk reduction in mortality of 44%. MERIT-HF trial led to FDA approval of metoprolol succinate in the treatment of heart failure
CAPRICORN (2001): Randomized, double-blind, placebo-controlled trial	To evaluate effects of carvedilol on mortality and morbidity in patients with reduced LVEF≤40% following an acute MI and already on an ACE-I (98%)	All cause mortality or CV hospitalizations: 35% in carvedilol group vs. 37% in placebo group, $p=0.296$, HR 0.92. All cause mortality: 12% in carvedilol group vs. 15% in placebo, $p=0.031$, HR 0.77. CAPRICORN showed a possible 24% reduction in all cause mortality with the use of carvedilol following acute MI with associated LV dysfunction

COPERNICUS (2001): Randomized, double-blind, placebo-controlled trial	To evaluate the effects of carvedilol on mortality in patients with severe heart failure already on diuretics (99%) and ACE-I/ARB (97%); NYHA functional class not specifically addressed in the trial	All cause mortality: 11.2% in the carvedilol group vs. 16.8% in the placebo group, $p = 0.00013$, RR 0.65. COPERNICUS demonstrated a 35% reduction in all cause mortality with the addition of carvedilol

Hydralazine and nitrates

V-HEFT (1986): Randomized, double-blind, parallel-group, placebo-controlled trial	To evaluate the effects of vasodilator therapy (isosorbide dinitrate (ISDN)/hydralazine) on mortality in patients with chronic heart failure	All cause mortality: 38.7% in ISDN/hydralazine group vs. 44% in placebo group, $p = 0.046$. 2-year cumulative mortality: 25.6% in ISDN/hydralazine group vs. 34.3% in placebo, $p < 0.028$, HR 0.66. Although at 2 years there was a possible 34% reduction in mortality, the all-cause mortality improvement with ISDN/hydralazine was of borderline significance. FDA did not approve this combination therapy for the treatment of heart failure
A-HeFT (2004): Randomized, double-blind, placebo-controlled trial	To evaluate the effects of combination ISDN and hydralazine on mortality in African-Americans with NYHA functional class III-IV heart failure already on medical therapy (90% on diuretics, 70% on ACE-I, 17% on ARBs)	All cause mortality: 6.2% in ISDN/hydralazine group vs. 10.2% in placebo group, $p = 0.01$, HR 0.57. First HF hospitalization: 16.4% in ISDN/hydralazine group vs. 24.4% in placebo, $p = 0.001$. A-HeFT trial showed mortality benefit of this drug combination in African American patients with heart failure

(continued)

TABLE 11.2 (Continued)

Trial (year): study design	Purpose	Primary outcome/important points
Digoxin		
DIG [13]: Randomized, double-blind, placebo-controlled trial	To study the effect of digoxin on mortality and morbidity in patients with heart failure with LVEF ≤45%; 94% on ACE-I, 82% on diuretics	All cause mortality: 34.8% in digoxin group vs. 35.1% in placebo group, $p = 0.80$, RR 0.99. HF-related hospitalizations: 26.8% in digoxin group vs. 34.7% in placebo group, $p < 0.001$, RR 0.72. The DIG trial showed no mortality benefit but showed a 28% reduction in HF-related hospitalizations

1. Angiotensin-converting enzyme inhibitors (ACE-I)

The long-term benefits of this class of drugs can be attributed to their effects on the renin-angiotensin-aldosterone system (RAAS). ACE-I function by inhibiting the enzyme that converts angiotensin I to angiotensin II, thereby preventing the negative downstream effects of the neurohormonal RAAS pathway caused by excess angiotensin II, aldosterone, and catecholamines. ACE-I have been shown to reverse the pathologic cardiac remodeling caused by progressive myocardial fibrosis, inflammation, and apoptosis associated with overstimulation of the RAAS pathway. Several randomized trials have established the benefit of ACE-I in patients with chronic LV dysfunction (Table 11.2). Consistently, ACE-I were shown to decrease mortality by approximately 20–25% at 1–5 years. Although low doses of an ACE-I should be used at first, over time, however, the dose should be gradually uptitrated to the optimal dosage used in the management of heart failure (Table 11.3). Because hyperkalemia and acute renal insufficiency can occur with ACE-I, close monitoring with labwork is advised after initiation or increase of an ACE-I. Small increases in creatinine levels (up to 30%) should be tolerated and expected, and the ACE-I should not be discontinued. If the creatinine increases by more than 30%, the ACE-I dose can be halved. However, if the creatinine level increases by more than 100%, the ACE-I should be held at that time. If hyperkalemia occurs, first discontinue any potassium supplementation, and if hyperkalemia continues to persist, then the ACE-I dose can be reduced. Other side effects of ACE-I are hypotension, cough, teratogenicity, and angioedema. For patients that develop a true ACE-inhibitor cough, angiotensin-II receptor blockers (ARBs) are an acceptable alternative. However, for patients who develop angioedema from an ACE-I, it is an absolute contraindication to use any type of ACE-I or ARB. Angioedema can occur within 2 weeks of initiation of an ACE-I or can present months to years after starting the medication.

2. Angiotensin-II receptor blockers (ARBs)

ARBs also work by targeting the RAAS pathway and function by inhibiting the angiotensin II type 1 receptors. ARBs act downstream of angiotensin-converting enzyme

TABLE 11.3 Drug dosing for optimal medical therapy for chronic heart failure

Drug	Start (mg)	Target (mg)	Max (mg)
ACE-inhibitors: titrate to target dose, as tolerated			
Captopril	6.25–12.5 tid	50 tid	100 tid
Enalapril	2.5–5 bid	10 bid	20 bid
Lisinopril	2.5–5 qday	40 qday or 20 bid	40 qday
Ramipril	1.25–2.5 bid	5 bid	10 bid
Quinapril	5 bid	20 bid	20 bid
Fosinopril	2.5 or 5 bid	20 bid	20 bid
Trandolapril	1 qday	4 qday	4 qday
Angiotensin Receptor Blockers (ARBs): titrate to target dose, as tolerated			
Candesartan	16 qday	32 qday	32 qday
Valsartan	80 qday	160 qday	320 qday
Aldosterone antagonists: titrate to target dose, as tolerated			
Spironolactone	12.5–25 qday	25 qday	50 bid
Eplerenone	50 qday	100 qday	100 qday
Beta-blockers: titrate to target dose, as tolerated			
Carvedilol	3.125 bid	25 bid (weight<85 kg) 50 bid (weight≥85 kg)	50 bid
Metoprolol succinate	25 qday	200 qday	200 qday
Bisoprolol	1.25 qday	10 qday	20 qday

TABLE 11.3 (continued)

Drug	Start (mg)	Target (mg)	Max (mg)
Hydralazine/nitrate combination: titrate to target dose, as tolerated			
Hydralazine	25–37.5 tid	75–100 tid	100 tid
Isosorbide dinitrate (Isordil)	10–20 tid	40 tid	40 tid
Isosorbide mononitrate (Imdur)	30 qday	120 qday	120 qday
BiDil (fixed-dose hydralazine-isosorbide dinitrate)	25/37.5 tid	50/75 tid	50/75 tid
Digoxin: reduce dose if low body mass index or renal insufficiency			
Digoxin	0.125–0.25 mg qday	Monitor digoxin levels, best outcomes in patients with levels <1 ng/mL	Not applicable
Diuretics: titrate to euvolemia			
Furosemide	10 qday (IV)	As required	1,000 qday (IV)
	20 qday (po)		240 bid (po)
Torsemide	10 qday	As required	200 qday
Bumetanide	10 qday	As required	10 qday
Metolazone	2.5 qday	As required	10 qday
Hydrochlorothiazide	25 qday	As required	50 qday
Chlorthalidone	12.5–25 qday	As required	100 qday

inhibitors and weaken the effects of angiotensin II. Clinical trials have shown ARBs to be equivalent to ACE-I in the management of heart failure. They remain acceptable alternatives in patients who are ACE-I intolerant, usually to the associated cough. Despite ARBs being better tolerated, they have the same side effect profile as ACE-inhibitors, with the exception of cough, and therefore, should be used and monitored in the same way as ACE-I. Although a logical hypothesis might be that combination therapy with an ACE-inhibitor and an ARB would provide greater inhibition of the RAAS pathway and increased benefit in heart failure patients, data to support this theory have been inconclusive. The CHARM-ADDED trial showed that the addition of an ARB to an ACE-inhibitor reduced heart failure hospitalizations and cardiac mortality by 15% compared to monotherapy with an ACE-I alone. However, in contrast, the VALIANT trial revealed no additional benefit in the use of combination therapy, and in fact, showed increased hypotension and hyperkalemia.

3. Aldosterone antagonists

The third class of therapeutic agents that target the RAAS pathway and provide a significant mortality reduction in patients with heart failure is aldosterone receptor antagonists, such as spironolactone and eplerenone. The benefit of these drugs is derived from the inhibition of aldosterone, an adrenal hormone produced through angiotensin II-dependent and -independent pathways. Aldosterone has been shown to cause fibrosis and adverse remodeling of the myocardium. The most common side effect of aldosterone antagonists is hyperkalemia, which can be exacerbated in patients with renal insufficiency or in those already taking an ACE-inhibitor or ARB. As a result, regular monitoring is required. In patients with creatinine 2.0–2.5 mg/dL or potassium 4.5–5 mg/day, the aldosterone antagonist should be started at a lower dose (12.5 mg/day or 25 mg every other day), and the potassium supplement should be discontinued or held. Aldosterone antagonists should be avoided in patients with a baseline creatinine >2.5 mg/dL or potassium ≥5.0 mEq/L. In addition, although spironolactone may also cause gynecomastia and galactorrhea, these side effects are rarely associated with eplerenone.

4. Beta-blockers

In addition to the RAAS inhibitors, beta-blockers are also essential to the management of chronic heart failure with LV systolic dysfunction through their actions on the neurohormonal axis. In heart failure, the sympathetic nervous system is chronically activated causing sustained stimulation of beta-receptors that eventually leads to a downregulation and desensitization of these beta-receptors to beta-adrenergic agonists. As a result, there is a reduced inotropic and chronotropic response of the myocardium to normal adrenergic stimulation. These effects are reversed with the initiation of beta-blockers as they help to upregulate beta 1-receptors and enhance cardiac contractility. Only carvedilol (Coreg), metoprolol succinate (Toprol XL), and bisoprolol have been approved for the treatment of chronic heart failure. Beta-blockers have consistently been shown to reduce mortality by approximately 25–45%. In general, beta-blockers should not be started in the setting of decompensated heart failure. It is recommended that patients be stable, clinically euvolemic, and already on an ACE-I or ARB prior to starting a beta-blocker. Beta-blockers should be initiated at low doses and slowly up-titrated every 2–4 weeks until goal dosages in the optimal management of heart failure are reached. Beta-blockers have a myriad of side effects, most commonly fatigue and dizziness/lightheadedness related to hypotension. Fatigue typically improves after 1–2 weeks of treatment, and in circumstances of recurrent hypotension, beta-1-selective agents, such as metoprolol succinate, may have lesser blood pressure-lowering effects than carvedilol, which has nonselective, alpha-1-receptor inhibition, as well. Beta-1-selective agents may also be better tolerated in patients with bronchospasm. Other adverse effects are bradycardia and worsening heart failure (i.e. increased fluid retention and congestion), which can occur given the negative inotropic effects of beta-blockers. Dose reduction and slower up-titration of beta-blockers, as well as more aggressive diuresis and salt restriction may be necessary to minimize these effects. Beta-blockers should be avoided in patients with advanced conduction system disease, unless a permanent pacemaker is present.

5. Hydralazine and nitrates

For patients intolerant to ACE-inhibitors or ARBs, combination therapy with hydralazine and nitrates is an acceptable alternative in the management of chronic heart failure as it improves symptoms and reduces mortality (V-HEFT I trial). Furthermore, this vasodilator combination therapy was shown to confer a 43% decrease in mortality in African Americans with advanced heart failure already on optimal medical therapy with an ACE-I/ARB and beta-blocker (A-HEFT trial). Based on these significant results, the combination of hydralazine and nitrates is recommended for the management of chronic heart failure in this population of patients. Side effects of hydralazine are reflex tachycardia and a lupus-like syndrome, whereas nitrates can causes headaches, hypotension, and tolerance after continuous use.

6. Diuretics

Diuretic therapy helps with symptomatic management in chronic heart failure by maintaining euvolemia in patients. Because overuse of diuretics is associated with electrolyte abnormalities and organ dysfunction (i.e. acute renal failure), only the lowest dose of diuretic needed to maintain euvolemia should be used. The loop diuretics furosemide (Lasix), torsemide (Demadex), and bumetanide (Bumex) are the most commonly used. Torsemide and bumetanide are more expensive loop diuretics but have better bioavailability and are more effective in diuretic-resistant patients. The conversion from oral furosemide to torsemide to bumetanide is about 40:20:1. In the case of intravenous-to-oral dose conversions, the intravenous and oral doses for both torsemide and bumetanide are equivalent, whereas the conversion from intravenous-to-oral furosemide is 1:2. If loop diuretics do not adequately prevent volume overload, a thiazide diuretic, such as metolazone (Zaroxolyn) or hydrochlorothiazide, can be added to assist with further diuresis. Thiazide diuretics work by inhibiting the reabsorption of $Na+/Cl-$ in the distal convoluted tubule, thereby allowing for increased diuresis. The effective combination of a loop diuretic with a thiazide can produce substantial volume depletion. As a result, it is recommended to use a thiazide with a loop diuretic for only short-term with close monitoring of electrolytes and renal function.

7. Digoxin

The use of digoxin in the management of chronic heart failure is controversial given its narrow therapeutic index and adverse reactions. As a result, it is often reserved for patients that have heart failure with concomitant atrial fibrillation, or for patients on optimal medical therapy who continue to be frequently hospitalized. The DIG trial showed that although digoxin did not improve mortality, it did decrease heart failure hospitalizations. Digoxin is a cardiac glycoside derived from the foxglove plant that functions as both a positive inotrope and a negative chronotropic agent. It increases intracellular calcium by blocking the Na-K-exchange ion channel, thereby increasing contractility. Digoxin levels < 1 ng/mL are desirable with toxicity occurring at levels greater than 2 ng/mL. As a result, digoxin should be used with caution in patients with renal insufficiency and in the elderly. Adverse events associated with digoxin have included cardiac arrhythmias (bidirectional VT, atrial tachycardia with AV block, atrial fibrillation with regular ventricular response), gastrointestinal symptoms, and neurological manifestations (i.e. visual changes/blurriness, dizziness, confusion, hallucinations). Hypokalemia and hypomagnesemia can exacerbate these negative effects, as well as lower the threshold for digoxin toxicity.

8. Other therapies in chronic heart failure with systolic dysfunction

(a) Cardiac resynchronization therapy (CRT): Up to one-third of patients with heart failure develop ventricular dyssynchrony (defined electrically as a QRS duration >120 ms, particularly those with a left bundle branch block morphology), which is associated with reduced cardiac efficiency. The benefits of biventricular pacemakers on mortality and morbidity in this subgroup of patients were evaluated in the COMPANION and CARE-HF trials. In these large, randomized studies,

CRT was associated with a definitive mortality bene-fit, as well as a reduction in hospitalizations in com-parison to patients receiving optimal medical therapy alone. The more recent MADIT-CRT trial also dem-onstrated a reduction in mortality and/or heart failure events in patients with heart failure. Biventricular pacemakers can consist of a right atrial lead with a right ventricular lead +/– ICD and epicardial left ven-tricular lead (placed through the coronary sinus). This allows biventricular pacemakers to resynchronize LV contraction and improve cardiac function. Based on data from the COMPANION and CARE-HF trials, CRT can be considered in chronic heart failure patients with dyssynchrony (QRS $\geq$ 120 ms), LVEF $\leq$ 35%, and NYHA functional class III-IV symp-toms despite being on optimal medical management. MADIT-CRT trial showed benefit of CRT in patients with LVEF $\leq$ 30%, QRS $\geq$ 130 ms, NYHA functional class I-II HF symptoms, and were in sinus rhythm.

(b) Implantable Cardiac Defibrillators (ICD): ICD implantation is frequently used in patients with chronic heart failure with systolic dysfunction for the primary prevention of sudden cardiac death from ventricular arrhythmias. The MADIT and MADIT-II trials dem-onstrated a survival benefit of ICD implantation in patients with ischemic cardiomyopathy with LVEF $\leq$ 30%. Results from the subsequent SCD-HEFT trial further showed a survival benefit of ICD in patients with nonischemic cardiomyopathy with LVEF $\leq$ 35%, as well. However, because patients with nonischemic cardiomyopathy often respond favorably to optimal medical therapy with LVEF improvement, at least a 3-month trial of optimal medical therapy (at least an ACE-I/ARB and beta blocker) in these patients must be attempted with LVEF remaining depressed despite medical management before ICD can be implanted. In addition, because the DINAMIT trial showed no mortality benefit for ICDs implanted within 40 days after an acute myocardial infarction, these patients with ischemic cardiomyopathy must wait at least 40 days before ICD implantation. Although the mortality benefit associated with ICD implantation has been established, in certain patients, ICD therapy may not be ideal given its huge cost and multiple risks. For example, in patients that are of an advanced age or have significant, life-shortening comorbidities, the survival benefit that ICD implantation can confer on these patients is reduced. Also, the risks associated with ICD implantation include inappropriate shocks, device infection, generator-site hematoma, cardiac rupture, and pneumothorax.

Heart Failure with Preserved Left Ventricular Ejection Fraction (Diastolic Heart Failure)

Heart failure with preserved ejection fraction (HFpEF) represents the other category of chronic heart failure. In fact, studies have shown that approximately one-half of patients with heart failure have a preserved ejection fraction. More commonly, HFpEF occurs in women and patients >65 years of age. Although it was initially thought that patients with HFpEF had improved survival outcomes, the mortality rates are actually similar in both types of heart failure.

HFpEF can be characterized by (1) normal or mildly abnormal systolic LV function (2) signs or symptoms of congestive heart failure and (3) evidence of diastolic dysfunction. HFpEF arises when myocardial relaxation or distensibility is disturbed leading to high cardiac filling pressures that are needed to maintain appropriate cardiac output. Common disorders that affect the viscoelastic properties or compliance of the LV are hypertension, LV hypertrophy, diabetes, obesity, and coronary artery disease. Other causes may be infiltrative processes (amyloid, sarcoid, hemochromatosis), hypertrophic cardiomyopathy, high output cardiac disorders (arteriovenous malformation, arteriovenous fistula, hyperthyroidism, anemia), and constrictive disease processes. Conditions such as atrial fibrillation and chronic renal insufficiency often can exacerbate diastolic heart failure.

Chief Complaint/Symptoms

The symptoms associated with HFpEF are identical to those of systolic heart failure that were previously mentioned. Oftentimes, a patient with preserved systolic function who is compensated will remain asymptomatic. However, dyspnea is typically the earliest symptom to occur.

Signs/Physical Examination

There are no specific clinical signs to distinguish systolic from diastolic heart failure. However, in general, heart failure patients with preserved systolic function more commonly present with acute or "flash" pulmonary edema with hypertension. On the contrary, patients with HFpEF can also have a slow and steady fluid accumulation presentation. In addition, when HFpEF occurs in the setting of constriction or restriction, these patients may present mainly with signs of right-sided heart failure, such as edema, ascites, abdominal distension, congestive hepatomegaly, and a positive hepatojugular reflex. Other signs that can be associated with pericardial constriction are Kussmaul's sign, which is paradoxical elevation of jugular venous pressure on inspiration, and Friedrich's sign, which is a "flickering" noted in the jugular venous pressure that represents a rapid "y" descent/short "y" duration.

Etiology

1. LV Hypertrophy (LVH): Systemic hypertension, hypertrophic cardiomyopathy, or LV outflow obstruction can cause

LV hypertrophy. The increased wall thickness associated with LVH reduces passive filling. Subendocardial ischemia can also be found with LVH and can interfere with active myocyte relaxation.

2. Coronary Artery Disease (CAD): As just mentioned, active myocyte relaxation can be diminished by ischemia, either acute or chronic. Chronic ischemia, scar tissue from a prior myocardial infarction, or pathologic remodeling of the myocardium lead to reduced LV compliance and impaired passive filling. In addition, ischemia can cause tachyarrhythmias, such as atrial fibrillation, that decrease diastolic filling time.

3. Restrictive cardiomyopathy: Myocardial and endomyocardial restrictive diseases can be categorized as being either infiltrative or noninfiltrative or can be classified as primary or secondary. Most myocardial infiltrative diseases are considered secondary restrictive cardiomyopathies, whereas myocardial noninfiltrative and endomyocardial diseases are primary restrictive cardiomyopathies. These diseases cause the heart to become rigid and resistant to ventricular filling during diastole.

(a) Myocardial infiltrative diseases/Secondary restrictive cardiomyopathies

(i) Amyloidosis: In amyloid heart disease, interstitial deposits (amyloid deposits/insoluble amyloid fibrils) replace normal cardiac myofilaments, thereby affecting myocardial contractility. The major types of amyloidosis are primary, secondary, familial, or senile. Primary amyloid is associated with multiple myeloma and is caused by overproduction of light-chain immunoglobulins from a monoclonal population of plasma cells. Secondary amyloid is typically associated with inflammatory conditions, such as rheumatoid arthritis, Crohn's disease, and tuberculosis. Lastly, familial and senile amyloidosis leads to overproduction of transthyretin. Endomyocardial biopsy is the gold standard for diagnosing amyloid heart disease (Congo red stain of amyloid deposits on histology). However, cardiac MRI has become an increasingly popular imaging modality used to detect cardiac amyloidosis. On cardiac MRI, a distinct pattern of late gadolinium enhancement along the subendocardium and myocardium is noted in cases of cardiac amyloid disease. Cardiac MRI for the diagnosis of cardiac amyloidosis yields a sensitivity of 80%, specificity of 94%, positive predictive value of 92%, and negative predictive value of 85%. Echocardiography can also be used in the diagnosis of cardiac amyloid. Typical echocardiographic findings associated with cardiac amyloidosis include a granular, sparkling appearance of thickened ventricular walls and significant biatrial enlargement. Patients with amyloid may have no evidence of LVH on EKG despite the presence of LVH on echocardiogram. The extent of wall thickness determines survival; in patients with increased wall thickness, the average survival is <6 months. Overall, however, cardiac amyloidosis has a poor prognosis as patients with a normal wall thickness have only an average survival of 2.4 years. Cardiac transplantation is contraindicated in patients with systemic amyloidosis.

(ii) Sarcoidosis: Infiltration of noncaseating graulomas with patchy scar formation in the heart characterizes sarcoidosis with cardiac involvement. In all patients with cardiac sarcoidosis, while it is clinically recognized in only 5% of patients, at autopsy, cardiac involvement is seen in 25% of patients. Myocardial restriction occurs as a result of the patchy scar formation, and the sarcoid granulomas cause conduction system disease that can result in sudden cardiac death from ventricular tachyarrhythmias or high-degree heart block. As a result, pacemaker placement is recommended in patients with cardiac sarcoidosis and conduction system disease, and ICD placement is recommended in the subset of patients with a history of VT. Because of the patchy nature of the disease, endomyocardial biopsy has a sensitivity of only 20–30% in the diagnosis of cardiac sarcoidosis. The presence of giant cells and noncaseating granulomas on biopsy confirms cardiac sarcoidosis. Echocardiography is not sensitive in the detection of cardiac sarcoid. In contrast, cardiac MRI is a highly sensitive method that can detect early cardiac sarcoid and can be used serially to monitor treatment response. Cardiac transplantation as a treatment for cardiac sarcoidosis is a possibility in certain patients.

(iii) Hemochromatosis: Primary hemochromatosis occurs from an autosomal recessive genetic abnormality that causes increased absorption of iron from the gastrointestinal tract, whereas secondary hemochromatosis is a result of iron overload from repeated blood transfusions. In both instances, the presence of excessive iron leads to iron deposition in the myocardium causing a restrictive cardiomyopathy. Treatment of hemochromatosis often is phlebotomy and chelation therapy.

(iv) Glycogen storage diseases: Gaucher's, Hurler's, and Fabry's diseases are the most common of these genetically transmitted diseases. Cardiac involvement is often characterized by LV wall thickness.

(b) Myocardial Noninfiltrative Disease/Primary Restrictive Cardiomyopathy

(i) Idiopathic restrictive cardiomyopathy: This condition can be inherited in an autosomal dominant pattern or can occur sporadically. It is associated with patchy endocardial fibrosis that is difficult to diagnose with endomyocardial biopsy. This interstitial fibrosis can result in variable hypertrophy that can be seen, along with biatrial enlargement and near-normal LV dimensions, on echocardiography. Mean survival time is 9 years. Cardiac transplantation is a treatment option for some patients.

(c) Endomyocardial   Diseases/Primary   Restrictive Cardiomyopathies

(i) Hypereosinophilic syndrome (Loeffler's endocarditis): As the name suggests, this restrictive cardiac disease occurs in the setting of eosinophilia where activated eosinophils release their cytoplasmic granular content that causes toxic damage and destruction to the endomyocardium. Subsequent endocardial thickening and obliteration of the cardiac apex occurs as a result. Another associated complication that can occur is a mural thrombus. As a result, anticoagulation, as well as corticosteroids, cytotoxic drugs, and typical heart failure medications are commonly used in treatment.

(ii) Carcinoid heart disease: The elevated concentration of serotonin and 5-hydroxyindoleacetic acid associated with untreated carcinoid syndrome leads to formation of lesions, typically in the right ventricular endocardium. These vasoactive substances can also affect the right-sided heart valves (carcinoid valvular disease).

4. Pericardial   constriction   (constrictive   pericarditis): Constrictive pericarditis is a result of chronic inflammation that causes the pericardium to become thickened by fibrosis, scarring, and/or calcification. Consequently, the pericardial space is obliterated in the process and diastolic function is adversely affected, as a result. The loss of pericardial compliance interferes with normal cardiac filling by placing a constraint on the heart. As the ventricles begin filling at the start of diastole, this external volume constraint causes pressures to rapidly increase causing ventricular filling to prematurely stop. An equalization of

pressures in all four cardiac chambers is typically seen with pericardial constriction. Common causes are mantle chest radiation, open-heart surgery, idiopathic or viral pericarditis, collagen vascular disease, end-stage renal disease/hemodialysis, malignancy, and tuberculosis. It is important to note that postcardiotomy and chest irradiation can result in pericardial constriction or restrictive cardiomyopathy. To help distinguish between constriction and restriction, echocardiography and right- and left- heart catheterizations are used. Findings on two-dimensional echocardiography with Doppler suggestive of constriction are septal bounce (rapid early diastolic filling); thickened, echogenic pericardium; and adherent pericardium to the myocardium

Treatment

Unlike in patients with systolic dysfunction, to date, there have been no large, randomized clinical trials of therapies that demonstrate a mortality benefit in patients with HFpEF. For example, the CHARM-preserved trial suggested candesartan therapy had a 15% relative risk reduction in hospitalizations; however, there was not a mortality benefit. As a result, there are no clear guidelines to direct optimal medical management in this group of heart failure patients. Therapy, therefore, is instead geared towards relief of symptoms, such as volume overload, and treatment of causative factors, such as hypertension, atrial fibrillation, and coronary artery disease.

For instance, diuretics should be used to control signs and symptoms of volume overload, such as pulmonary congestion and peripheral edema. Simultaneously, strict restriction on fluid and sodium intake should be implemented to further prevent volume overload.

In addition, in those patients with atrial fibrillation, rapid ventricular rates are poorly tolerated by further impedance of diastolic filling. Medications such as beta-blockers and calcium channel blockers are helpful in reducing the heart rate, thereby allowing improved diastolic filling. Interestingly, there is little data to support the hypothesis that the conversion of atrial fibrillation to sinus rhythm improves outcomes in patients with HFpEF even though atrial fibrillation often leads to decompensation in patients with diastolic dysfunction.

In the large subset of patients with HFpEF and coexisting hypertension, systolic and diastolic blood pressures should be treated aggressively according to the Joint National Committee (JNC) 7 guidelines. Treatment of hypertension has been shown to diminish cardiac hypertrophy, improve ventricular relaxation and distensibility, and subsequently improve diastolic filling.

In those patients with coronary artery disease causing chronic ischemia and associated diastolic dysfunction, coronary revascularization can be considered, along with lipid-lowering agents, antiplatelet therapy, and beta-blockade.

Contrary to most patients with diastolic dysfunction who face a dismal prognosis, patients with diastolic dysfunction caused by constrictive pericarditis can be treated with pericardiectomy. Unfortunately, despite similarities in presentation, patients with restrictive cardiomyopathies do not have a curative treatment and fall into the general category of patients with HFpEF where medical therapies provide only symptomatic relief and can only slow down the progression of disease.

Acute Decompensated Heart Failure

There are several precipitants that can exacerbate chronic heart failure, either with systolic dysfunction or preserved ejection fraction, and cause an acute decompensated state (Table 11.4).

Treatment should first be geared towards identifying and potentially reversing any underlying cause. The medical therapies used in the acute setting are with the goal of improving symptoms associated with respiratory and circulatory compromise. Hemodynamic monitoring should be considered as treatments are optimized for organ perfusion and normalization of cardiac filling pressures and function.

TABLE 11.4 Common causes of acute decompensated heart failure

Myocardial ischemia

Acute myocarditis

Infection/sepsis

Acute valvular disease

Hypertension (malignant, emergency, crisis)

Arrhythmia (atrial fibrillation)

Substance abuse/toxins

Noncompliance (dietary/sodium, medication)

Acute pulmonary embolism (acute right heart failure)

Treatment

1. Oxygenation
   In acute decompensated heart failure, oxygen saturation should be maintained at least ≥90%. Positive airway ventilation and/or intubation may be necessary to achieve this goal.
2. Vasodilators
   Acute decompensated heart failure in the setting of elevated blood pressures often presents with acute or "flash" pulmonary edema caused by increased vascular resistance and poor diastolic filling from diminished left ventricular relaxation. Vasodilators, such as nitroglycerin, are first-line drug therapy in these instances but should not be used in patients in cardiogenic shock.
3. Diuretics
   Diuretics provide not only a vasodilatory effect but can reduce intravascular volume, which oftentimes helps to relieve the acute presentation of pulmonary edema in decompensated states. With diuretic therapy, 66% of patients have improved symptoms by 24 h and 80% of patients by 3 days or at time of discharge. Diuretics are commonly administered intravenously with close monitoring of electrolytes, net fluid balance, and daily weights. In cases with associated renal insufficiency, ultrafiltration can be used as an alternative to pharmacologic diuresis to assist with fluid removal in volume overloaded states.

4. Inotropes

Acute decompensated heart failure with hemodynamic compromise may warrant the need for inotropic therapy to improve tissue perfusion. Both intravenous dobutamine and milrinone can accomplish this through their ability to increase cardiac output. However, results from trials, such as the OPTIME-CHF and ADHERE trials, do not support the routine use of inotropes because mortality and morbidity are not reduced and there is actually an increase in adverse events. Persistent hypotension, myocardial ischemia, and cardiac arrhythmias have been noted. In some cases, vasopressors, such as norepinephrine, dopamine, and vasopressin are temporarily used to treat the associated hypotension with inotropic use.

5. Mechanical Support

Intra-aortic balloon pumps (IABP) can be used in patients with cardiogenic shock to provide temporary hemodynamic stability. An IABP helps to reduce afterload, augment cardiac output, and decease myocardial oxygen requirement. Other devices that can be used in the setting of acute cardiogenic shock are percutaneous ventricular assist devices and left ventricular assist devices (LVAD), which will be addressed later in this chapter.

Classification of Heart Failure

There are three main classification systems in the assessment of heart failure: New York Heart Association (NYHA) functional classification, American College of Cardiology and American Heart Association (ACC/AHA) staging system, and the Killip classification. The NYHA functional classification system is the most commonly used method to describe signs and symptoms of heart failure (Table 11.5).

The ACC/AHA staging system describes heart failure as a progression of disease (Table 11.6).

The Killip classification system is often employed in patients after acute coronary syndromes or can be helpful in describing patients with heart failure who require placement of a pulmonary artery catheter (Table 11.7).

TABLE 11.5 New York Heart Association functional classification

Class I	+Cardiac disease; no limitation/symptoms with physical activity
Class II	+Cardiac disease; slight limitation/symptoms with moderate exertion/physical activity; comfortable at rest
Class III	+Cardiac disease; marked limitation/symptoms with minimal exertion/physical activity; comfortable at rest
Class IV	+Cardiac disease; inability to perform physical activity; symptoms at rest

TABLE 11.6 ACC/AHA staging system

Stage A	No structural heart disease; high risk for developing heart failure
Stage B	+Structural heart disease; no symptoms of heart failure
Stage C	+Structural heart disease; +prior or current symptoms of heart failure amenable to therapy
Stage D	End-stage heart failure requiring advanced treatment (i.e. ventricular assist device, transplantation, or palliative care)

TABLE 11.7 Killip classification

Class I	Warm and dry; PCWP < 18 mmHg, CI > 2.2 L/min/m^2
Class II	Warm and wet; PCWP > 18 mmHg, CI > 2.2 L/min/m^2
Class III	Cold and dry; PCWP < 18 mmHg, CI < 2.2 L/min/m^2
Class IV	Cold and wet; PCWP > 18 mmHg, CI < 2.2 L/min/m^2

These three classification models provide an accurate assessment of patients with heart failure and are another standard used by health care providers to reliably estimate prognosis and mortality rate. For example, a patient classified as NYHA functional class IV has a 1-year survival rate of between 30% and 50%.

Prognosis

There are several predictors that can be utilized to accurately assess survival in patients with heart failure. The Seattle Heart Failure Model is a risk-prediction tool that incorporates these factors, some of which are NYHA class, age, LV ejection fraction, and cardiac dyssynchrony, and provides the ability to calculate survival probability in a patient with heart failure.

Diagnostic Testing

We have discussed the clinical presentations and etiologies of both chronic and acute heart failure. This section will focus on accurately establishing the diagnosis of heart failure upon initial evaluation of a patient with presenting symptoms (as described earlier in this chapter) suggestive of heart failure. The algorithm below is a reasonable, stepwise approach towards making the diagnosis of new-onset heart failure.

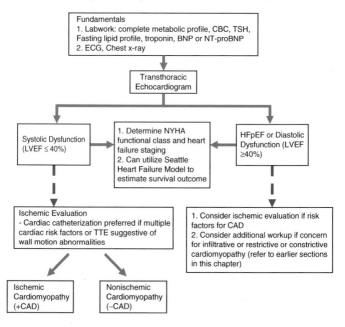

The initial evaluation should begin with obtaining basic laboratory values, that includes complete blood count, comprehensive metabolic profile, thyroid function tests, fasting lipid profile, troponin level, and in some instances, a B-type natriuretic peptide level. A BNP or NT-proBNP level can be helpful in making the diagnosis of heart failure, however, keeping in mind multiple variables (i.e. age, gender, BMI, renal function, medical therapy) can influence and confound the interpretation. Regardless, BNP or NT-proBNP levels are useful in ruling out heart failure as it has a negative predictive value of up to 90% when the level is <300 pg/mL.

An electrocardiogram and chest x-ray should also be attained to evaluate for ischemia, infarct, or arrhythmias, as well as for pulmonary edema, cardiomegaly, or other factors that could be causing dyspnea. Afterwards, if necessary, a transthoracic echocardiogram can be considered to assess LV systolic and diastolic function, chamber enlargement, wall thickness, valvular abnormalities, or pericardial effusion/tamponade. From this point, focus can then be directed towards determining the etiology of the heart failure to look for reversible causes.

Special Topics in Heart Failure

Advanced treatment with mechanical assist devices and/or cardiac transplantation can be considered in patients with end-stage heart failure. We will briefly focus on left ventricular assist devices (LVADs) and cardiac transplantation.

Left Ventricular Assist Devices (LVADs)

LVADs are circulatory support devices that extract oxygenated blood from either the left atrium or left ventricle and directs flow of the blood through a pulsatile or continuous-flow generator that then directs flow of blood out of the aorta. LVADs can be short-term or used as long-term devices as bridge to transplant, bridge to recovery, or destination therapy. For LVADs being used for destination therapy, the REMATCH trial showed a 48% relative risk reduction of mortality in patients with end-stage heart failure not eligible for cardiac transplant that received LVAD (pulsatile HeartMate XVE) compared to the group treated medically. When LVADs are used as a bridge to transplant, 70–80% of patients with an LVAD are successfully bridged to transplantation, compared to only 36% of patients on inotropic therapy. Currently, based on results from the HeartMate II trial, the smaller and more efficient, continuous-flow LVADs are being used more commonly than the pulsatile devices as they were shown to have a 2-year survival of 58% compared to 24% in the pulsatile flow group.

Cardiac Transplantation

Heart transplantation remains the gold standard for treatment of end-stage heart failure; however, the number of available organs is limited. Survival rates after heart transplantation are 85% at 1 year, 70% at 5 years, and 50% at 10 years, respectively. Malignancy and coronary artery vasculopathy are some of the complications associated with transplant that limit survival.

The United Network for Organ Sharing (UNOS), a national, nonprofit organization, along with local organ procurement organizations (OPO), allocate organs for transplantation in the United States, maintain organ transplantation waiting lists, and evaluate potential organ donors. Screening and evaluation for transplant consideration is extensive. Some absolute contraindications to transplant are irreversible pulmonary hypertension and systemic illness that will limit survival. Once a patient is accepted as a potential candidate for cardiac transplantation by a UNOS-certified transplant program, the potential recipient is given a status level on the UNOS list based on specified criteria. Status 1A is given the highest priority.

Suggested Reading

1. Abraham WT, Adams KF, Fonarow GC, et al. In-hospital mortality in patients with acute decompensated heart failure requiring intravenous vasoactive medications: an analysis from the Acute Decompensated Heart Failure National Registry (ADHERE). J Am Coll Cardiol. 2005;46:57–64.

2. Bardy GH, Lee KL, Mark DB, et al. Amiodarone or an implantable cardioverter-defibrillator for congestive heart failure. N Engl J Med. 2005;352:225–37.

3. Bristow MR, Saxon LA, Boehmer J, et al. Cardiac-resynchronization therapy with or without an implantable defibrillator in advanced chronic heart failure. N Engl J Med. 2004;350(21):2140–50.

4. CIBIS-II Investigators. The cardiac insufficiency bisoprolol study II (CIBIS-II): a randomized trial. Lancet. 1999;353:9–13.

5. Cleland JGF, Daubert JC, Erdmann E, et al. The effect of cardiac resynchronization on morbidity and mortality in heart failure. N Engl J Med. 2005;352:1539–49.

6. Cohn JN, Archibald DG, Ziesche S, et al. Effect of vasodilator therapy on mortality in chronic congestive heart failure. Results of a veterans administration cooperative study. N Engl J Med. 1986; 314(24):1547–52.

7. Cohn JN, Tognoni G. Valsartan heart failure trial investigators. A randomized trial of the angiotensin-receptor blocker valsartan in chronic heart failure. N Engl J Med. 2001;345:1667–75.

8. CONSENSUS Trial Study Group. Effects of enalapril on mortality in severe congestive heart failure results of the Cooperative North Scandinavian Enalapril Survival Study (CONSENSUS). N Engl J Med. 1987;316(23):1429–35.

9. Crow S, John R, Boyle A, et al. Gastrointestinal bleeding rates in recipients of nonpulsatile and pulsatile left ventricular assist devices. J Thorac Cardiovasc Surg. 2009;137:208–15.

10. Cuculich PS, Kates AM, editors. Cardiology subspecialty consult, vol. 2. Philadelphia: Wolters Kluwer/Lippincott Williams and Wilkins; 2009. p. 19–23, 112–161.

11. Cuff MS, Califf RM, Adams KF, et al. Short-term intravenous milrinone for acute exacerbation of chronic heart failure. JAMA. 2002; 287(12):1541–7.

12. Dargie HJ et al. Effect of carvedilol on outcome after myocardial infarction in patients with left-ventricular dysfunction: the CAPRICORN randomized trial. Lancet. 2001;357:1385–90.

13. Digitalis Investigation Group. The effect of digoxin on mortality and morbidity in patients with heart failure. N Engl J Med. 1997;336(8): 525–33.

14. Felker GM, Benza RL, Chandler AB, et al. Heart failure etiology and response to milrinone in decompensated heart failure: results from the OPTIME-CHF study. J Am Coll Cardiol. 2003;41:997–1003.

15. Goldhaber JI, Hamilton MA. Role of inotropic agents in the treatment of heart failure. Circulation. 2010;121:1655–60.

16. Granger CB, McMurray JJ, Yusuf S, et al. Effects of candesartan in patients with chronic heart failure and reduced left-ventricular systolic function intolerant to angiotensin-converting-enzyme inhibitors: the CHARM-Alternative trial. Lancet. 2003;362:772–6.

17. Griffin BP, Topol EJ, editors. Manual of cardiovascular medicine. 3rd ed. Philadelphia: Wolters Kluwer/Lippincott Williams and Wilkins; 2009. p. 105–90.

18. He J, Ogden LG, Bazzano LA, et al. Risk factors for congestive heart failure in US men and women: NHANES I epidemiologic follow-up study. Arch Intern Med. 2001;161(7):996–1002.

19. Ho KK, Anderson KM, Kannel WB, et al. Survival after the onset of congestive heart failure in Framingham Heart Study subjects. Circulation. 1993;88(1):107–15.

20. Hohnloser S, Kuck KH, Dorian P, et al. Prophylactic use of an implantable cardioverter-defibrillator after acute myocardial infarction. N Engl J Med. 2004;351:2481–8.

21. Hunt S, Abraham WT, Chin MH, et al. ACC/AHA 2005 Guideline Update for the diagnosis and management of chronic heart failure in the adult: a Report of the American College of Cardiology/American Heart Association Task Force on Practice Guidelines. Circulation. 2005;112:154–235.

22. Januzzi Jr JL, Camargo CA, Anwaruddin S, et al. The N-terminal pro-BNP investigation of dyspnea in the emergency department (PRIDE) study. Am J Cardiol. 2005;95(8):948–54.

23. Levy WC, Mozaffarian D, Linker DT, et al. The seattle heart failure model: prediction of survival in heart failure. Circulation. 2006;113:1424–33.

24. Libby P, Bonow RO, editors. Braunwald's heart disease: a textbook of cardiovascular medicine. 8th ed. Philadelphia: WB Saunders; 2008. p. 509–727.

25. Lindenfeld J, Mann DL, et al. Executive summary: HFSA 2010 comprehensive heart failure practice guideline. J Card Fail. 2010;16(6):475–539.

26. McKee PA, Castelli WP, McNamara PM, et al. The natural history of congestive heart failure: the Framingham study. N Engl J Med. 1971;285(26):1441–5.

27. McMurray JJ, Ostergren J, Swedberg K, et al. Effects of candesartan in patients with chronic heart failure and reduced left-ventricular systolic function taking angiotensin-converting-enzyme inhibitors: the CHARM-Added Trial. Lancet. 2003;362:767–71.

28. MERIT-HF Study Group. Effect of metoprolol CR/XL in chronic heart failure: Metoprolol CR/XL Randomized Intervention Trial in Congestive Heart Failure (MERIT-HF). Lancet. 1999;353:2001–7.

29. Moss AJ, Hall WJ, Cannom DS, et al. Cardiac-resynchronization therapy for the prevention of heart-failure events. N Engl J Med. 2009;361(14):1329–38.

30. Moss AJ, Hall WJ, Cannom DS, For the Multicenter Automatic Defibrillator Implantation Trial Investigators. Improved survival with an implanted defibrillator in patients with coronary disease at high risk for ventricular arrhythmia. N Engl J Med. 1996;335(26): 1933–40.

31. Moss AJ, Zareba W, Hall WJ, et al. Prophylactic implantation of a defibrillator in patients with myocardial infarction and reduced ejection fraction. N Engl J Med. 2002;346(12):877–83.

32. Nohria A, Mielniczuk LD, Stevenson LW. Evaluation and monitoring of patients with acute heart failure syndromes. Am J Cardiol. 2005;96(6):32–40.

33. Packer M, Coats AJ, Fowler MB, et al. Effect of carvedilol on survival in severe chronic heart failure. N Engl J Med. 2001;344: 1651–8.

34. Pfeffer MA, Braunwald E, Moye LA, et al. Effect of captopril on mortality and morbidity in patients with left ventricular dysfunction after myocardial infarction. N Engl J Med. 1992;327(10):669–77.

35. Pitt B, Remme W, Zannad F, et al. Eplerenone, a selective aldosterone blocker, in patients with left ventricular dysfunction after myocardial infarction. N Engl J Med. 2003;348(14):1309–21.

36. Pitt B, Zannad F, Remme WJ. The effect of spironolactone on morbidity and mortality in patients with severe heart failure. Randomized Aldactone Evaluation Study Investigators. N Engl J Med. 1999; 341(10):709–17.

37. Rose EA, Gelijns AC, et al. Long-term mechanical left ventricular assistance for end-stage heart failure. N Engl J Med. 2001;345(20):1435–43.

38. Ryden L, Armstrong PW, Cleland JGF, et al. Efficacy and safety of high-dose lisinopril in chronic heart failure patients at high cardiovascular risk, including those with diabetes mellitus. Eur Heart J. 2000;21(23):1967–78.

39. Slaughter MS. Hematologic effects of continuous flow left ventricular assist devices. J Cardiovasc Transl Res. 2010;3(6):618–24. Epub 2010 Sep 11.

40. Slaughter MS, Rogers JG, Milano CA, et al. Advanced heart failure treated with continuous-flow left ventricular assist device. N Engl J Med. 2009;361:1–11.

41. SOLVD Investigators. Effect if enalapril on survival in patients with reduced left ventricular ejection fractions and congestive heart failure. N Engl J Med. 1991;325(5):293–302.

42. Steinhart B, Thorpe KE, Ahmed BM, et al. Improving the diagnosis of acute heart failure using a validated prediction model. J Am Coll Cardiol. 2009;54(16):1515–21.
43. Taylor AL, Ziesche S, Yancy C, et al. African-American heart failure trial investigators. Combination of isosorbide dinitrate and hydralazine in blacks with heart failure. N Engl J Med. 2004;351(20): 2049–57.
44. Young JB, Abraham WT, Stevenson LW, For the VMAC Study Group. Results of the VMAC trial: vasodilation in the management of acute congestive heart failure. Circulation. 2000;102:2794.
45. Yusuf S, Pfeffer MA, Swedberg K, et al. Effects of candesartan in patients with chronic heart failure and preserved left-ventricular ejection fraction: the CHARM-Preserved Trial. Lancet. 2003;362: 777–81.
46. Zannad F, McMuray JV, Krum H, et al. Eplerenone in patients with systolic heart failure and mild symptoms. N Engl J Med. 2011;364: 11–21.

Chapter 12
Vascular Diseases – Peripheral/Aorta

Craig R. Narins, Jason D. Pacos, and Theodore I. Hirokawa

Lower Extremity Peripheral Arterial Disease

Prevalence and Implications

Peripheral arterial disease (PAD) is a common yet vastly underdiagnosed condition that is associated with substantial morbidity and mortality. Because atherosclerosis is a systemic disease, the presence of PAD, whether symptomatic or not, is associated with a two- to fourfold increase in the risk of myocardial infarction, stroke and cardiovascular death [1–3]. More timely diagnosis of PAD in the primary care setting has the potential not only to improve quality of life by helping to alleviate the lifestyle-impairing symptoms often associated with

C.R. Narins (✉)
Department of Cardiology and Vascular Surgery,
University of Rochester School of Medicine,
Rochester, NY, USA
e-mail: craig_narins@urmc.rochester.edu

J.D. Pacos
Department of Cardiology, University of Rochester Medical Center,
Rochester, NY, USA

T.I. Hirokawa
Department of Surgery, Highland Hospital,
Rochester, NY, USA

J.D. Bisognano et al. (eds.), *Manual of Outpatient Cardiology*, 325
DOI 10.1007/978-0-85729-944-4_12,
© Springer-Verlag London Limited 2012

the disease, but also to identify individuals at high risk for cardiac and cerebrovascular events providing the opportunity to initiate effective life-saving therapies at an earlier stage [4]. In the large PARTNERS initiative, patients from 350 medical practices throughout the United States who had risk factors for atherosclerosis underwent screening, and PAD was detected among 29% of individuals [5]. In less than half of cases was the patient's primary physician previously aware of the presence of PAD, and 55% of those with PAD already had manifestations of cardiovascular disease affecting other organ systems.

Symptoms

Lower extremity PAD is associated with a wide potential spectrum of symptoms, ranging from asymptomatic disease to limb-threatening ischemia (Fig. 12.1). Obstructive PAD can be detected while still asymptomatic by the use of non-invasive tests such as the ankle-brachial index (ABI), which is discussed in detail below. Intermittent claudication represents the symptom classically associated with lower extremity PAD and is described as a cramping or burning sensation in the lower extremities that occurs predictably with ambulation and is relieved by rest [6]. Generalized weakness or fatigue of the affected extremity during ambulation is also

Lower Extremity PAD
Spectrum of Disease

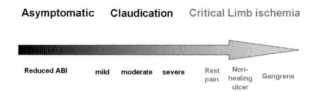

FIGURE 12.1 Spectrum of symptoms associated with lower extremity PAD

frequently described. The location of discomfort in the lower extremities usually correlates with the site of disease in the arterial system. Obstruction of more proximal vessels (the abdominal aorta or iliac arteries) generally produces claudication symptoms of the hip, buttock, and thigh muscles, while disease involving more distal vessels such as the femoral and popliteal arteries typically manifests as claudication of the calf muscles. It is important to recognize that PAD often presents with atypical or unusual symptoms, which can make diagnosis more difficult [7]. For example, in the PARTNERS study, only 11% of patients with PAD described classic claudication symptoms.

The severity of claudication can be measured subjectively by standardized questionnaires assessing functional status and quality of life, or objectively by a treadmill walking test that measures the distances a patient is able to walk prior to the onset of pain ("initial claudication distance") and the distance before the pain intensity forces them to stop ("absolute claudication distance") [8]. Patients with milder degrees of claudication often maintain the ability to walk long distances with only mild discomfort, while more severely affected individuals may be able to take only a few steps before needing to stop and rest. Therapy to alleviate symptoms is usually initiated when the symptoms become "lifestyle-limiting," which represents a subjective threshold that varies substantially from individual-to-individual. For example, an active patient may be greatly frustrated by claudication symptoms that occur only when engaged in strenuous exercise, whereas a more sedentary individual with substantial comorbidities may not be impaired by claudication that occurs after walking only a short distance. Symptoms of intermittent claudication often progress slowly or remain stable for many years even without therapy.

The presence of critical limb ischemia (CLI) constitutes an emergency in which the degree of arterial perfusion becomes inadequate to maintain tissue integrity, and the risk of limb loss is substantial [9]. Manifestations of CLI include ischemic lower extremity pain at rest, non-healing ulceration or infection involving the distal extremities, or the presence of frank gangrene.

Patients with diabetes mellitus are especially predisposed to CLI and resultant limb loss. When CLI is present or suspected, urgent referral to a vascular specialist is essential.

Differential Diagnosis

A variety of disease processes other than PAD can result in lower extremity discomfort with ambulation. Musculoskeletal conditions, such as lumbar spinal stenosis or degenerative joint disease of the lower back, hips or knees can produce pain with walking. Neuropathic conditions also should be considered [10].

An all too common scenario in clinical practice is for patients with PAD to be misdiagnosed and mistreated for a suspected musculoskeletal etiology for their symptoms. Many vascular specialists have unfortunately encountered patients who have undergone orthopedic procedures for symptoms that were in fact related to vascular insufficiency that could have been detected by a proper pulse exam.

Physical Exam

The primary components of the vascular exam include inspection of the extremities and palpation/auscultation of the peripheral pulses. Cutaneous changes including thinning of the skin, loss of hair, and foot discoloration are sometimes noted with lower extremity arterial insufficiency, however these findings have poor sensitivity and specificity for PAD [11]. Careful examination of ankles and feet including the inter-digital spaces for evidence of skin breakdown or ulceration is essential for patients with known or suspected PAD. Regular examination of the feet is especially important among individuals with diabetes, who are not only at much greater risk for infection resulting in limb loss, but often have sensory neuropathy that impairs their ability to sense the pain that may accompany early skin breakdown [12].

The focus of a proper vascular exam is careful palpation of the upper and lower extremity pulses. The brachial, radial, ulnar, femoral, popliteal, dorsalis pedis and posterior tibial pulses should be assessed bilaterally for intensity and equality. Absence or relative reduction in pulse intensity indicates the presence and location of obstructive disease. The lower extremity vascular exam should also include palpation of the abdominal aorta and iliac arteries for aneurysm, and auscultation over the aorta and femoral arteries for bruits suggestive of stenosis.

Diagnostic Testing

Ankle-Brachial Index

The ABI is a quick and accurate test that can be performed in any office or medical setting. The test is essentially an extension of the physical exam, and provides such powerful diagnostic and prognostic information that all practitioners should feel comfortable with its performance and interpretation. The ABI is the ratio of the blood pressure at the ankle to the brachial artery blood pressure, which in healthy individuals are equivalent. In the presence obstructive lower extremity PAD, the blood pressure at the ankle of the affected extremity will be reduced relative to that of the brachial artery, resulting in a decreased ABI (Fig. 12.2).

To measure the ABI, a blood pressure cuff and a handheld Doppler device are used [13]. With the patient resting in the supine position, the cuff is paced on the upper arm and the position of brachial artery is located with the Doppler probe. The cuff is inflated to occlude the artery, and then deflated until the Doppler signal returns, marking the brachial systolic pressure. The process is repeated on the contralateral arm, and the higher of the two brachial artery pressures (right or left) is used for the ABI calculation. The cuff is then placed around the lower calf on each lower extremity and the above process is repeated using the Doppler probe to determine the

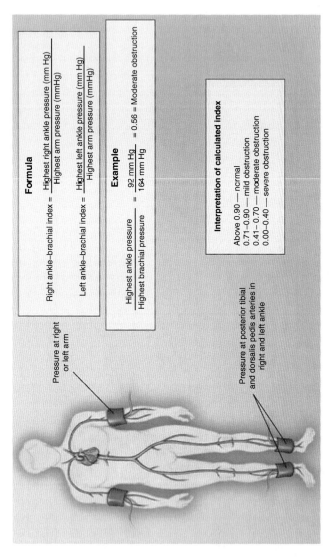

Formula

Right ankle–brachial index = $\dfrac{\text{Highest right ankle pressure (mm Hg)}}{\text{Highest arm pressure (mmHg)}}$

Left ankle–brachial index = $\dfrac{\text{Highest left ankle pressure (mm Hg)}}{\text{Highest arm pressure (mmHg)}}$

Example

$\dfrac{\text{Highest ankle pressure}}{\text{Highest brachial pressure}} = \dfrac{92 \text{ mm Hg}}{164 \text{ mm Hg}} = 0.56 = \text{Moderate obstruction}$

Interpretation of calculated index

Above 0.90 — normal
0.71–0.90 — mild obstruction
0.41–0.70 — moderate obstruction
0.00–0.40 — severe obstruction

Pressure at right or left arm

Pressure at posterior tibial and dorsalis pedis arteries in right and left ankle

FIGURE 12.2 Performance and interpretation of the ABI (Adapted from White [6] with permission)

dorsalis pedis and posterior tibial artery systolic pressures. The ABI is calculated for each lower extremity individually by dividing the highest systolic pressure (dorsalis pedis or posterior tibial) measured on that limb by the highest brachial artery pressure.

Traditionally, an ABI between 0.9 and 1.3 has been considered normal. An ABI < 0.9 is indicative of obstructive PAD, and progressively lower ABI values usually correspond to greater disease severity. ABI values of > 1.3 are considered non-diagnostic, and result from the presence of heavy calcification of the distal lower extremity arteries that renders the vessels "non-compressible" during inflation of the blood pressure cuff. Measurement of the toe-brachial index (TBI), which requires specialized equipment and therefore referral to a vascular laboratory, can be helpful in better assessing patients with an ABI > 1.3 for the presence of obstructive PAD [14]. Among individuals with clinical symptoms suggestive of intermittent claudication who have a normal ABI at rest, repeating the ABI immediately following exercise is often useful [15]. The patient is asked to walk until their typical lower extremity symptoms occur, and the ABI is checked. This frequently unmasks the presence of a stenosis, as the blood pressure distal to the obstruction often is unable to rise to the same degree as that of the proximal vessels during exercise, resulting in a drop in the ABI.

Imaging Studies

The presence of intermittent claudication and a reduced ABI are typically sufficient to confirm the presence of symptomatic PAD. Detailed imaging studies including duplex ultrasonography, computerized tomographic or magnetic resonance angiography (CTA or MRA), or invasive angiography can be used in instances when the diagnosis remains uncertain, and can help to more precisely determine the extent and location of disease when surgical or percutaneous revascularization is being contemplated.

Therapy

There are two distinct goals of therapy once the diagnosis of PAD is made: (1) prevention of cardiovascular events, and; (2) treatment of the local symptoms of PAD.

Prevention of Cardiovascular Events

Because the vast majority of individuals with PAD ultimately die from a cardiac event or stroke, patients with PAD, even if asymptomatic, should undergo aggressive lifestyle modification and medical therapy aimed at preventing such events. Simply performing a revascularization procedure to treat a patient's claudication symptoms without also addressing their risk for future cardiovascular events is a shortsighted approach that constitutes a major disservice to the patient [16].

An individual with PAD carries the same risk for future cardiac events as a patient who has already suffered a myocardial infarction (MI). Angiographic studies have demonstrated that up to 80% of individuals with PAD have concomitant coronary artery disease. The presence of PAD, therefore, should be viewed as a coronary artery disease equivalent, and all patients with PAD should be treated with the same secondary prevention strategies used to treat patients following a MI (Table 12.1) [17]. Such measures include smoking cessation, hypertension control with a target of <140/90 (or <130/80 if diabetes or renal insufficiency are present), and lipid-lowering therapy, preferably with HMG-CoA reductase inhibitor therapy to achieve a goal LDL-cholesterol level of <70 mg/dL [18–20]. While conflicting efficacy data exists, current ACC/AHA Guidelines recommend aspirin therapy for all individuals with documented PAD [21–23]. ACE inhibitor therapy appears especially beneficial among individuals with PAD. Among the >4,000 patients with PAD who were enrolled in the HOPE trial of ramipril versus placebo, ramipril therapy was associated with a significant 35% relative reduction in the incidence of MI, stroke, or cardiovascular death during follow-up [24, 25]. Beta-blocker therapy, once thought to be

TABLE 12.1 ACC/AHA recommendations for the diagnosis and management of PAD

History and exam

1. Ask at risk patients about walking impairment, claudication, ischemic rest pain, and the presence of non-healing wounds.

2. Perform comprehensive pulse examination and/or measurement of the ABI and inspection of the feet in at risk patients.

General approach to patients with asymptomatic PAD

1. Anti-platelet therapy

2. Lipid lowering therapy (preferably using statin with goal LDL < 70 mg/dL)

3. Hypertension treatment per current national guidelines

4. Diabetes treatment per current national guidelines

5. Smoking cessation

General approach to patients with intermittent claudication

1. All of the above measures for asymptomatic PAD should be initiated

2. Full vascular physical examination, including measurement of the ABI

3. The ABI should be measured after exercise if the resting ABI is normal.

4. Consider revascularization ONLY if significant functional impairment AND a reasonable likelihood of symptomatic improvement are present should revascularization be performed.

5. Prior to revascularization, patients should:

   (a) Receive information regarding exercise therapy and pharmacotherapy

   (b) Receive comprehensive risk factor modification and antiplatelet therapy

   (c) Have lesion anatomy favoring low procedural risk and a high probability of initial and long-term success.

---

contraindicated among patients with PAD given the potential for unopposed alpha-receptor stimulation and peripheral vasoconstriction, is not only safe but also appears beneficial for the prevention of cardiovascular events among individuals with PAD [26, 27].

Unfortunately, appropriate preventative therapies remain woefully underutilized among individuals with PAD. In the PARTNERS study of outpatients with PAD, for example, only 43% of patients with PAD were receiving anti-platelet therapy, 50% were being treated with lipid-lowering therapy, and only 52% of smokers had received smoking cessation counseling [5].

Treatment of PAD Symptoms

For patients with lifestyle-limiting claudication, a variety of treatment options exist. Exercise therapy has the potential to provide substantial symptomatic benefits [28]. In order to be effective, exercise therapy must occur in a supervised setting and be performed on a consistent basis at least 3 times per week for a minimum duration of 12 weeks. The patient walks to their absolute claudication distance, recovers, and then repeats the process for 30–45 min. The mechanism by which exercise therapy is effective is not clearly defined, but it is postulated that exercise may stimulate collateral vessel formation or alter individual pain thresholds. While exercise therapy can provide similar or even superior functional benefits compared to medical therapy or revascularization, insurance coverage for this effective treatment remains inconsistent.

At present, cilostazol (Pletal®) represents the only effective FDA approved medical treatment for claudication in the United States [29]. Cilostazol is a phosphodiesterase III inhibitor that is administered at a dose of 100 mg twice a day. The medication has several physiological effects including anti-platelet and vasodilator properties; however its mechanism of action in alleviating the symptoms of claudication remains unknown. Because other phosphodiesterase III inhibitors have been associated with increased mortality among patients with advanced heart failure, cilostazol is contraindicated in the setting of congestive heart failure of any severity. Among patients with claudication, cilostazol has been associated with relative increases in maximum walking distance of 40–60%, however in clinical practice the drug's effectiveness is unpredictable and highly variable, and some patients obtain minimal or no benefit.

Revascularization therapy, performed using endovascular (usually angioplasty and/or stenting) or surgical techniques, represents another effective approach for treating properly selected patients lifestyle-limiting claudication. In general, endovascular therapy is associated with the most durable results when used for shorter length lesions in larger caliber more proximal vessels such as the iliac arteries, although experience, equipment, techniques, and results all continue to improve steadily [30].

Acute Arterial Insufficiency

Sudden loss of perfusion to one of the lower extremities is an emergency situation that is classically heralded by the "five Ps" on history and exam (pain, pallor, pulselessness, parasthesias and paralysis affecting the affected extremity). Acute peripheral arterial occlusion is usually a result of a cardioembolic event, often related to atrial fibrillation. Prompt recognition of the clinical symptoms with immediate referral to a vascular specialist for revascularization is critical for limb salvage. Revascularization is performed either via open surgical embolectomy or by using endovascular techniques including local catheter-directed infusion of thrombolytic agents directly into the clot, often coupled with aspiration of thrombus.

Renovascular Disease

Diagnosis

Renal artery stenosis (RAS) is a relatively uncommon finding among individuals with hypertension, with a prevalence of 5% [31]. Because hypertension is a very common condition and because the effectiveness of renal artery revascularization remains unclear, widespread screening for RAS among individuals with hypertension is not recommended. Even so, evaluation for RAS remains worthwhile in certain higher-risk settings, including refractory hypertension despite multiple antihypertensive medications, presentation with a hypertensive crisis, "flash" pulmonary edema in the setting of normal left ventricular function (especially if hypertension or azotemia are also present), renal insufficiency in patients with known coronary or PAD, or when acute renal failure develops after initiation of ACE inhibitor therapy.

While over 90% of cases RAS are attributable to atherosclerotic disease, fibromuscular dysplasia (FMD) is another potential etiology. FMD is an idiopathic process affecting the arterial wall that can result in RAS, and classically presents as difficult-to-control hypertension in younger to middle aged women [32].

When RAS is suspected, duplex ultrasound, CTA, or MRA represent the preferred diagnostic tests. The accuracy of renal ultrasonography for detecting RAS is highly operator dependent. CTA and MRA generally have better sensitivity and specificity than ultrasound for the detection of RAS, however both carry risks related to contrast exposure among individuals with renal insufficiency. Neither captopril renal scintigraphy nor selective renal vein renin assessment, once considered cornerstones in the diagnosis of RAS, are currently recommended because of their poor specificity and sensitivity [17]. Invasive renal angiography remains the gold standard for the diagnosis of renal artery stenosis, and should be considered if non-invasive imaging studies are non-diagnostic or equivocal.

Renal Artery Stenting

With current techniques, renal artery stenting is associated with technical success rates approaching 100%. Uncertainty remains, however, as to which subset of patients with RAS are likely to benefit from stenting. Older retrospective studies suggested that about 70% of patients with hypertension who underwent RAS had improved blood pressure control following the procedure, and approximately 70% of patients who underwent RAS in the setting of renal insufficiency had improvement or stabilization of renal function following stenting. The more recent ASTRAL trial results, however, have called the efficacy of renal stenting into question [33]. In ASTRAL, 806 patients with hypertension and/or renal insufficiency were randomized to renal stenting plus medical therapy versus medical therapy alone. After 27 months, there were no significant differences between the treatment groups with respect to blood pressure control, renal function, incidence of vascular events, or mortality. The design of the trial has been widely criticized for including a large number of lower risk patients, which may have resulted in underestimation of the potential benefits of stenting [34]. For example, 40% of patients who underwent stenting in ASTRAL did not in fact have severe RAS (defined as a stenosis severity of >70%), and the mean diastolic blood pressure among all enrolled subjects was only 76 mmHg at enrollment.

Given the uncertain benefits of renal stenting at present, use of this therapy is currently restricted to higher risk individuals. Renal artery stenting remains indicated for individuals presenting with sudden-onset pulmonary edema in the setting of hypertension and normal left ventricular function. Also, renal revascularization is appropriate for patients with refractory hypertension in the setting of FMD. Balloon angioplasty (usually without the need for stent placement) is highly effective in this setting. Renal stenting should also be considered for patients with progressive renal insufficiency and severe bilateral RAS. Among patients with RAS and severe truly refractory hypertension despite maximal doses of multiple antihypertensive medications, stenting also should be considered.

Subclavian Artery Stenosis

The subclavian artery supplies the upper extremity, vertebral artery, and internal mammary artery, hence potential symptoms related to a proximal stenosis of the subclavian artery include upper extremity claudication, vertebrobasilar insufficiency related to "subclavian steal," and angina related to myocardial ischemia in instances when the internal mammary artery has been used as coronary bypass graft [17].

Subclavian artery stenosis or occlusion is frequently asymptomatic, as spontaneous development of collateral circulation is often sufficient to meet the metabolic demands of the upper extremity. Atherosclerotic disease is responsible for subclavian stenosis in most instances, although large vessel vasculitis can periodically affect the subclavian arteries. Interestingly, Subclavian stenosis far more commonly involves the left (rather than the right) subclavian artery.

Subclavian stenosis should be suspected if a discrepancy between pulse intensity or blood pressure is detected between the upper extremities, and the diagnosis can be confirmed if necessary by ultrasound, CTA, or MRA. For patients with symptoms of lifestyle-limiting upper extremity claudication, subclavian steal syndrome, or myocardial ischemia related to internal mammary graft insufficiency, stent implantation is the treatment of choice and is associated with high technical and clinical success rates [35]. If stent placement is unfeasible or unsuccessful, carotid-to-subclavian artery bypass represents a more invasive but highly effective alternate means of revascularization.

Diseases of the Aorta

Abdominal Aortic Aneurysm (AAA)

AAA is typically a manifestation of atherosclerotic disease of the aorta, and is defined as enlargement of the abdominal aorta to greater 3 cm in diameter [36]. Among the strongest risk factors for aortic aneurysm are male gender, advanced age, tobacco use, and history of AAA in a 1st degree relative. Among one high-risk population of white male US veterans who smoked and were between 50 and 79 years of age, the prevalence of AAA was 5.9%.

Aneurysm rupture is associated with mortality rates of up to 90%, thus early detection of AAA is of paramount importance. Unfortunately, because aortic aneurysms typically remain asymptomatic until the time of rupture, early diagnosis is typically difficult. The sensitivity and specificity of the physical exam for early detection of AAA are poor even in experienced hands, and aneurysms are most often discovered as an incidental finding during imaging studies performed for other indications. Given the occult nature of aneurysms coupled with the dire consequences of rupture, screening for AAA is recommended for high-risk individuals. In the US, Medicare will reimburse for a single ultrasound exam to screen for AAA among: (1) men aged 65–75 who have smoked >100 cigarettes in their life, or (2) individuals with a family history of AAA in a 1st degree relative.

When an AAA is detected early, surveillance with serial abdominal ultrasound or CTA studies is recommended every 6–12 months to monitor aneurysm growth. While variable, aneurysms from 3.0 to 5.5 cm in size typically grow at a rate of 0.2–0.3 cm per year, and larger aneurysms tend to grow more rapidly. Natural history studies have demonstrated a low likelihood of rupture (1% per year) for aneurysms < 5.0 cm in diameter (Figs. 12.3 and 12.4). Because the risks associated with aneurysm repair typically exceed the likelihood of spontaneous rupture for smaller aneurysms, current guidelines caution against repairing an asymptomatic AAA smaller than 5 cm in diameter. If symptoms or findings suggestive of rupture are present, emergent repair is indicated regardless of aneurysm size [37–39].

When aneurysm diameter reaches a threshold of 5.5 cm, the likelihood of rupture increases rapidly and repair is indicated. Open surgical aneurysm repair is typically curative but is associated with substantial morbidity, as well as overall mortality rates in the 5% range. Endovascular aneurysm repair (EVAR) provides a less invasive approach with lower procedural complications than open repair, and is feasible for a substantial proportion of patients with AAA contingent upon individual anatomical constraints. Among properly selected patients, EVAR is associated with good immediate and long-term success rates [40].

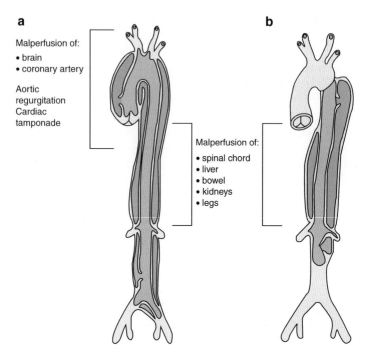

a

Malperfusion of:
- brain
- coronary artery

Aortic
regurgitation
Cardiac
tamponade

b

Malperfusion of:
- spinal chord
- liver
- bowel
- kidneys
- legs

FIGURE 12.3 Normal aorta

Thoracic Aortic Aneurysm (TAA)

The thoracic aorta extends from the aortic valve to the diaphragm, and can be subdivided into four segments: the aortic root, the ascending aorta, the aortic arch, and the descending thoracic aorta. The normal diameter of the aorta tapers from approximately 3.5 cm at the aortic root to approximately 2.5 cm at the level of the diaphragm. A variety of pathological processes can lead to dilation of the thoracic aorta, including aortic valve disease, atherosclerosis, medial degeneration of the vascular wall, vasculitis or inflammatory conditions such as giant cell arteritis, Takayasu arteritis, or ankylosing spondylitis, congenital conditions such as Marfan or Ehlers Danlos Syndrome, or infectious disorders.

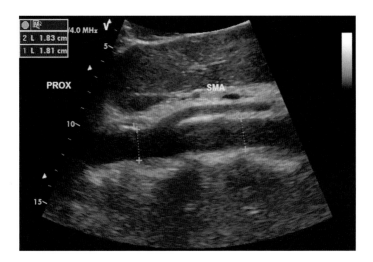

FIGURE 12.4 Small AAA with mural thrombus

As with AAA, dilation of the thoracic aorta is usually asymptomatic, and TAA is often discovered incidentally. Screening for TAA via CTA or MRA is recommended for the high-risk groups listed in Table 12.2. For patients with Marfan syndrome, an echocardiogram is recommended at the time of diagnosis and every 6 months thereafter to determine the aortic root and ascending aortic diameters. Imaging frequency can be reduced to annually if stability of the aortic diameter is subsequently documented [38].

Once the diagnosis of TAA is established, Beta-blocker therapy is recommended for all patients to reduce wall stress. Blood pressure management to meet or exceed JNC-7 guidelines is also recommended (favoring therapy with an angiotensin converting enzyme inhibitor or angiotensin receptor blocker), as is statin therapy with a goal LDL < 70 mg/dL and smoking cessation. Serial imaging to monitor aneurysm size is performed every 6–12 months, and surgical or endovascular aneurysm repair is indicated when any of the thresholds outlined in Table 12.2 are met.

TABLE 12.2 ACC/AHA recommendations for screening for and treatment of Thoracic Aortic Aneurysm

Indications to perform screening for TAA

1. Family history of TAA in a first degree relative

2. Bicuspid aortic valve,

3. Takayasu or giant cell arteritis.

4. Marfan syndrome, or other congenital syndrome associated with TAA (e.g. Loeys-Dietz Syndrome, Turner Syndrome)

Indications for Thoracic Aortic Aneurysm repair

1. Aneurysm diameter ≥ 5.5 cm

2. Rate of aneurysm growth > 0.5 cm/year (even if the absolute diameter remains < 5.5 cm)

3. Thoracoabdominal aneurysm > 6.0 cm (aneurysm extending from thoracic to abdominal aorta)

4. Aneurysm diameter > 4.0–5.0 cm in an individual with Marfan syndrome or other genetic disorder predisposing to TAA

5. Patient requiring aortic valve surgery with an aortic diameter > 4.5 cm

6. Symptomatic TAA of any size

Aortic Dissection

An aortic dissection is a partial thickness tear of the aorta, and occurs when layers of the aortic wall become disrupted and separate from each other [41]. Dissection typically results in the sudden onset of chest or back pain that is often described as "tearing" in nature, and is often overlooked as a potential etiology for acute chest pain. According to the Stanford classification system, a type A aortic dissection involves the ascending thoracic aorta and usually requires urgent surgical repair because of a high risk of rupture if left unrepaired, and a type B dissection is confined to the aortic arch and/or descending aorta and usually can be managed

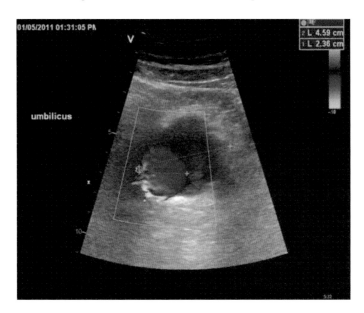

FIGURE 12.5 Stanford Type A (**a**) and Type B (**b**) aortic dissection and their potential associated complications (Adapted from Golledge and Eagle [41] with permission)

medically (Fig. 12.5). CTA, MRA, or transeophageal echo are all well-established non-invasive modalities for confirming the presence of dissection.

The initial management of acute dissection is aimed at reducing aortic wall stress through rapid control of blood pressure and heart rate using intravenous beta-blocker therapy, supplemented with other agents as necessary. Surgical consultation should be obtained once the diagnosis of aortic dissection is made, regardless of its location. Treatment of dissection involving the ascending aorta requires urgent open surgical repair. Acute dissection involving the descending aorta should be managed medically unless life-threatening complications develop, such as organ malperfusion, progression of dissection, enlarging aneurysm, or inability to control blood pressure or other symptoms.

References

1. Ankle Brachial Index C. Ankle brachial index combined with Framingham risk score to predict cardiovascular events and mortality: a meta-analysis. JAMA. 2008;300(2):197–208.
2. Golomb BA, Dang TT, Criqui MH. Peripheral arterial disease: morbidity and mortality implications. Circulation. 2006;114(7):688–99.
3. Diehm C, Allenberg JR, Pittrow D, Mahn M, Tepohl G, Haberl RL, et al. Mortality and vascular morbidity in older adults with asymptomatic versus symptomatic peripheral artery disease. Circulation. 2009;120(21):2053–61.
4. Perlstein TS, Creager MA, Perlstein TS, Creager MA. The ankle-brachial index as a biomarker of cardiovascular risk: it's not just about the legs. Circulation. 2009;120(21):2033–5.
5. Hirsch AT, Criqui MH, Treat-Jacobson D, Regensteiner JG, Creager MA, Olin JW, et al. Peripheral arterial disease detection, awareness, and treatment in primary care. JAMA. 2001;286(11):1317–24.
6. White C. Intermittent claudication. N Engl J Med. 2007;356(12): 1241–50.
7. McDermott MM, Greenland P, Liu K, Guralnik JM, Criqui MH, Dolan NC, et al. Leg symptoms in peripheral arterial disease: associated clinical characteristics and functional impairment. JAMA. 2001;286(13):1599–606.
8. Hiatt WR, Hirsch AT, Regensteiner JG, Brass EP. Clinical trials for claudication. Assessment of exercise performance, functional status, and clinical end points. Circulation. 1995;92(3):614–21.
9. Varu VN, Hogg ME, Kibbe MR. Critical limb ischemia. J Vasc Surg. 2010;51(1):230–41.
10. Norgren L, Hiatt WR, Dormandy JA, Nehler MR, Harris KA, Fowkes FG. Inter-society consensus for the management of peripheral arterial disease (TASC II). J Vasc Surg. 2007;45(Suppl S):S5–67.
11. McGee SR, Boyko EJ. Physical examination and chronic lower-extremity ischemia: a critical review. Arch Intern Med. 1998;158(12):1357–64.
12. Cheer K, Shearman C, Jude EB. Managing complications of the diabetic foot. BMJ. 2009;339:1304–7.
13. Grenon SM, Gagnon J, Hsiang Y, Grenon SM, Gagnon J, Hsiang Y. Video in clinical medicine. Ankle-brachial index for assessment of peripheral arterial disease. N Engl J Med. 2009;361(19):e40.
14. Brooks B, Dean R, Patel S, Wu B, Molyneaux L, Yue DK. TBI or not TBI: that is the question. Is it better to measure toe pressure than ankle pressure in diabetic patients? Diabet Med. 2001;18(7): 528–32.
15. Stein R, Hriljac I, Halperin JL, Gustavson SM, Teodorescu V, Olin JW. Limitation of the resting ankle-brachial index in symptomatic patients with peripheral arterial disease. Vasc Med. 2006;11(1):29–33.

16. Mukherjee D, Lingam P, Chetcuti S, Grossman PM, Moscucci M, Luciano AE, et al. Missed opportunities to treat atherosclerosis in patients undergoing peripheral vascular interventions: insights from the University of Michigan Peripheral Vascular Disease Quality Improvement Initiative (PVD-QI2). Circulation. 2002;106(15):1909–12.

17. Hirsch AT, Haskal ZJ, Hertzer NR, Bakal CW, Creager MA, Halperin JL, et al. ACC/AHA 2005 practice guidelines for the management of patients with peripheral arterial disease. Circulation. 2006;113(11):e463–654.

18. Chobanian AV, Bakris GL, Black HR, Cushman WC, Green LA, Izzo Jr JL, et al. The seventh report of the Joint National Committee on prevention, detection, evaluation, and treatment of high blood pressure: the JNC 7 report. JAMA. 2003;289(19):2560–72.

19. Mehler PS, Coll JR, Estacio R, Esler A, Schrier RW, Hiatt WR. Intensive blood pressure control reduces the risk of cardiovascular events in patients with peripheral arterial disease and type 2 diabetes. Circulation. 2003;107(5):753–6.

20. Heart Protection Study Collaborative G. Randomized trial of the effects of cholesterol-lowering with simvastatin on peripheral vascular and other major vascular outcomes in 20,536 people with peripheral arterial disease and other high-risk conditions. J Vasc Surg. 2007;45(4):645–54.

21. Berger JS, Krantz MJ, Kittelson JM, Hiatt WR. Aspirin for the prevention of cardiovascular events in patients with peripheral artery disease: a meta-analysis of randomized trials. JAMA. 2009;301(18):1909–19.

22. Clagett GP, Sobel M, Jackson MR, Lip GY, Tangelder M, Verhaeghe R. Antithrombotic therapy in peripheral arterial occlusive disease: the seventh ACCP conference on antithrombotic and thrombolytic therapy. Chest. 2004;126(3 Suppl):609S–26.

23. McDermott MM, Criqui MH. Aspirin and secondary prevention in peripheral artery disease: a perspective for the early 21st century. JAMA. 2009;301(18):1927–8.

24. Ostergren J, Sleight P, Dagenais G, Danisa K, Bosch J, Qilong Y, et al. Impact of ramipril in patients with evidence of clinical or subclinical peripheral arterial disease. Eur Heart J. 2004;25(1):17–24.

25. Yusuf S, Sleight P, Pogue J, Bosch J, Davies R, Dagenais G. Effects of an angiotensin-converting-enzyme inhibitor, ramipril, on cardiovascular events in high-risk patients. N Engl J Med. 2000;342(3):145–53.

26. Radack K, Deck C. Beta-adrenergic blocker therapy does not worsen intermittent claudication in subjects with peripheral arterial disease. A meta-analysis of randomized controlled trials. Arch Intern Med. 1991;151(9):1769–76.

27. Narins CR, Zareba W, Moss AJ, Marder VJ, Ridker PM, Krone RJ, et al. Relationship between intermittent claudication, inflammation, thrombosis, and recurrent cardiac events among survivors of myocardial infarction. Arch Intern Med. 2004;164(4):440–6.

28. McDermott MM, Ades P, Guralnik JM, Dyer A, Ferrucci L, Liu K, et al. Treadmill exercise and resistance training in patients with peripheral arterial disease with and without intermittent claudication: a randomized controlled trial. JAMA. 2009;301(2):165–74.

29. Chi YW, Lavie CJ, Milani RV, White CJ. Safety and efficacy of cilostazol in the management of intermittent claudication. Vasc Health Risk Manag. 2008;4(6):1197–203.

30. Mahmud E, Cavendish JJ, Salami A. Current treatment of peripheral arterial disease: role of percutaneous interventional therapies. J Am Coll Cardiol. 2007;50(6):473–90.

31. Dworkin LD, Cooper CJ. Renal-artery stenosis. N Engl J Med. 2009;361(20):1972–8.

32. Olin JW, Pierce M. Contemporary management of fibromuscular dysplasia. Curr Opin Cardiol. 2008;23(6):527–36.

33. ASTRAL Investigators. Revascularization versus medical therapy for renal-artery stenosis. N Engl J Med. 2009;361(20):1953–62.

34. George JC, White CJ. Renal artery stenting: lessons from ASTRAL (Angioplasty and Stenting for Renal Artery Lesions). JACC Cardiovasc Interv. 2010;3(7):786–7.

35. Sixt S, Rastan A, Schwarzwalder U, Burgelin K, Noory E, Schwarz T, et al. Results after balloon angioplasty or stenting of atherosclerotic subclavian artery obstruction. Catheter Cardiovasc Interv. 2009;73(3): 395–403.

36. Metcalfe D, Holt PE, Thompson M. The management of abdominal aortic aneurysms. BMJ. 2011;342:644–9.

37. Chaikof EL, Brewster DC, Dalman RL, Makaroun MS, Illig KA, Sicard GA, et al. The care of patients with an abdominal aortic aneurysm: the society for vascular surgery practice guidelines. J Vasc Surg. 2009;50(4 Suppl):S2–49.

38. Hiratzka LF, Bakris GL, Beckman JA, Bersin RM, Carr VF, Casey Jr DE, et al. American College of Cardiology Foundation/American Heart Association Task Force on Practice G. 2010 ACCF/AHA/ AATS/ACR/ASA/SCA/SCAI/SIR/STS/SVM guidelines for the diagnosis and management of patients with Thoracic Aortic Disease. Circulation. 2010;121(13):e266–369.

39. Moll FL, Powell JT, Fraedrich G, Verzini F, Haulon S, Waltham M, et al. Management of abdominal aortic aneurysms clinical practice guidelines of the European society for vascular surgery. Eur J Vasc Endovasc Surg. 2011;41 Suppl 1:S1–58.

40. Greenhalgh RM, Powell JT. Endovascular repair of abdominal aortic aneurysm. N Engl J Med. 2008;358(5):494–501.

41. Golledge J, Eagle KA. Acute aortic dissection. Lancet. 2008; 372(9632):55–66.

Part III
Approach to the Patient

Chapter 13
Approach to the Patient with Chest Pain

Benjamin R. McClintic and Robert L. Rosenblatt

Introduction

Despite significant advances in both diagnostic and therapeutic modalities in the last few decades, a chief complaint of chest pain still presents the clinician with a challenging management situation. Chest pain can indicate serious and immediately life-threatening underlying pathology but can also be due to common and benign processes. This dichotomy makes prompt and accurate identification of chest pain etiologies important from patient care, medical-legal, and cost-effectiveness standpoints. And it is a frequent patient complaint: chest pain is the most common cause for emergency room visits in adult males and in females over the age of 65 (second most common in younger adult women) [1]. Chest pain is also commonly encountered in the outpatient setting, although there is a lower likelihood of life-threatening etiologies such

B.R. McClintic (✉)
Division of Cardiology, Department of Medicine,
University of Rochester Medical Center, Rochester, NY, USA
e-mail: benjamin_mcclintic@urmc.rochester.edu

R.L. Rosenblatt
Division of Cardiology Department of Medicine,
University of Rochester Medical Center, Rochester, NY, USA
email: robert_rosenblatt@urmc.rochester.edu

J.D. Bisognano et al. (eds.), *Manual of Outpatient Cardiology*,   349
DOI 10.1007/978-0-85729-944-4_13,
© Springer-Verlag London Limited 2012

as acute myocardial infarction, pulmonary embolism, etc. as compared to the emergency department [2].

From a patient care and liability standpoint, proper identification of patients at high risk for adverse events is paramount so that appropriate hospital admission and management can be initiated. Despite the best efforts of clinicians, 2–8% of patients presenting to emergency departments with acute myocardial infarction are inappropriately sent home. These patients have almost twice the short-term mortality of their hospitalized counterparts [3]. Conversely, the majority of patients presenting to the emergency department or to their primary care physician with a complaint of chest pain do not have a life-threatening underlying etiology for their pain. Extensive diagnostic workup of these patients drives up costs and increases the risk of iatrogenic harm. This chapter will describe the initial clinical approach to a patient presenting with chest pain and specifically focus on differential diagnosis and risk stratification as well as some individual management issues related to specific causes of chest pain.

The majority of the literature is focused on the evaluation of chest pain in the inpatient setting. This chapter will focus on this information and try to apply it when possible to the outpatient setting.

Pathophysiology

An understanding of the clinical presentations for various etiologies of chest pain requires a basic knowledge of the physiologic pathways of visceral pain sensation. In general, damage to visceral organs such as heart and esophagus will stimulate afferent sensory fibers that run in autonomic nerves and synapse on the dorsal root ganglia of the upper thoracic spinal segments. These fibers are only able to transmit chronic/aching types of pain and the sensation is referred to the surface area of the body that is served by those thoracic nerve roots. The origin of this type of visceral pain is often difficult for the patient and clinician to localize. In contrast, pain originating in the parietal pleura, pericardium, and peritoneum is usually localized directly over the affected area because parietal pain sensations are transmitted directly into the local spinal nerves and do not travel along autonomic pathways [4].

Ischemic cardiac pain begins with free nerve endings that serve as sensory receptors in the myocardium (primarily epicardium). These nerve endings do not seem to be stimulated by mechanical mechanisms such as ventricular stretch given that processes which dilate the ventricle (acute ventricular failure, valvuloplasty, etc.) do not usually cause pain. Therefore, myocardial sensory receptors are thought to be stimulated by chemical mediators such as bradykinin and adenosine, which are released during myocardial ischemia [5]. Afferent impulses from the myocardium then travel along autonomic nerve fibers (both sympathetic and parasympathetic) to dorsal root ganglia. Many of the signs and symptoms of bradycardia, hypotension, diaphoresis, and nausea associated with myocardial damage result from vagal stimulation from afferent fibers of the vagus nerve, which are located primarily in the inferior cardiac wall [6].

Clinical Presentation and Differential Diagnosis

Initial Risk Stratification

When a patient presents to either the emergency department or outpatient provider with a complaint of chest pain, it is essential to first identify the patient's risk of having a serious, life-threatening event. The most serious (and life threatening) diagnoses in this category are acute coronary syndrome, aortic dissection, and pulmonary embolism. Some common clinical features of each of these entities as well as a broader differential diagnosis for acute chest pain can be found in Table 13.1. Prompt recognition and hospitalization for aggressive workup and management is essential in such cases, although the majority of patients presenting with chest pain will not have one of these diagnoses. Depending on

TABLE 13.1 Differential diagnosis of acute chest pain

	Helpful clinical features
Cardiovascular	
Angina	Retrosternal chest pressure, squeezing, heaviness. Associated with exertion or emotional stress, relieved by rest or nitroglycerin. Usually between 2 and 20 min in duration.
Aortic stenosis	Similar features as for angina, but with late-peaking systolic murmur radiating to carotids. May be associated with syncope or signs of left heart failure.
Pericarditis	Sharp, retrosternal, pleuritic chest pain lasting hours to days. May be associated with friction rub and may be alleviated by leaning forward.
Aortic dissection	Sudden onset of tearing, ripping chest pain radiating to back. Associated with underlying hypertension.
Pulmonary embolism	Ipsilateral pleuritic pain associated with dyspnea, tachycardia, possible cor pulmonale. May have irritative cough or hemoptysis or present with syncope. Usually sudden onset.
Pulmonary	
Pneumonia/pleuritis/pleural effusion	Pleuritic pain, lateralizing to side of infection/inflammation. May be associated with fevers, dyspnea, cough. Exam with pleural rub, consolidation, or dullness to percussion.
Asthma/COPD exacerbation	Chest "tightness" associated with more prominent findings of dyspnea, tachypnea and diffuse wheezing.
Spontaneous pneumothorax	Sudden onset of pleuritic pain. Unilateral and associated with dyspnea. More common in thin, young males or patients with emphysematous disease. Decreased breath sounds and hyperresonance on side of pneumothorax.
Chest wall	
Muscle spasm/strain	Associated with prior increased physical activity/weight lifting. Pain variable in character but usually reproducible with palpation.

TABLE 13.1 (continued)

	Helpful clinical features
Costochondritis	Sharp, sudden onset pain that is short in duration. May be reproducible with palpation.
Herpes zoster	Sharp, burning, superficial neuropathic pain. May have allodynia, vesicular rash on exam. Unilateral dermatomal distribution.
Rib fracture	Prior trauma or known metastatic disease of bone. Point tenderness over affected rib(s). Pain is usually pleuritic.
Cervical/thoracic nerve root compression	Intermittent neuropathic pain often associated with neck movement or position. Usually unilateral.

Gastrointestinal

Mediastinitis/ esophageal rupture	Often preceded by esophageal procedure or forceful vomiting. Pt. may have fever, associated septic shock. Symptoms vary from burning chest discomfort to severe dyspnea.
Esophageal reflux	Burning pain, often associated with nausea, belching. Usually worse at night and after large meals. Alleviated by antacids.
Esophageal spasm	Sudden onset, sharp, retrosternal pain. May be relieved by nitroglycerine and exacerbated by cold liquids. Sometimes associated with dysphagia.
Pancreatitis	Sharp epigastric pain, usually constant and prolonged. Exacerbated by food and often associated with nausea/vomiting. Alcohol and gallstones are risk factors.
Peptic ulcer	Sharp or burning epigastric pain. Often relieved by food or antacids. May be associated with occult GI bleeding or massive acute blood loss.

Psychogenic

Anxiety/panic disorder	May be unable to distinguish from anginal pain, but usually has atypical features such as prolonged duration and no exertional component. Should be a diagnosis of exclusion at initial workup.

the respiratory and hemodynamic stability of the patient, a thorough history and physical exam may not be possible or appropriate in the acute setting, and immediate treatment to stabilize the patient may be the necessary first step.

The initial approach to the hemodynamically stable patient presenting with acute chest pain should include a history, physical exam, and ECG. Unless a noncardiac diagnosis is clear based on these initial steps, then cardiac biomarkers should be drawn as soon as possible. The resultant clinical and laboratory features can then be used to stratify patients into low, intermediate, or high likelihood of having an acute coronary syndrome secondary to coronary artery disease. Table 13.2 describes specific features of the history, exam, ECG, and biomarkers that the ACC/AHA guidelines delineate in their initial risk stratification paradigm [7].

History

A thorough and detailed symptom history should be obtained by the provider on initial presentation, and should include:

- Features of the pain (onset, quality, location, radiation, exacerbating/alleviating factors, and timing).
- Associated symptoms (nausea, vomiting, diaphoresis, dyspnea, lightheadedness, syncope, etc.).
- Precipitating events (excessive exertion, long periods of immobilization, trauma, recent medical procedure, repeated vomiting, etc.).
- Comorbidities (especially prior CAD, hypertension, diabetes mellitus, thrombophilia or prior episode of venous thromboembolism, malignancy, etc.).
- Social and family factors (tobacco use, cocaine or other stimulant use, alcohol use, family history of CAD or PE, etc.).

Multiple studies have examined the predictive value of clinical criteria for identifying acute coronary syndrome in the patient presenting with undifferentiated chest pain [6–9].

TABLE 13.2 Likelihood that signs and symptoms represent an ACS secondary to CAD

Feature	High likelihood Any of the following:	Intermediate likelihood Absence of high-likelihood features and presence of any of the following:	Low likelihood Absence of high- or intermediate-likelihood features but may have:
History	Chest or left arm pain or discomfort as chief symptom reproducing prior documented angina	Chest or left arm pain or discomfort as chief symptom	Probable ischemic symptoms in absence of any of the intermediate likelihood characteristics
	Known history of CAD, including MI	Age greater than 70 years Male sex Diabetes mellitus	Recent cocaine use
Examination	Transient MR murmur, hypotension, diaphoresis, pulmonary edema, or rales	Extracardiac vascular disease	Chest discomfort reproduced by palpation
ECG	New or presumably new, transient ST-segment deviation (1 mm or greater) or T-wave inversion in multiple precordial leads	Fixed Q waves	T-wave flattening or inversion less than 1 mm in leads with dominant R waves
		ST depression 0.51 mm or T-wave inversion greater than 1 mm	Normal ECG
Cardiac markers	Elevated cardiac TnI, TnT, or CK-MB	Normal	Normal

Modified with permission from Braunwald et al. [30]; Adapted with permission from Anderson et al. [7]
ACS acute coronary syndrome, *CAD* coronary artery disease, *CK-MB* MB fraction of creatine kinase, *ECG* electrocardiogram, *MI* myocardial infarction, *MR* mitral regurgitation, *TnI* troponin I, *TnT* troponin T

Historical features that were most predictive of ACS included chest pain that radiated to one or both arms or shoulders as well as pain that worsened with exertion (likelihood ratios of 2.3–4.7). Characteristics of chest pain that reduced the likelihood of ACS included stabbing quality, pleuritic or positional nature of the pain, and pain that was reproducible by palpation (likelihood ratios of 0.2–0.3) [6]. Although nausea, vomiting, and diaphoresis are often associated with chest pain caused by cardiac ischemia, these symptoms are not predictive of ACS [8]. Also, patients with cardiac and noncardiac causes of chest pain respond equally well to nitroglycerin administration, and this response is not useful in differentiating causes of chest pain [10]. To date, no single historical feature or combination of symptoms alone has proven adequate to rule out cardiac ischemia or other serious causes of chest pain without further diagnostic testing.

Physical Examination

In general, the physical examination does not contribute significantly to the discrimination between acute coronary syndrome and noncardiac causes of chest pain. However, some findings may help identify other causes of chest pain and certain features have been found to correlate with ACS. Hypotension (LR 3.1), a third heart sound (LR 3.2), and pulmonary crackles (LR 2.1) all increase the likelihood that the patient is experiencing an acute coronary syndrome, but these findings may also indicate other etiologies of the chest pain [6]. In patients presenting with acute aortic dissection, 32% will have an aortic insufficiency murmur, 15% will have a pulse deficit, 8% will have cardiac shock or tamponade, 7% will have acute heart failure, and 5% will have signs of stroke [11].

Despite the overall poor diagnostic performance of most physical exam findings when used alone, common associations between certain findings and specific causes of chest pain should be known to the provider evaluating the patient and may help indicate an underlying etiology. Prominent and new murmurs should make the provider think of cardiac ischemia, endocarditis, or aortic dissection, while a cardiac friction rub should bring pericarditis to mind. The presence of bruits indicates peripheral arterial disease and increases the patient's risk of having coronary arterial disease. Unilateral extremity swelling, focal wheezes, and elevated JVP may indicate acute pulmonary embolism and/or right heart failure, while other abnormal lung sounds may indicate decompensated left heart failure (bibasilar crackles), pneumonia (rhonchi, egophony), pleural effusion (decreased breath sounds, dullness to percussion, pleural rub), pneumothorax (decreased breath sounds and hyperresonance) or bronchoconstriction (diffuse wheezes). Chest pain that is reproducible to palpation suggests a musculoskeletal cause of chest wall pain while epigastric tenderness may indicate a gastrointestinal etiology. Again, no single physical exam finding alone is sufficient to make a definitive diagnosis of a cause for chest pain, and the interpretation of exam findings must be done in the context of the entire clinical picture.

Electrocardiogram

This section will focus on the aspects of the ECG that are most important in the evaluation of a patient presenting with acute chest pain. For a more general discussion about ECG interpretation, see Chap. 2.

Given its utility in triaging and risk-stratifying patients with chest pain, current ACC/AHA guidelines specify that a 12-lead ECG should be obtained within 10 min of presentation to the emergency department [12]. Although such specific guidelines do not exist for the patient presenting to an office visit, it is prudent to obtain an ECG in this setting and have a system in place for prompt interpretation. A completely normal initial ECG should be followed by serial ECGs at approximately 10 min intervals if the patient has ongoing chest pain and the clinical presentation is consistent with ACS because ECG findings of ischemia may evolve over time. Also, if a prior ECG tracing is available it can be helpful in identifying new abnormalities.

A patient with no prior history of coronary artery disease and an initial ECG without ischemic changes has a 2% risk of having an acute myocardial infarction. This risk is 4% in patients with a prior history of CAD. However, in a patient with new ST-segment elevation of 1 mm or more, the risk of an acute myocardial infarction is approximately 80%, and emergency coronary reperfusion therapy is warranted. The prevalence of acute myocardial infarction in patients with new ST-segment depression or T-wave inversion is approximately 20%, and so further monitoring, workup, and possibly reperfusion therapy are also indicated in these patients [13]. Q waves of ≥0.03 s in two contiguous leads without ST-segment or T wave changes indicate prior MI, but taken alone only confer intermediate risk that a given episode of acute chest pain is due to ACS (see Table 13.2) [7].

Despite its central role in the acute evaluation of chest pain, the ECG has several limitations. It has a relatively low sensitivity for the diagnosis of ACS, with only 20–30% of initial ECGs showing ischemic changes in patients having an acute myocardial infarction [14]. Also, even though traditional teaching states that pulmonary embolism will result in classic ECG findings ("S1Q3T3"…a prominent S wave in lead 1, Q wave in lead 3, and T wave inversion in lead 3), ECG is actually of little utility in the diagnosis of acute pulmonary embolism. The most common findings are nonspecific, and include sinus tachycardia (42%) and incomplete right bundle branch block (7%), while the classic finding of S1Q3T3 can be a sign of acute cor pulmonale from any cause and is equally prevalent in patients with and without pulmonary embolism [15]. ECG is similarly unhelpful in establishing the diagnosis of acute aortic dissection. Patients presenting with aortic dissection may have ischemic changes (15%), nonspecific ST and T wave changes (42%) or normal findings (31%) [11].

Cardiac Biomarkers

In addition to clinical history, physical exam, and ECG, measurement of serum markers for myocardial injury is needed to accurately risk stratify patients with angina-type pain according to the guidelines proposed by the ACC/AHA and outlined in Table 13.2. Several different assays for cardiac ischemia are available, but the most accurate and commonly used are cardiac troponin I and troponin T as well as creatine kinase-MB. Until recent years, CK-MB was used in addition to cardiac troponin measurement because it was thought that additional diagnostic accuracy was conferred by doing so. Current recommendations obviate the need for checking CK-MB in the setting of undifferentiated acute chest pain given its inferiority in sensitivity, specificity, and prognostic value as compared to cardiac troponins [16]. However, given that troponins remain elevated for 5–7 days after myocardial injury and CK-MB starts trending down by 24 h, it may still have value in the assessment of periprocedural injury or reinfarction.

In a patient presenting with symptoms consistent with ACS, cardiac troponins should be checked on presentation and then rechecked 6–8 h later to establish whether they are trending up or down. In most patients, a single set of cardiac troponins does not rule out myocardial infarction because levels do not start to rise until approximately 6 h after the onset of symptoms. However, if a patient presents after 8 or more hours of symptoms, a single measurement may be sufficient to rule out myocardial infarction [7, 12]. Multiple point-of-care tests on whole blood for cardiac troponins are now available and may facilitate faster risk stratification of patients. These tests vary in sensitivity as compared to many of the serum tests used, and so the provider must be aware of these differences when using them for clinical decision making.

Faced with a positive cardiac troponin test result, the provider must interpret this result in its clinical context. While it is generally accepted that a cardiac troponin value above the 99th percentile of the upper reference limit does indicate some degree of myocardial necrosis, such a positive value does not inform the clinician about the underlying cause for myocardial injury. Criteria for myocardial infarction include at least one elevated cardiac troponin along with at least one of the following: symptoms of cardiac ischemia, ECG changes indicative of new ischemia, or imaging evidence of new

TABLE 13.3 Selected causes of elevated cardiac troponins

• Acute coronary syndrome	• Sepsis	• Apical ballooning syndrome
• Acute and chronic heart failure	• Hypothyroidism	• Cardioversion
	• Hypertension	• Rhabdomyolysis
• Trauma (contusion, cardiac ablation, cardiac surgery, etc.)	• Acute aortic dissection	• Hypotension
	• Pericarditis	• Severe burns
• Renal disease	• Myocarditis	• Cardiac Infiltrative Diseases
• Pulmonary embolism	• Endocarditis	• Transplant vasculopathy
• Cerebrovascular accident	• Drug toxicities (e.g., chemo)	• GI bleeding

regional wall motion abnormality [17]. A basic knowledge of other (non-thrombotic) causes for troponin elevation is also necessary for the clinician to appropriately interpret such elevations. See Table 13.3 for a list of differential diagnoses of elevated cardiac troponins not associated with ACS [18, 19]. One such cause that is commonly encountered is end stage renal disease. This is one situation in which cardiac troponin I and troponin T are not equivalent: 15–53% of patients with end-stage renal disease will have elevated troponin T in the absence of any clinical evidence for acute myocardial infarction, while less than 10% of these patients will have elevated troponin I [7]. In these situations, serial troponin measurements demonstrating a rise and fall is most helpful in determining a diagnosis of acute myocardial infarction.

Atypical Chest Pain

Typical angina is classically described as deep, aching discomfort or pressure in the chest or arm that is brought on by exertion or emotional stress and relieved within minutes by rest or nitroglycerin. Many patients will describe this pain as "squeezing," "pressure," or "heaviness," although some may report a sharp or burning sensation. Episodes of typical angina usually last between 2 and 20 min, and the patient may have a difficult time localizing the discomfort due to the physiology of visceral sensation described earlier in this chapter. Autonomic symptoms such as diaphoresis and nausea may also be present but ACC/AHA guidelines also describe other, less classic symptoms that should be considered "anginal equivalents." These include jaw, neck, shoulder, arm, ear, back, or epigastric discomfort, or dyspnea without discomfort, which are brought on by exertion and relieved with rest or nitroglycerin [7].

"Atypical" chest pain is an entity that often confounds clinicians and can lead to missed diagnoses of myocardial ischemia or alternatively may lead to unnecessary testing. The term refers to angina-like pain that differs from typical angina in one or more characteristics such as timing, location, or quality. ACC/AHA guidelines list the following symptom characteristics as *not* being typical for myocardial ischemia [7]:

- Pleuritic pain (i.e., sharp or knifelike pain brought on by respiratory movements or cough)
- Primary or sole location of discomfort in the middle or lower abdominal region
- Pain that may be localized at the tip of one finger, particularly over the left ventricular apex or a costochondral junction
- Pain reproduced with movement or palpation of the chest wall or arms
- Very brief episodes of pain that last a few seconds or less
- Pain that radiates into the lower extremities

Despite the fact that some of the above symptom characteristics may make cardiac ischemia less likely in any given patient presenting with acute chest pain, ACS can certainly present in an atypical fashion and the presence of these features does not entirely exclude the diagnosis. Furthermore, the lack of chest pain symptoms does not exclude a diagnosis of ACS: in a large registry of over 400,000 patients with confirmed acute myocardial infarction, 33% did not have any chest, neck, or jaw discomfort on presentation [20]. Populations that more commonly present with atypical or absent chest pain in the setting of ACS include women and diabetics, and these populations are at higher risk of having unrecognized cardiac ischemia as a result [21]. Clinicians need to have a higher degree of suspicion in these subgroups in order to prevent missed diagnoses.

Chronic Chest Pain

Multiple diagnoses can lead to chronic, recurrent chest pain symptoms, but one of the most common reasons is chronic stable angina. By definition, this entity consists of typical anginal symptoms (described above) that are present and unchanging for weeks to months to years. Chronic stable angina is caused by myocardial ischemia during increased myocardial oxygen demand in the setting of fixed coronary artery stenoses. This is in contrast to *unstable* anginal symptoms, which are of more recent onset or frequency, or are increasing in intensity ("crescendo" angina). Unstable angina is part of the spectrum of ACS, and is much more likely to be due to an acute coronary plaque event (rupture, erosion, etc.). It is extremely important for the practicing clinician to distinguish between these two types of angina, as the short term prognosis and management are quite different.

By the time most patients have been labeled with "chronic stable angina" they have already undergone exercise stress testing and may have had coronary angiography to better define the extent of their CAD. For the outpatient provider who encounters a patient with symptoms of chronic angina and no prior workup, a stepwise diagnostic approach is appropriate. This should consist first of a resting ECG in the office setting to confirm that there is no evidence of active ongoing ischemia. Pathologic Q waves may provide clues about previously unrecognized myocardial infarctions. If there is no ECG evidence of acute ischemia and the patient denies any resting or unstable chest pain symptoms, it is reasonable to proceed with noninvasive testing on an outpatient basis. Individual patient characteristics will help decide which stress test is most appropriate, but results of all available tests can help to further risk stratify patients with chronic angina and also assist in the decision about whether to proceed to coronary angiography, which remains the gold standard for diagnosis of CAD [22]. Chapters 4 and 5 describe stress testing and coronary evaluation in more detail, and may be helpful when deciding which diagnostic modality to use in a given patient with chronic stable angina.

The two primary goals of treatment for the patient with chronic stable angina are symptom relief and risk factor modification to prevent progression of disease. First-line therapy for symptom relief continues to be β-blockers, and evidence for this is even stronger in patients with prior myocardial infarction [23]. Other traditional therapies for symptom management include nitrates and calcium channel blockers, and these can be added on if β-blockers alone fail to relieve symptoms. A newer agent, ranolazine, is a sodium channel inhibitor that may be effective as second-line therapy for patients who continue to experience anginal symptoms after traditional agents have been tried. However, ranolazine is metabolized by CYP3A4, and a full understanding of possible drug-drug interactions and side effects is necessary before prescribing this medication to patients. Despite optimal medical therapy, some patients will continue to have debilitating symptoms of chronic angina. These patients are often best served by coronary revascularization and may experience significant symptom improvement. Patients who have failed optimal medical therapy and are not candidates for revascularization are considered to have refractory angina. These patients may benefit from less common therapies, such as spinal cord stimulation, enhanced external counterpulsation, and other modalities [24].

Once reasonable relief of angina symptoms has been achieved, the provider should focus efforts on risk factor modification in order to help prevent disease progression.

The ACC/AHA guidelines suggest that all patients with chronic stable angina should undergo smoking cessation counseling, participate in moderate aerobic exercise as tolerated, and have a goal BMI of 18.5–24.9 kg/m². Providers should focus on maintaining good glucose control in diabetics, blood pressure control according to JNC7 guidelines (with ACE-inhibitors as a first-line choice), and lipid management. For a patient with established CAD, the goal LDL should be less than 100 mg/dL, and preferably less than 70 mg/dL. All patients with chronic stable angina should also be given an antiplatelet agent (recommendation is for 75–162 mg of aspirin per day) and continued on this indefinitely [23].

Chest Pain in the Outpatient Setting

Most of the literature and guidelines regarding evaluation and management of chest pain are geared toward the inpatient or emergency department setting. In many ways, encountering a complaint of chest pain in the office poses a more difficult problem for the provider because continuous monitoring, rapid return of test results, and resuscitation tools are not as readily available. In this setting the initial history and physical exam, as well as their clinical context, become even more important. The clinician should first determine the patient's baseline probability of having coronary disease, as this will significantly affect his/her interpretation of historical features of chest pain described by the patient. Traditionally, the Framingham Risk Score is used to easily calculate a patient's 10-year risk of developing coronary heart disease. This risk score takes into account gender, age, total cholesterol, HDL cholesterol, systolic blood pressure, treatment for hypertension, and cigarette smoking [25]. Many free electronic calculators are available to quickly determine the 10-year Framingham CHD risk at the point of care. Other traditional risk factors, such as family history, kidney disease, and diabetes also need to be taken into account. Only after the patient's baseline risk for CHD has been determined can a symptom of chest pain be truly taken in context. For example, a young otherwise healthy patient who presents with atypical or non-anginal quality chest pain who has a normal EKG would be very low risk when compared to an older individual with multiple risk factors, such as diabetes mellitus who complains of fairly typical angina. It is essential in the outpatient setting to put the symptoms in the context of the patient and their risk factors. The history is key in the evaluation: if a high-risk patient presents to your office with signs or symptoms suggestive of unstable or rapidly accelerating angina, or other worrisome complaints, referral to the emergency department may be warranted.

The initial outpatient evaluation should always include a detailed history and physical exam, 12 lead EKG and referral for basic imaging such as a chest x-ray and essential lab work such as a CBC. The physical exam, when normal, is not often times helpful, but when there is a pertinent finding such as a pericardial friction rub or critical aortic stenosis murmur it can be very useful in determining the etiology of the patient's chest pain and referral for additional imaging such as echocardiography may be warranted. The history is also important in determining the appropriate work-up for someone who presents with chest pain. If a high-risk patient presents with signs and symptoms suggestive of stable or accelerating angina, referral for cardiac catheterization may be warranted. If the symptoms are somewhat atypical and sound like chronic stable angina then further risk stratification with non-invasive stress testing may be appropriate.

As helpful as traditional risk predictors such as Framingham can be, a significant proportion of coronary heart disease remains unexplained by traditional risk factors. This is especially true in certain subsets of the population, most notably in women, whose often atypical chest pain symptoms lead to underdiagnosed coronary disease. In the outpatient setting, novel predictors of risk may help to further stratify a patient's pretest probability of having coronary disease. C-reactive protein is one such marker, and has shown to be an independent predictor of risk for cardiovascular disease in women [26].

In addition there is recent data that elevation of C-reactive protein alone may be an important predictor of increased cardiac risk even in patients with "acceptable" lipid profiles; this is especially true in patients with a family history of CAD [27]. In patients with a family history of premature CHD, it may be helpful to check a lipoprotein(a) level, as this independently correlates with increased CHD risk [28]. Also, as described in more detail in Chap. 5, coronary artery calcium scoring measured by computed tomography has been shown to represent subclinical coronary artery disease and predict future coronary events [29]. Multiple other novel markers for CHD, such as amyloid A, homocysteine, retinal microvascular abnormalities, etc., are continually being developed and investigated. And while any new test should only be used with a thorough understanding of the evidence, subsets of the population who would otherwise be deemed "low risk" by traditional scoring systems may benefit from further risk stratification. Women and "low risk" patients with a strong family history of premature CHD are particular populations to target.

After a reasonable pretest probability for CHD has been established in the outpatient presenting with chest pain, the history and physical exam become extremely important in deciding on further management. In general, there are three management strategies that can be pursued for outpatients with chest pain: (1) immediate referral to an emergency department, (2) further workup for CHD (possibly including stress testing) as an outpatient, or (3) reassurance that CHD is not a likely cause of the patient's chest pain with a plan for further workup of other potential causes for his/her symptoms. As detailed earlier in this chapter, symptoms or exam findings consistent with immediately life-threatening diagnoses such as ACS, pulmonary embolism, and aortic dissection should prompt immediate emergency department evaluation. In these cases further delay to take a more thorough history or do more testing is unwarranted and potentially harmful to the patient. If alarm features (such as multiple underlying risk factors for CHD, crescendo or resting symptoms, etc.) are not present, then further outpatient workup can be considered. In the low risk patient with atypical chest pain and no other high risk features on history or exam, stress testing should not be pursued because the vast majority of these patients will either have a negative test or a false positive that begets further testing and its associated risks. Again, a higher suspicion for CHD is needed in women and patients with a strong family history, and further risk stratification may be warranted. Ideal patients for outpatient stress testing are those with intermediate risk for CHD who have stable chest pain symptoms. Chap. 4 provides further detail about stress testing modalities and test selection.

Often times adolescents and young adults are referred for outpatient evaluation of chest pain. This is generally a low-risk patient population where the prevalence of life threatening conditions is rather low. It is important to have a general knowledge of some of the more serious causes of chest pain in the young adult. The differential includes: anomalous coronary artery, left ventricular outflow obstruction (of any etiology), hypertrophic cardiomyopathy, and potentially serious rhythm disturbances. Again, the history and physical exam and basic diagnostic testing such as EKG and chest x-ray are very useful; ambulatory holter monitoring and referral for more sophisticated imaging such as echocardiography, CT coronary angiography or even cardiac MRI may be warranted based on the initial evaluation.

Conclusions and Management Recommendations

The patient presenting to either the emergency department or outpatient setting with acute chest pain continues to pose a diagnostic and management challenge. As detailed earlier in this chapter, the general provider should first focus energy on the detection of serious underlying causes for chest pain, such as ACS, pulmonary embolism, and aortic dissection. Since acute coronary syndrome is the most common life-threatening cause of chest pain, a systematic approach to risk stratification should be used to minimize missed diagnoses as well as overuse of the healthcare system. Multiple clinical risk scores have been developed and validated to aid the clinician in this venture, and these generally include a combination of history, exam, and ECG findings and may also include cardiac biomarkers [13, 14]. A reasonable approach is to stratify the patient into three risk categories as defined by the ACC/AHA and outlined in Table 13.2. This is much easier to do in the emergency department setting because cardiac biomarkers can be drawn and results received quickly while the patient is being monitored. However, point-of-care testing for cardiac troponins may soon make this aspect of risk stratification more accessible to the outpatient clinician.

Once a patient's risk for ACS has been defined, there are three general management strategies that the clinician can pursue. First, the patient at high risk for having ACS should be admitted and be considered for urgent or emergent therapy by a cardiologist. This may include anticoagulation, arrhythmia management, and probable coronary evaluation and revascularization. Second, the intermediate or low risk patient (again, as defined in Table 13.2) can be admitted to a dedicated chest pain unit (CPU) or observation unit. These units serve to provide further risk assessment in a rapid and cost-effective manner and usually involve accelerated diagnostic protocols that are based on serial ECGs, cardiac biomarkers, and clinical monitoring. The patient that has a negative initial workup for cardiac ischemia can then undergo provocative testing either prior to discharge or within 72 h of leaving the hospital [12]. The most common test used in CPUs remains standard exercise treadmill testing, but imaging tests such as stress echocardiography or myocardial perfusion imaging may give additional information in low-to intermediate- risk patients. See Chap. 4 for a further description of these diagnostic modalities.

Finally, a third management strategy is available to the outpatient, office-based clinician. As discussed earlier, many patients with chest pain (both ongoing as well as resolved) can be worked up on an outpatient basis. Identification of patients who are appropriate for outpatient management depends on their baseline risk for underlying cardiac disease as well as their symptoms and physical exam in the context of their presentation. All patients should receive an EKG during their office visit, but other simple tests such as chest x-ray, CBC, and other basic labwork are often warranted during the initial evaluation to help identify other noncardiac causes for a patient's chest pain complaints. Further cardiac risk stratification with novel markers such as CRP, lipoprotein(a), coronary artery calcium scoring, and others may be warranted. Further outpatient evaluation/risk stratification with stress testing, echocardiography or other imaging modalities may be necessary in the appropriate patient. Finally, particular attention should be paid to certain subsets of patients. These include women, who are more likely to present with atypical symptoms, as well as adolescents and young adults, who despite their low risk may be presenting with one of the potentially life-threatening conditions described above.

References

1. Niska R, Bhuiya F, Xu J. National hospital ambulatory medical care survey: 2007 emergency department summary. Natl Health Stat Report. 2010;26:1–32.
2. Buntinx F, Knockaert D, Bruyninckx R, et al. Chest pain in general practice or in the hospital emergency department: is it the same? Fam Pract. 2001;18(6):586–9.
3. Pope JH, Aufderheide TP, Ruthazer R, et al. Missed diagnoses of acute cardiac ischemia in the emergency department. N Engl J Med. 2000;342(16):1163–70.
4. Guyton AC, Hall JE. Visceral pain. Textbook of medical physiology. 9th ed. Philadelphia: Saunders; 1996. p. 615–6.
5. Foreman RD. Mechanisms of cardiac pain. Annu Rev Physiol. 1999;61:143–67.
6. Panju AA, Hemmelgar BR, Guyatt GH, Simel DL. Is this patient having a myocardial infarction? JAMA. 1998;280(14):1256–63.
7. Anderson JL, Adams CD, Antman EM, et al. ACC/AHA 2007 guidelines for the management of patients with unstable angina/

non-ST elevation myocardial infarction: a report of the American College of Cardiology/American Heart Association Task Force on Practice Guidelines (Writing Committee to Revise the 2002 Guidelines for the Management of Patients With Unstable Angina/Non–ST-Elevation Myocardial Infarction), developed in Collaboration with the American College of Emergency Physicians, the Society for Cardiovascular Angiography and Interventions, and the Society of Thoracic Surgeons. [published correction appears in *J* Am Coll Cardiol. 2008;51:974]. J Am Coll Cardiol. 2007;50:e1–157.

8. Goodacre S, Locker T, Morris F, Campbell S. How useful are clinical features in the diagnosis of acute, undifferentiated chest pain? Acad Emerg Med. 2002;9:203.

9. Swap CJ, Nagurney JT. Value and limitations of chest pain history in the evaluation of patients with suspected acute coronary syndromes. JAMA. 2005;294:2623–9.

10. Shry EA, Dacus J, Van De Graaff E, et al. Usefulness of the response to sublingual nitroglycerin as a predictor of ischemic chest pain in the emergency department. Am J Cardiol. 2002;90:1264–6.

11. Hagan PG, Nienaber CA, Isselbacher EM, et al. The International Registry of Acute Aortic Dissection: new insights into an old disease. JAMA. 2000;283:897–903.

12. Amsterdam EA, Kirk JD, Bluemke DA, et al. Testing of low risk patients presenting to the emergency department with chest pain: a scientific statement from the American Heart Association. Circulation. 2010;122:1756–76.

13. Lee TH, Goldman L. Evaluation of the patient with acute chest pain. NEJM. 2000;342:1187–95.

14. Kontos MC, Diercks DB, Kirk JD. Emergency department and office-based evaluation of patients with chest pain. Mayo Clin Proc. 2010;85(3):284–99.

15. Chan TC, Vilke GM, Pollack M, Brady WJ. Electrocardiographic manifestations: pulmonary embolism. J Emerg Med. 2001;21(3):263–70.

16. Eggers KM, Oldgren J, Nordenskjold A, Lindahl B. Diagnostic value of serial measurement of cardiac markers in patients with chest pain: limited value of adding myoglobin to troponin I for exclusion of myocardial infarction. Am Heart J. 2004;148:574–81.

17. Thygesen K, Alpert JS, White HD, et al. Universal definition of myocardial infarction. Circulation. 2007;116:2634–53.

18. Kelley WE, Januzzi JL, Christenson RH. Increases of cardiac troponin in conditions other than acute coronary syndrome and heart failure. Clin Chem. 2009;55(12):2098–112.

19. Saenger AK, Jaffe AS. The use of biomarkers for the evaluation and treatment of patients with acute coronary syndromes. Med Clin North Am. 2007;91:657–81.

20. Canto JG, Shlipak MG, Rogers WJ, et al. Prevalence, clinical characteristics, and mortality among patients with myocardial infarction presenting without chest pain. JAMA. 2000;283(24):3223–9.
21. Jones ED, Slovis CM. Pitfalls in evaluating the low-risk chest pain patient. Emerg Clin North Am. 2010;28:183–201.
22. Kones R. Recent advances in the management of chronic stable angina I: approach to the patient, diagnosis, pathophysiology, risk stratification, and gender disparities. Vasc Health Risk Manag. 2010;6:635–56.
23. Fraker TD, Fihn SD. 2007 Chronic Angina Focused Update of the ACC/AHA 2002 Guidelines for the Management of Patients With Chronic Stable Angina: a Report of the American College of Cardiology/American Heart Association Task Force on Practice Guidelines Writing Group to Develop the Focused Update of the 2002 Guidelines for the Management of Patients with Chronic Stable Angina. Circulation. 2007;116:2762–72.
24. Kones R. Recent advances in the management of chronic stable angina II: anti-ischemic therapy, options for refractory angina, risk factor reduction, and revascularization. Vasc Health Risk Manag. 2010;6:749–74.
25. Grundy SM, Becker D, Clark LT, Cooper RS, Other Members of the National Cholesterol Education Program Expert Panel. Third report of the NCEP on detection, evaluation, and treatment of high blood cholesterol in adults (adult treatment panel III) executive summary. Bethesda: National Heart, Lung, and Blood Institute/National Institutes of Health; 2001.
26. Ridker PM, Hennekens CH, Buring JE, Rifai N. C-reactive protein and other markers of inflammation in the prediction of cardiovascular disease in women. N Engl J Med. 2000;342:836–43.
27. Ridker PM, Danielson E, Fonseca FAH, et al. Rosuvastatin to prevent vascular events in men and women with elevated C-reactive protein. N Engl J Med. 2008;359:2195–207.
28. Clarke R, Peden JF, Hopewell JC, et al. Genetic variants associated with Lp(a) lipoprotein level and coronary disease. N Engl J Med. 2009;361:2518–28.
29. Budoff MJ, Achenbach S, Blumenthal RS, et al. Assessment of coronary artery disease from cardiac computed tomography: a scientific statement from the American Heart Association Committee on Cardiovascular Imaging and Intervention, Council on Cardiovascular Radiology and Intervention, and Committee on Cardiac Imaging, Council on Clinical Cardiology. Circulation. 2006;114:1761–91.
30. Braunwald E, Mark DB, Jones RH, et al. Unstable angina: diagnosis and management. Rockville: Agency for Health Care Policy and Research and the National Heart,Lung, U.S.Public Health Service, U.S. Department of Health and Human Service; 1994. AHCPR publication no 94-0602 (124).

Chapter 14
Syncope, Work Up and Management

Menachem Wakslak and David T. Huang

Introduction

Syncope, like headaches and chest pain, has the frustrating property of being an extremely common symptom for which the significance runs the gamut from benign nuisance to ominous harbinger. When evaluating syncope the care provider therefore should not dismiss it lightly, and at the same time avoid excessive utilization of health care resources in the work up of these patients.

Syncope represents 1–1.5% of all visits to the emergency department, 10% of outpatient visits and up to 6% of hospital admissions. It is important to note that syncope is a symptom and not a diagnosis. Syncope is very common with approximately 40% of the population experiencing syncope at some point in their life-time. In addition, the evaluation of syncope places a large burden on the healthcare system with an estimated cost of $2 billion attributable to only hospitalized evaluation of syncope [1]. To achieve a proper balance

M. Wakslak (✉)
Department of Cardiology, Maimonides Medical Center,
Brooklyn, NY, USA
e-mail: mwakslak@gmail.com

D.T. Huang
Department of Cardiology, University of Rochester Medical Center,
Rochester, NY, USA

J.D. Bisognano et al. (eds.), *Manual of Outpatient Cardiology*,   373
DOI 10.1007/978-0-85729-944-4_14,
© Springer-Verlag London Limited 2012

of appropriate work up and management of patients with syncope without over utilization of health care resources and expenditure entails a practice that applies the science as well as the art to the diagnosis and treatment congruent with the presentation.

Despite the commonplace nature of syncope the workup and evaluation of syncope is far from straightforward and may potentially be confusing, and frustrating for the patient as well as the healthcare provider.

These difficulties stem from several sources. Understanding these difficulties can help the care providers to avoid pitfalls in the evaluation of patients with syncope and to be more understanding and sympathetic towards the patients as well.

1. The experience of syncope is often traumatic and scary for the victim and witnesses; "Syncope is like dying but then you wake up" [2] and can appear eerily similar to sudden death. This can make an accurate description of the event difficult to obtain and also adds an emotional layer to the evaluation of syncope, often prompting the examiner to err to the side of caution, "just to be sure".

2. The definition of syncope as well as the terminology used to describe the different etiologies and the pathophysiology of syncope is often imprecise and overlapping further confusing the evaluation.

3. In almost all instances the symptom of syncope precedes the medical evaluation. At the time of the work up the patient is almost by definition an asymptomatic patient. As a result, when evaluating for syncope we are not looking for the cause of syncope but rather an abnormality on exam or testing that might be sufficient to explain the syncopal episode. Even when such an abnormality is identified it is often only presumptive, with varying degrees of certainty, that the abnormality has actually caused the syncopal episode.

4. While there are a great number of tests which are useful in the exclusion of disease entities causing syncope, there is no single gold standard test for the diagnosis of syncope.

Any particular test in any given patient may be of variable yield so that the practitioner is often uncertain of which tests to order for which patient.

In this chapter an attempt will be made to clarify some of these difficulties with regard to the evaluation of syncope. A stepwise approach will be outlined with a logistical progression of workup and specific considerations during a workup of patients with syncope will be emphasized. Syncope will be defined and the common causes of syncope will be discussed. The pathophysiology of some of the causes of syncope will be addressed with an emphasis on clarifying some of the common and confusing terms. Emphases on risk stratification, focused testing based on the results of history and physical examination, along with the treatment for syncope will then be discussed.

Definition

It is important to recognize that the term "syncope" is not in and of itself a diagnosis, rather it can represent any number of different disease states. Nor is it just the name of a symptom synonymous with the term "loss of consciousness". Syncope is defined as a transient loss of consciousness due to transient global cerebral hypoperfusion characterized by rapid onset, short duration, and spontaneous complete recovery [3]. This definition although complex encapsulates several important features of syncope. It is an attempt to place syncope in the context of the broader spectrum of entities which may lead to a transient loss of consciousness and thereby facilitate an organized approach to a patient being evaluated for syncope.

Loss of consciousness – this basic component of syncope allows us to differentiate syncope from other entities which may superficially resemble syncope but in which there was no true loss of consciousness, such as drop attacks, falls, psychogenic pseudo syncope, and transient ischemic attacks (TIA).

These entities can often easily be differentiated on the bases of the history but can be confused with syncope when the patient or witnesses are unable to provide an accurate history.

Cerebral hypoperfusion – this aspect of the definition approaches the basic pathophysiological mechanism common to all causes of syncope. While loss of consciousness can be a result of trauma, seizures, metabolic derangements, such as hypoxia or hypoglycemia, or vertebrobasilar TIA; the loss of consciousness of syncope is due to a drop in systemic blood pressure and resultant cerebral hypoperfusion.

Evaluation

Although it is helpful and reassuring to diagnose the etiology of syncope in all patients, it is important to realize that this is an unrealistic goal of an initial evaluation, especially in an urgent setting. Even after an extensive evaluation in a specialized syncope clinic, 25% [4] of patients will not have a definitive cause of syncope identified. Nevertheless, the initial evaluation immediately following a syncopal episode is particularly critical, both because the historical events are still fresh in the patient's mind and because transient abnormalities on physical exam are more likely to be noted during that proximate time.

The aim of the initial evaluation should therefore involve risk stratification and identify those patients who have a high likelihood of a serious adverse event in the near future and require a more intense immediate evaluation. Patients who are assessed to be at lower risk can be reassured to a degree and their workup can be evaluated in a more routine manner. The initial history and physical examination can often point the way to the more likely causes and guide the way to the most effective testing in the future. The evaluation should also involve inspection and noting any injuries sustained during the episode which may need attention independent of the etiology of syncope.

Step 1 – Determine Whether the Patient Experienced an Episode of Syncope

In answering this question it is critical to obtain a thorough history while keeping in mind the different components of the definition of syncope as well as the competing causes of a transient loss of consciousness and its mimics.

Was There Loss of Consciousness?

While the answer to this question is usually straight forward, it is common for some people, especially the elderly to be unable to clearly recall if there was true lost consciousness. If loss of consciousness is clearly documented to be absent during the event, then it is appropriate to consider alternative diagnoses such as, mechanical fall, TIA or Vertigo.

Was the Recovery Spontaneous and Complete and of Short Duration?

Metabolic states such as hypoglycemia or intoxication do not tend to reverse themselves and if they do, the time course is usually prolonged. This aspect of syncope serves also to distinguish stroke and resuscitated cardiac arrest in which the recovery is not spontaneous and often not complete. It is common however for people who experience neurally mediated syncope to report feeling fatigued, often for hours or even days.

Was the Event Due to Transient Global Cerebral Hypoperfusion?

Obviously the answer to this question is not easily obtainable. In particular differentiating syncope from epileptic seizures is a common diagnostic dilemma. Syncope which results from a decrease in cerebral perfusion can lead to hypoxic convulsions and can mimic an epileptic seizure. These convulsions tend to be somewhat different in that the seizures associated with syncope tend to be brief <15 s and they never precede the loss of consciousness. Several historical features have been demonstrated to be suggestive of epileptic seizures and these include (1) tongue biting, (2) a sense of déjà vu or an aura before a spell, (3) an association with emotional stress, (4) urinary or bowel incontinence, and (5) having no memory of a spell after it ends [5].

Causes of Syncope

Once an episode of transient loss of consciousness has been sub-classified as syncope, there are several different etiologies, listed below, which might be the cause of syncope and the remainder of the evaluation should focus on an attempt to identify a specific cause or to exclude particularly dangerous causes (see Fig. 14.1).

Reflex Mediated Syncope

The most common cause of syncope is reflex syncope, also known as neurally mediated syncope or neurocardiogenic syncope which has been subdivided into cardioinhibitory syncope and vasodepressor syncope. The prognosis of this group of disorders is generally benign although the impact on quality of life of recurrent syncope can be profound [6].

The pathogenesis of this reflex is incompletely understood and may vary depending on the patient and the clinical scenario. Simplistically, this group of disorders results from an inappropriate reflex which results in a decrease in vascular tone with a consequent drop in blood pressure (vasodepressor) and/or heart rate with a profound bradycardia (cardioinhibitory). This occurs as a result of a sudden increase in vagal efferent activity and sympathetic withdrawal. The particular stimulus which triggers this reflex in each patient is quite variable and is the basis for further sub-classification of reflex mediated syncope.

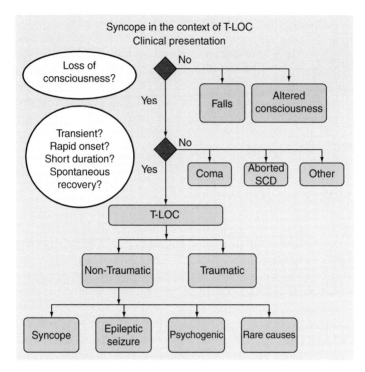

FIGURE 14.1 Context of transient loss of consciousness (*T-LOC*). *SCD* sudden cardiac death (Moya [3]. With permission from Elseiver)

Vasovagal syncope or "the common faint" refers to reflex mediated syncope which occurs as a result of emotional or orthostatic stress such as having blood drawn, extreme fear or being startled, as well as prolonged standing particularly in a warm environment A.K.A "church syncope".

Situational syncope in which an assortment of particular scenarios result in reflex mediated syncope. Often, a particular patient will experience syncope in only one of these situations. Some examples of stimuli that may precipitate syncope are blood draws, coughing, swallowing, defecating, urinating, post prandial state and the post exercise state.

Carotid sinus syndrome refers to an exaggerated response to carotid manipulation and a resultant drop in blood pressure and heart rate causing syncope. While syncope caused by this abnormal reflex may follow inadvertent carotid manipulation such as from a tight collar while turning one's heads or during shaving, this entity also refers to a syndrome in those patients in whom an otherwise negative work up for syncope reveals an abnormal response to carotid massage.

Orthostatic Hypotension

This is defined as a significant decrease in blood pressure (at least 20 mmHg fall in systolic pressure or at least a 10 mmHg fall in diastolic pressure) upon 2–5 min of quiet standing associated with symptoms of cerebral hypoperfusion [3]. As a result a patient with orthostasis will suffer from syncope after assuming a standing position. Orthostatic hypotension is much more common in older patients. Like reflex mediated syncope, this condition does not independently convey an increased risk although it seems to identify a sicker population of patients with more comorbidity. While patients with reflex mediated syncope can be thought of as having an abnormally exuberant reflexive response to a stimulus, patients with orthostatic hypotension have a failure of the normal sympathetic response to the standing position and the resultant pooling of blood in the lower extremities. This autonomic failure may be a primary disorder or may be associated with other disease states such as Diabetes Mellitus or Parkinson's disease and can also commonly be a result of prescription medications, particularly antihypertensive medications.

Cardiac Syncope

This is caused by a decrease in cardiac output resulting from a primary cardiac issue. This can be an arrhythmia, either extreme bradycardia or tachycardia, or due to a structural problem resulting in pump failure like a massive heart attack, pulmonary embolus or obstructive disease like severe aortic stenosis or severe pulmonary hypertension. Cardiac syncope conveys a dramatically increased risk of all-cause mortality with the prognosis often related to the underlying disease [6].

Step 2 – Obtain Background and Detailed History of the Event

In order to approach history taking in the work up of syncope in an organized fashion, it may be helpful to divide the history into chronological segments.

Background

Is there a personal history of heart disease?

Is there a history of prior syncopal events and if so when was the first event and how often have they recurred? A long history of recurrent syncope may suggest a benign etiology, though not always.

A directed review of systems can help ensure a thorough history and not miss pertinent aspects. For example associated conditions which might predispose to peripheral neuropathy such as diabetes or Parkinson's disease should be addressed. Medication history is always critical as some may lead to hypotension or be proarrhythmic. Recently, emphasis has been placed on medications that lead to prolonged QT in susceptible individuals. Some of the more often encountered offending medications include antihistamines, antifungals, and even some antibiotics. Finally, family history is another critical aspect including a family history of sudden death or hereditary arrhythmias.

Events Immediately Preceding the Episode

What position was the patient in? Did the event occur with activity? What were the surrounding circumstances? (e.g. prolonged standing in a hot crowded room)

Events at the Onset of the Episode

Was the event preceded by nausea, vomiting, clammy feeling, diaphoresis? Was there a preceding aura? Was there associated heart racing or palpitations?

Events During the Episode

Eyewitness observation from others can be very helpful for further description of the events and, if available, should be included as part of the history. Did the patient fall suddenly or slowly slump over? Was there associated injury? How long was the loss of consciousness? Were there associated seizure-like movements, tongue biting or loss of urine or stool?

Events After the Episode

Did the patient feel normal immediately after the event or was there residual confusion, lethargy or weakness?

Step 3 – Examine the Patient for Signs That May Suggest a Cause for Syncope

A full examination is mandatory in the evaluation of patients with syncope; however, targeted findings of specific signs that may suggest a cause for syncope should be noted.

Orthostatic hypotension, especially with reproduction of syncope or near syncope on having the patient stand up can be a very helpful finding. Keeping in mind that when one is examining a patient in the emergency department immediately following an episode of syncope the patient may have already received a significant amount of fluid. Carotid sinus massage should be performed in all patients greater than age 40 (after having excluded an ipsilateral carotid bruit) and if it results in a >3 s ventricular pause or >50 mmHg drop in systolic blood pressure is diagnostic of carotid sinus hypersensitivity. Cardiac auscultation may reveal evidence of an obstructive lesion such as aortic stenosis, hypertrophic obstructive cardiomyopathy or an atrial myxoma. Some of the physical findings may be dynamic; therefore, auscultation with maneuvers such as Valsalva, squatting should be included.

An EKG is a critical part of the work up of syncope and may reveal suggestions of an arrhythmic cause for syncope such as Long QT, WPW, or pathologic AV block. An EKG may also demonstrate evidence of outflow obstruction such as hypertrophic cardiomyopathy. Although relatively rare, these should not be missed due to the prognosis related to some of these findings.

With careful attention to details, in approximately 40% of cases a cause for syncope will be identified based on the initial history and physical examination or EKG [7].

Some important scenarios can be considered diagnostic of a cause for syncope as suggested by the 2009 European Guidelines [3].

Vasovagal syncope is diagnosed if syncope is precipitated by emotional or orthostatic stress and is associated with the typical prodromal symptoms of nausea, vomiting, sweating, a feeling cold or tiredness.

Situational syncope is diagnosed if syncope occurs during or immediately after a typical situation like coughing, sneezing, while swallowing, post micturation or post exercise.

Orthostatic syncope is diagnosed when syncope occurs after standing up and there is documentation of orthostatic hypotension.

Arrhythmia related syncope is diagnosed by ECG when there is:

Profound sinus bradycardia
Mobitz II second or third degree AV block
Alternating left and right bundle branch block
Ventricular tachycardia or rapid paroxysmal supraventricular tachycardia
Non-sustained episodes of polymorphic VT and long QT interval
Pacemaker malfunction with cardiac pauses

Cardiac ischemia related syncope is diagnosed when syncope presents with ECG evidence of acute ischemia, while it is often considered a potential cause of syncope is not as common as traditionally taught. Cardiac Arrhythmias related to ischemia that lead to syncope are mostly due to polymorphic VT or heart block due to ischemic insult of the atrioventricular conduction system or Bezold-Jarisch reflex. ECG at rest post event often does not show evidence of ischemia though a transmural myocardial scar (Q waves) may be evident. Provocative testing with exercise treadmill testing should be considered if initial evaluation is suggestive of coronary artery disease.

Other cardiovascular syncope is diagnosed when syncope presents in patients with prolapsing atrial myxoma, severe aortic stenosis, pulmonary hypertension, pulmonary embolus, or acute aortic dissection.

Step 4 – Stratify According to Risks

Among the 40% or so of patients in whom a diagnosis will be found on initial evaluation, a decision to admit the patient will be based on the need to facilitate the prompt initiation of treatment as driven by the perceived risks of recurrent syncope events. For example, patient with drug related long QT and syncope consistent with an arrhythmic etiology should be observed until the drug wears off or the corrected QT interval normalizes. Patients in whom a cardiovascular or arrhythmic cause for their syncope is identified will almost universally need to be admitted for definitive treatment whereas patients who are diagnosed with reflex mediated syncope can likely be safely discharged.

In the patients in whom a diagnosis is not reached a decision about the short-term risk for adverse events should guide a decision to admit for further work up. This assessment has two components.

The first is to identify the type of patient who is most likely to suffer from a serious adverse event. There have been several risk scores devised based on both retrospective and prospective observational studies in an emergency setting which

Older age and associated comorbidities*

Abnormal ECG†

Hct < 30 (if obtained)

History or presence of heart failure, coronary artery disease, or structural heart disease

*Different studies use different ages as threshold for decisionmaking. Age is likely a continuous variable that reflects the cardiovascular health of the individual rather than an arbitrary value.

†ECG abnormalities, including acute ischemia, dysrhythmias, or significant conduction abnormalities.

FIGURE 14.2 Factors that lead to stratification as high risk for adverse outcome

attempt to quantify the risk of short term events based on clinical characteristics. Based on these studies the American College of Emergency Physicians [1] has devised a simple list of characteristics which place a victim of syncope at increased risk (see Fig. 14.2).

In addition, certain historical features of the specific syncopal episode can suggest a higher risk patient. These include syncope during exertion, syncope while supine, and a family history of sudden death in patients with a history of cardiovascular disease.

Test Selection

Whether a decision to admit or to evaluate as an outpatient is made the next step in the evaluation of syncope of unknown etiology is to obtain those tests which are likely to lead to a diagnosis.

Echocardiography, stress testing, electrocardiographic monitoring, carotid ultrasound, head CT, electrophysiological study and tilt table testing are some of the commonly ordered tests in the evaluation of syncope. It is not uncommon for the same patient to undergo a majority of these tests and still not have a diagnosis. Judicious use of directed testing here is called for rather than reflexive testing in these settings to avoid much of this inappropriate testing.

The following represents a typical recommended approach to testing in syncope.

Echocardiography represents the cornerstone of the cardiac evaluation of syncope and is indicated in any patient with a history of cardiac pathology or any finding on physical or EKG that suggests cardiac disease. Although it is only rarely, as in the case of severe aortic stenosis or an atrial myxoma, that echocardiography can definitively diagnose the cause of syncope it is invaluable with regards to risk stratification. The absence of structural heart disease on echocardiography can be reassuring that a life threatening tachyarrhythmia is less likely the cause of syncope. At the same time the finding of significant heart disease and in particular a reduced ejection fraction marks a patient as high risk, prompting a more aggressive approach to diagnosis and treatment.

The next step in our diagnostic tree is electrocardiographic and symptom correlation. The only way to better ascertain an arrhythmic cause of syncope is to correlate ECG monitor findings at the time of syncope. Given the unpredictable nature of syncope, this often requires prolonged electrocardiographic monitoring. There are several types of available monitoring which range from externally applied 24–48 h of continuous monitoring with a Holter monitor, or up to 30 days with a continuous loop recorder either a patient activated event monitor or commercially available home telemetry continuous monitor. In patient with events which are more rare or in patients unable to use external monitors, an implantable subcutaneous monitor can be implanted, this can provide data for up to several years. The particular type of monitoring is dependent on the frequency of symptoms. A finding of a normal rhythm at the time of syncope is as valuable as an abnormal rhythm in ruling in or ruling out an arrhythmic cause of syncope.

Invasive electrophysiological study, in which catheters are threaded into the heart via the femoral vein and the heart, is electrically stimulated in an attempt to evaluate the patients propensity to develop sustained ventricular arrhythmias and in which the conduction system is measured for evidence of significant disease and a tendency towards heart block, is utilized in those patients with abnormal hearts. In particular it is of value in those patients whose ejection fraction is significantly reduced or who have structural heart disease (ARVD) at potential risk of sudden cardiac death but not below the values for which an implantable cardioverter defibrillator would be indicated independently of syncope for the primary prevention of sudden cardiac death.

Tilt table testing is a noninvasive test in which a patient lies on a table which is then tilted to 60–70°. As a patient is maintained in that position for 30–40 min there is the potential to elicit a vasovagal response, due to the orthostatic stress, in those patients who are predisposed to reflex mediated syncope. There is a substantial incidence of false positive and false negative test results related to tilt table testing. Therefore its diagnostic yield is often not significantly better than a good history and physical evaluation. Furthermore, it is important to note that a positive tilt table test does not necessarily rule out other causes of syncope. If concerns for other potential causes, such as tachyarrhythmias related to structural heart disease, further testing should be pursued.

Carotid dopplers, although commonly ordered, are not beneficial in the routine evaluation of syncope unless there are focal neurological signs of a TIA or stroke. Similarly CT scans of the head are only useful if there is a focal neurological sign or if there is concern of head trauma as a result of the syncopal event [3].

Treatment

In most cases where a cardiac cause of syncope has been identified the treatment is usually self-evident. Pacemaker implantation for a brady-arrhythmia, an ICD for syncope due to ventricular tachy-arrhythmias either clinical diagnosis or suspicion in patient with a high risk substrate, surgery for valvular causes of syncope and aortic dissection and anticoagulation for pulmonary embolism are a few of the more common therapies. The treatment of vasovagal syncope as well as orthostatic hypotension is somewhat more complex.

Part of the foundation for treatment of reflex mediated syncope involves education, explaining the mechanism of vagal syncope as well as its benign prognosis. Simply pointing out the situational triggers which lead to syncope, like standing outside in the heat, and common sense advice like lying down when the patient feels like they will lose consciousness, often may effectively reduce the incidence of syncope. Patients should also be counseled to maintain adequate salt and water intake with a target intake of 2–3 L and 10 g of sodium daily.

While several medications which have shown variable success in the treatment of vasovagal syncope none have shown consistent results and as a result none can be recommended conclusively in the prevention of reflex mediated syncope.

Physical counter pressure maneuvers in which a person with recurrent syncope performs either leg crossing, handgrip, or arm tensing when they feel a syncopal episode is imminent was successful in reducing the rate of recurrent syncope by 40% in a selected group of young patients who were known to have prodromal symptoms before syncope [8].

In the treatment of orthostatic hypotension the single most important step is a careful review of medications and the discontinuation of any offending agents which might be stopped. Some examples of common offending agents which do not typically proffer an independent antihypertensive survival benefit are alpha blockers, nitrates and diuretics. Depending on the severity of the symptoms associated with orthostatic hypotension it is sometimes necessary to tolerate a higher than optimal supine blood pressure in order to prevent debilitating orthostatic symptoms.

Like reflex mediated syncope orthostatic hypotension also responds to lifestyle measures including liberalized fluid and salt intake, pressure stockings which prevent the peripheral pooling of blood upon standing, sleeping on a bed with an elevated head (i.e. the head of the bed is propped up on cinder blocks) is believed to encourage volume retention during the night. This tilt training may be trialed for more resistant cases but its efficiency is not universal. Both Midodrine, a direct alpha agonist, and fludrocortisode, a mineralocorticoid with volume expanding properties, have been shown to improve symptoms in orthostatic hypotension.

In summary, syncope can be a challenging and frustrating entity to diagnose and to treat. With a systematic approach it is hoped that those patients at high risk will be identified and treated in a prompt fashion. Recognizing patients with high risk causes, (arrhythmic, cardiac outflow obstruction, acute pulmonary embolus, etc.) is a main goal for care providers who evaluate these patients. Nevertheless, less life threatening causes will encompass the bulk of the causes of syncope. Proper triage with appropriate risk stratification as guided by directed strategies should comprise the approach of those patients. While reflex mediated syncope and orthostatic hypotension are relatively benign in their prognosis, the treatment is challenging but can be immensely satisfying given their detrimental impact on quality of life.

References

1. Huff JS, Decker WW, Quinn JV, et al. Clinical policy: critical issues in the evaluation and management of adult patients presenting to the emergency department with syncope. Ann Emerg Med. 2007;49(4):431–44. http://www.ncbi.nlm.nih.gov/pubmed/17371707 Accessed March, 2011.
2. Engel GL. Psychologic stress, vasodepressor (vasovagal) syncope, and sudden death. Ann Intern Med. 1978;89(3):403–12. Available at: http://www.ncbi.nlm.nih.gov/pubmed/99068. Accessed 13 Jan, 2011.
3. The Task Force for the Diagnosis and Management of Syncope of the European Society of Cardiology (ESC), Moya A, Sutton R, Ammirati F, et al. Guidelines for the diagnosis and management of syncope (version 2009). Eur Heart J. 2009;30(21):2631–71. Available at: http://www.ncbi.nlm.nih.gov/pubmed/19713422. Accessed March, 2011
4. Alboni P, Brignole M, Menozzi C, et al. Diagnostic value of history in patients with syncope with or without heart disease. J Am Coll Cardiol. 2001;37(7):1921–8. Available at: http://www.ncbi.nlm.nih.gov/pubmed/11401133. Accessed March, 2011

5. Sheldon R, Rose S, Ritchie D, et al. Historical criteria that distinguish syncope from seizures. J Am Coll Cardiol. 2002;40(1):142–8. Available at: http://www.ncbi.nlm.nih.gov/pubmed/12103268. Accessed March, 2011

6. Sample S. The new England Journal of Medicine Incidence and prognosis of syncope. English Journal. 2002;347(12):878–85.

7. Linzer M, Yang EH, Iii NAME, Wang P. Clinical guideline diagnosing syncope part 1: value of history, physical examination, and electrocardiography. Ann Inter Med. 1997;126(15):989–96.

8. van Dijk N, Quartieri F, Blanc J-J, et al. Effectiveness of physical counterpressure maneuvers in preventing vasovagal syncope: the Physical Counterpressure Manoeuvres Trial (PC-Trial). J Am Coll Cardiol. 2006;48(8):1652–7. Available at: http://www.ncbi.nlm.nih.gov/pubmed/17045903. Accessed 29 Mar, 2011.

Chapter 15
Palpitations

Matthew Jonovich and Burr Hall

Introduction

Palpitations are a common, unpleasant sensory symptom characterized by a conscious awareness of an abnormal heartbeat [1]. Patient description of palpitations is variable but often include forceful, rapid or irregular beating, the feeling of fluttering, the perception of pauses, or a pounding sensation in the chest or neck. Palpitations are one of the most common complaints reported by outpatients who present to internists and cardiologists [2]. One study of 500 medical encounters demonstrated 16% of visits were prompted by a chief complaint of palpitations [3]. In most cases, the cause of palpitations is benign but in rare instances this symptom is a manifestation of a potentially life-threatening arrhythmia. The physician's concern of missing a serious, treatable condition may lead to the overuse of diagnostic testing and unnecessary referrals that consume considerable healthcare resources but yield little diagnostic or therapeutic value

M. Jonovich (✉)
Division of Cardiology, Department of Medicine,
University of Rochester Medical Center, Rochester, NY, USA
e-mail: mathew_jonovich@urmc.rohester.edu

B. Hall
Division of Electrophysiology, Department of Medicine
University of Rochester Medical Center, Rochester, NY, USA

J.D. Bisognano et al. (eds.), *Manual of Outpatient Cardiology*, 391
DOI 10.1007/978-0-85729-944-4_15,
© Springer-Verlag London Limited 2012

[4]. In this chapter, we discuss a differential diagnosis, the common clinical presentations in the adult patient and a guide to the evaluation, appropriate diagnostic testing and treatment of the patient with palpitations.

Differential Diagnosis

Palpitations can occur from a myriad of causes that are both cardiac and non-cardiac in origin (Table 15.1). While cardiac disorders are a common cause of palpitations it is essential to remember palpitations are a symptom and often occur in the absence of cardiac arrhythmia or disease. In a prospective cohort study of 190 consecutive patients who presented to a university medical center with palpitations Weber and Kapoor identified a cause in 84% of the patients [5]. Of these patients, 43% had palpitations attributed to a cardiac cause (40% arrhythmia, 3% other cardiac causes), 31% had palpitations caused by anxiety or panic disorder, 6% had palpitations caused by street drugs, prescription or over-the-counter medications and 4% had palpitations from noncardiac causes (thyrotoxicosis, anemia, fever, pregnancy and mastocytosis) [5]. In 16% of patients no specific cause of the palpitations was identified despite extensive diagnostic testing. A cardiac etiology was more common in patients presenting to the emergency department as compared to those patients seen in the outpatient setting. (47% vs. 21%). Psychiatric etiologies were more common in the medical clinic compared to the emergency department (45% vs. 27%). Cardiac etiologies may also be more common among patients who present to a specialist due to prescreening [6]. Weber and Kapoor identified four independent predictors of a cardiac etiology of palpitations: Male gender, description of an irregular heartbeat, history of heart disease and event duration greater than 5 min [5]. In patients with zero predictors, none had a cardiac etiology, compared to 26%, 48% and 71% of patients with one, two and three predictors respectively [5]. Of note, despite the relatively high prevalence of cardiac disorders in the study population the short-term prognosis was excellent.

TABLE 15.1 Differential diagnosis of palpitations

Cardiac 43%	Psychiatric 43%	Miscellaneous 10%
Arrhythmia (40%)	Generalized	**Drugs or medication**
Atrial	anxiety	**(6%)**
Paroxysmal atrial	Panic disorder	Alcohol
fibrillation/flutter	Hypochondriasis	(use or withdrawl)
Paroxysmal atrial	Major	A-agonists
tacycardia	depression	Amphetamines
Supraventricular	Somatization	Anticolinergic B-blockers
tachycardia		(withdrawal) agents
Premature		Caffeine
supraventricular		Cocaine
contractions		Epinephrine
Multifocal atrial		Digitalis
tachycardia		Theophylline
Wolff-Parkinson-		Vasodilators (Nitrates)
White syndrome		**Metabolic disorder**
Sick Sinus Syndrome		Hyperthyroidism
Bradycardia-		Hypoglycemia
Tachycardia syndrome		Hypo/hypercalcemia
Sinus tachycardia		Hypo/hyperkalemia
Ventricular		Hypo/hypermagnesemia
Premature ventricular		Pheochromocytoma
contractions		**High cardiac output**
Ventricular tachycardia		**states**
Nonarrhythmic cardiac		Anemia
causes (3%)		Arteriovenous fistula
Mitral valve prolapse		BeriberiFever
Valvular heart disease		Paget's disease
(AS, AI)		Pregnancy
Atrial myxoma		Mastocytosis
Pacemaker-mediated		
tachycardia		
CHF		
Congenital heart		
disease		
Atrial septal defect		
Patent ductus		
arteriosus		
Ventricular septal		
defect		
Pericarditis		
Cardimyopathy		
Aortic aneurysm		

Data from Weber and Kapoor [4]

At 1 year of follow up only three deaths occurred, all in women over age 70 and none of the deaths were sudden or related to the etiology of the palpitations [5].

Common Presentations: Symptoms and Circumstances

Patient description of palpitations is highly variable but some specific and common symptoms can be useful in narrowing the broad differential diagnosis [4]. To this end the practitioner must elicit a detailed description of the sensation associated with the palpitation.

Flip Flopping in the Chest

The sensation of the heart stopping and starting again is frequently described as producing a pounding or "Flip-Flopping". This type of palpitation is often caused by premature atrial or ventricular contractions. The sensation that the heart has stopped comes from the compensatory pause following a premature contraction. The characteristic pounding or flip-flopping sensation is attributed to the more forceful systolic contraction following the pause.

Rapid Fluttering in the Chest

The feeling of rapid fluttering in the chest suggests a sustained tachyarrhythmia such as ventricular tachycardia, supraventricular arrhythmia or sinus tachycardia. An irregular tachycardia suggests atrial fibrillation while a regular tachycardia is consistent with sinus or reentrant tachycardia.

Pounding in the Neck

A pounding feeling in the neck suggests atrioventricular dissociation. The independent contraction of the atria and ventricles results in occasional atrial contraction against a closed tricuspid and mitral valve [4]. This produces "cannon" A waves or intermittent increases in the A wave of the jugular venous pulse. The cause of cannon A waves may be benign (premature ventricular contractions) or serious (complete heart block, ventricular tachycardia) etiologies. Rapid and regular pounding in the neck suggests a reentrant supraventricular tachycardia. Atrioventricular nodal tachycardia is the most common form of paroxysmal AVT and is three times more common in women than men [7].

Circumstances

The circumstances during which palpitations manifest are often helpful in identifying the underlying cause.

Palpitations Associated with Anxiety or Panic

When palpitations occur in the context of anxiety or panic the patient may struggle to determine whether the feeling of anxiety or panic preceded or resulted from the palpitations. Panic disorder was diagnosed as the cause of palpitations in 20% of patients in one study [8]. Another study demonstrated 31% of patients had palpitations caused by anxiety or panic disorder [4]. Of note, 13% of patients in the same study had palpitations attributed to more than one etiology. Although there is good evidence psychiatric disorders are a common cause of palpitations, this diagnosis should be reserved until arrhythmic causes have been excluded.

Palpitations During Catecholamine Excess

Onset of palpitations with sympathetic stimulation and catecholamine excess that occurs during exercise can suggest supraventricular (most commonly sinus tachycardia) or ventricular tachyarrhythmias. Studies have demonstrated that

benign nonsustained supraventricular and ventricular premature beats are more common than sustained arrhythmias after
exercise. The incidence of ventricular arrhythmias is more
common in patients with underlying structural heart disease
with a rare exception. For example, idiopathic ventricular
tachycardia can occur during exercise in patients with structurally normal hearts. This disorder most often presents in the
second and third decades of life with associated palpitations,
dizziness, or syncope [9]. Supraventricular tachyarrhythmias
(often atrial fibrillation) may be induced during exercise or
immediately following exercise when the withdrawal of catecholamines is coupled with increased vagal tone [10]. Finally,
palpitations occurring at times of catecholamine surge from
emotionally startling experiences can be indicative of a long
QT syndrome. This rare inherited abnormality of myocardial
repolarization can trigger polymorphic ventricular tachycardia during emotional stress or exercise [11].

Positional Palpitations

Body position at the time of palpitations can provide insight
into the etiology. Atrioventricular nodal tachycardia (AVnRT)
often occurs when a patient stands up after bending over and
may terminate upon lying down. Some patients report a pounding sensation when they are lying supine or in the left lateral
decubitus position [4]. This symptom may be the result of
premature beats that occur more frequently at slow heart
rates when a person is resting in bed.

Sudden Onset Palpitations

The onset of palpitations can also be a very useful clue as
to the underlying etiology. Reentrant arrhythmias such as
AVNRT and orthodromic reciprocating tachycardia (ORT)
usually have a sudden onset and offset. Palpitations that start
more gradually with a slow steady acceleration and then
deceleration of heart rate are often indicative of an

automatic rather than reentrant etiology such as atrial or sinus tachycardia.

Initial Diagnostic Evaluation

When evaluating a patient with symptomatic palpitations the clinician's primary goal should be to detect and identify the presence of organic heart disease or other precipitating causes [12]. The initial evaluation of the patient should include a detailed history, physical examination, 12-lead electrocardiogram and consideration of limited laboratory testing.

History

The history should include a qualitative description of the character of the palpitations, a quantitative description of the frequency, duration and triggers, associated symptoms or situations, drug or medication use, comorbid illness and age of onset. Often the patient describes characteristics of the palpitations can help identify the etiology. Previously discussed examples include "flip-flopping" (PACs, PVCs), "rapid fluttering" (atrial or ventricular arrhythmias, including sinus tachycardia), and "pounding sensation in the neck" (AV dissociation, AVNRT). The caregiver should make particular effort to elicit high risk clinical features that warrant urgent, aggressive diagnostic evaluation (Table 15.2). The presence of these symptoms should prompt the rapid evaluation of the patient's cardiac structure and function with an echocardiogram.

Physical Exam

Physicians typically do not have the opportunity to examine the patient during an episode of palpitations. The physical examination primarily serves to determine the presence of cardiovascular abnormalities or other medical disorders that

TABLE 15.2 High risk clinical features

High risk feature	Possible diagnosis
Presyncope or syncope	Hemodynamically significant and potentially serious arrhythmia (Ventricular tachycardia)
	Valvular heart disease (Aortic stenosis)
	Structural heart disease (Hypertrophic cardiomyopathy)
Chest pain/angina	Myocardial ischemia (either primary or precipitated by increased oxygen demand from a tachyarrhythmia)
Family history of sudden cardiac death	Cardiomyopathy, long QT-syndrome

may be associated with palpitations. A careful cardiovascular examination may reveal murmurs, extra heart sounds or cardiac enlargement. Identification of a midsystolic click suggests mitral valve prolapsed, a condition commonly associated with palpitations due to supraventricular arrhythmia, ventricular premature contractions or non-sustained ventricular tachycardia. The presence of a harsh holosystolic murmur at the left sternal border that increases with Valsalva maneuver suggests hypertrophic obstructive cardiomyopathy. Identification of an extra heart sound (S3) or displaced and diffuse point of maximal impulse (PMI) provides clinical evidence of a dilated cardiomyopathy and heart failure which raise the possibility of ventricular tachycardia as well as atrial fibrillation. These findings warrant an echocardiogram to define patient's cardiac structure and function. In patients who report palpitations with exercise, a brisk walk in the office may provide adequate sympathetic activation and increased catecholamines to reveal an arrhythmia or unmask a murmur exacerbated by increased heart rate and cardiac output. Finally, the broader physical exam should include inspection for thyrotoxicosis (goiter, nervousness, heat intolerance), evidence of illicit drug use or presence of other serious illness that may be culprit.

12-Lead Electrocardiogram (ECG)

A 12-lead ECG evaluation is indicated in all patients who complain of palpitations. If the patient is experiencing palpitations at the time of the ECG the physician may be able to confirm the diagnosis of arrhythmia. Absent active palpitations the ECG can still provide insight into underlying structural and electrical abnormalities that could precipitate arrhythmias. The presence of a short PR interval and delta waves suggest ventricular preexcitation and predisposes a patient to supraventricular tachycardia (Wolff–Parkinson–White syndrome) [4]. Left ventricular hypertrophy with deep septal Q waves in I, aVL and V4 through V6 suggests hypertrophic obstructive cardiomyopathy. Left ventricular hypertrophy and left atrial enlargement indicated by a negative terminal P-wave in V1 > 40 ms in duration suggests a patient is predisposed to atrial fibrillation [4]. The presence of Q waves in two or more contiguous leads is consistent with prior myocardial infarction and warrants a more extensive search for non-sustained or sustained ventricular tachycardia. A prolonged QT interval and abnormal T-wave morphology may suggest the presence of a congenital long-QT syndrome (Fig. 15.1). Any bradycardia can be accompanied by ventricular premature depolarizations causing the perception of palpitations. Complete heart block in particular can be associated with ventricular premature depolarizations or a prolonged QT interval and torsades de pointes.

Laboratory Testing

There exists no evidence based guidelines to direct the use of laboratory testing in the evaluation of patients with palpitations. However, limited testing to rule out anemia and infection (complete blood count), electrolyte imbalance (chemistry panel) and thyroid dysfunction (TSH) is reasonable. Consider toxicology screening as guided by clinical suspicion.

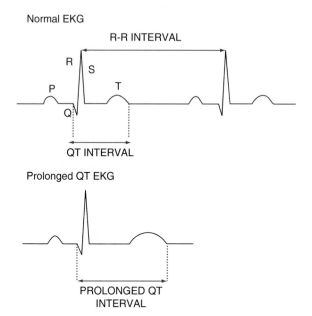

Fig. 15.1 Normal vs. Prolonged QT Interval

Expanded Diagnostic Evaluation

Most patients with palpitations do not have a life threatening condition. In patients at low risk for coronary heart disease who have non-sustained palpitations without associated symptoms such as dizziness or syncope, a negative physical examination and unremarkable ECG findings, no further evaluation is required in most cases. However, patients with recurrent symptoms may suffer from decreased quality of life. If symptoms persist, are poorly tolerated or the patient needs the reassurance of a documented benign cause of their palpitations use of ambulatory monitoring is a reasonable next step. Further diagnostic testing should be pursued in patients when the initial diagnostic evaluation (history, physical examination, ECG) suggests an arrhythmic cause and in those who are at high risk for an arrhythmia. High risk patients who need ECG monitoring include those with organic heart disease or any myocardial abnormality that could predispose them to arrhythmias [13]. ECG evidence of myocardial scar from prior myocardial infarction, idiopathic dilated cardiomyopathy, clinically significant regurgitant or stenotic valves and hypertrophic cardiomyopathies all are associated with the development of ventricular tachycardia and require ambulatory monitoring [4]. Patients with a family history of arrhythmia, syncope, or sudden death may also be at higher risk and likewise warrant ambulatory monitoring.

Ambulatory Monitoring

The expanded diagnostic work-up of patients with persistent symptoms, documented arrhythmia or those considered "high risk" should begin with ambulatory monitoring. Ambulatory ECG monitoring devices record the heart's electrical activity over a prespecified time period in the outpatient setting. When appropriately utilized they are an immensely useful tool in the diagnosis of palpitations. The duration of data collection and the invasiveness of the recording device spans a broad range with specific indications and diagnostic yields for each type presented below.

Continuous ECG Monitors

The Holter monitor continuously and simultaneously records two or three electrocardiographic leads for a monitoring period of 24 or 48 h while the patient keeps a diary detailing the timing and characteristics of symptoms. Analysis of the recording allows diagnosis of an arrhythmia while correlation with the symptoms diary helps to establish a clinical cause and effect relationship. Often Holter monitors can identify asymptomatic arrhythmias of little or no clinical significance. Holter monitors typically are the most expensive of the monitoring devices due to their continuous data collection requiring timely analysis. In addition they are limited by the short duration of monitoring and as a result have a diagnostic yield ranging from 33% to 35% [13].

Continuous Loop Event Monitors

Continuous-loop event monitors record data continuously but only save data for the preceding and subsequent 2 min after the patient manually activates the monitor. This reliance on the patient to trigger data acquisition means asymptomatic arrhythmias or those occurring during sleep go uncaptured. Loop recorders which are smaller than Holter monitors, may be worn for longer periods of time (typically 2 weeks) and the event driven nature of the recording provides a more focused, relevant data stream [19]. Consequently, event recorders provide a higher diagnostic yield (ranging from 66–83%) and achieve better cost efficacy than Holter Monitors [13, 14, 19]. One prospective trial showed that 87% of patients had diagnostic transmissions within the first 2 weeks of using a transtelephonic event monitor [14]. Patients must have the mental and physical ability to activate the loop recorder and therefore loop recorders may not be the diagnostic modality of choice when attempting to elucidate the etiology of palpitations that are associated with syncopal episodes.

Implantable Loop Recorder

An implantable loop recorder (ILR) is the most invasive ambulatory ECG monitor but provides the longest, most robust data stream. The ILR is a subcutaneous monitoring device implanted on the left anterior chest wall that stores events when the device is activated automatically by programmed criteria or manually by magnet application. An ILR may be used in selected patients with infrequent, symptomatic palpitations or those with unexplained syncope.

Selection of an Ambulatory Monitoring Device

The appropriate selection of an ambulatory ECG monitoring device relies on prudent clinical judgment made in the context of the patient's description of their palpitations. Holter monitoring for 24–48 h is most appropriate in patients who have daily palpitations. A review of six studies of patients with palpitations found Holter monitors had a diagnostic yield of 33–35% compared to 66–83% for transtelephonic event monitors [15]. An implantable loop recorder should only be utilized by a cardiologist for the electrophysiologic evaluation of particularly cryptogenic palpitations.

Stepwise Diagnostic Approach to Palpitations

The evaluation of patients with palpitations always begins with a thorough history, physical examination and 12-lead electrocardiography. In patients with no evidence of heart disease and non-sustained, well-tolerated palpitations reassurance *or* ambulatory monitoring is appropriate. If the palpitations are sustained or poorly tolerated, ambulatory monitoring is indicated. If the initial evaluation suggests organic heart disease and the palpitations are non-sustained, ambulatory monitoring is recommended. If the palpitations are sustained or poorly tolerated (suggesting hemodynamic instability) and there is evidence of heart disease, an urgent referral to a cardiologist for an electrophysiologic study is warranted [4].

Management of Palpitations

If a patient is diagnosed with a noncardiac, psychiatric, or nonarrhythmic cardiac etiology of palpitations, the underlying condition is managed according to the diagnosis [13]. In patients with arrhythmia-induced palpitations, the most common arrhythmias diagnosed on ambulatory monitoring is benign atrial or ventricular ectopic beats associated with normal sinus rhythm [14, 16]. A significant proportion of patients with palpitations have ventricular premature contractions or episodes of non-sustained ventricular tachycardia that in the setting of a structurally normal heart are not associated with increased mortality [17]. In this instance the caregiver should provide education and reassure the patient the diagnosis is not life threatening. Patients should be advised to abstain from caffeine, stimulants, alcohol, herbal supplements and foods or stressful situations known to trigger or potentiate the palpitations. If frequent supraventricular or ventricular ectopy causes significant symptoms, treatment with a beta blocker may be initiated. Antiarrhythmic medications should not be used as first line therapy given the potential proarrhythmic effect. Antiarrhythmic medications may be a reasonable therapy if the cause of a patient's palpitations is determined to be from documented atrial fibrillation or atrial tachycardia. Coronary and organic heart disease should be ruled out before the administration of any antiarrhythmic drug. The identification of sustained supraventricular or ventricular arrhythmias palpitations warrants referral to a specialist for pharmacologic or invasive electrophysiologic management of arrhythmias [4]. Most regular supraventricular tachycardias and an increasing portion of ventricular tachycardias can be treated and cured with radiofrequency ablation [18].

Summary

In the overwhelming majority of outpatients with a complaint of palpitations the cause is benign and extensive, costly investigation is unwarranted. A detailed history and physical exam with special attention to high risk characteristics can identify the subset of patients at risk for serious cardiac causes of palpitations who warrant more extensive diagnostic investigation.

References

1. Mayou R, Sprigings D, Birkhead J, Price J. Characteristics of patients presenting to a cardiac clinic with palpitation. QJM. 2003;96(2):115–23.
2. Extra heart beats: usually benign…but not always. Harv Heart Lett. 2001;11(17):5–6.
3. Kroenke K, Arrington ME, Mangelsdorff AD. The prevalence of symptoms in medical outpatients and the adequacy of therapy. Arch Intern Med. 1990;150:1685.

4. Zimetbaum P, Josephson ME. Evaluation of patients with palpitations. N Engl J Med. 1998;338:1369.
5. Weber BE, Kapoor WN. Evaluation and outcomes of patients with palpitations. Am J Med. 1996;100:138–48.
6. Mayou R, Sprigings D, Birkhead J, Price J. Characteristics of patients presenting to a cardiac clinic with palpitation. QJM. 2003;96:115.
7. Josephson ME, Wellens HJJ. Differential diagnosis of supraventricular tachycardia. Cardiol Clin. 1990;8:411–42.
8. Barsky AJ, Cleary PD, Coeytaux RR, Ruskin JN. Psychiatric disorders in medical outpatients complaining of palpitations. J Gen Intern Med. 1994;9:306–13.
9. Varma N, Josephson ME. Therapy of "idiopathic" ventricular tachycardia. J Cardiovasc Electrophysiol. 1997;8:104–16.
10. Coumel P. Clinical approach to paroxysmal atrial fibrillation. Clin Cardiol. 1990;13:209–12.
11. Zipes DP, Jalife J, editors. Cardiac electrophysiology: from cell to bedside. Philadelphia: W.B. Saunders; 1995. p. 788–811.
12. Yalamanchili, Madhuri et al. Evaluation of Palpitations: Etiology and Diagnostic Methods. Hosp Physician 2003;53–8.
13. Abbott A. Diagnostic approach to palpitations. Am Fam Physician. 2005;71:743–50.
14. Kinlay S, Leitch JW, Neil A, Chapman BL, Hardy DB, Fletcher PJ, et al. Cardiac event recorders yield more diagnoses and are more cost-effective than 48-hour holter monitoring in patients with palpitations. A controlled clinical trial. Ann Intern Med. 1996;124(1 pt 1):16–20.
15. Zimetbaum PJ, Josephson ME. The evolving role of ambulatory monitoring in general clinical practice. Ann Intern Med. 1999;130: 848–56.
16. Zimetbaum PJ, Kim KY, Josephson ME, Goldberger AL, Cohel DJ. Diagnostic yield and optimal duration of continuous-loop event monitoring for the diagnosis of palpitations. A cost-effectiveness analysis. Ann Intern Med. 1998;128:890–5.
17. Kennedy HL, Whitlock JA, et al. Long-term follow-up of asymptomatic healthy subjects with frequent and complex ventricular ectopy. N Engl J Med. 1985;312:193–7.
18. Guidelines for Clinical Intracardiac Electrophysiological and Catheter Ablation Procedures. A report of the American College of Cardiology/American Heart Association Task Force on practice guidelines. (Committee on Clinical Intracardiac Electrophysiologic and Catheter Ablation Procedures). Developed in collaboration with the North American Society of Pacing and Electrophysiology. Circulation 1995; 92:673.
19. Zimetbaum PJ, Kim KY, Ho KK, Zebede J, Josephson ME, Goldberger AL. Utility of patient-activated cardiac event recorders in general clinical practice. Am J Cardiol. 1997;79:371–2.

Chapter 16
New Murmur

Angelo J. Pedulla and Bryan Henry

Introduction

The stethoscope is a symbol that has universally represented the physician for centuries. It is a tool that embodies what "doctoring" has been perceived to be by many. The ausculta- tion of the heart and its components, in conjunction with the other portions of the physical exam, allows us to integrate the data obtained from each sense. Compilation of this data yields a working diagnosis and ultimately, a plan of care. As medicine has been infused with complicated, advanced, and often expensive testing, the stethoscope has remained a simple and effective device. In the right hands, it yields vast amounts of information regarding myocardial, pericardial, vascular, and valvular function. It is worn with pride by caregivers as a constant, connecting the plight of the past with successes of today.

This chapter is designed to provide a general understanding of the sounds of the cardiovascular system, most notably the

A.J. Pedulla (✉)
Department of Cardiology,
University of Rochester Medical Center, Rochester, NY, USA
e-mail: angelo_pedulla@urmc.rochester.edu

B. Henry
Department of Cardiology, Finger Lakes Cardiology Associates,
University of Rochester, NY, USA

J.D. Bisognano et al. (eds.), *Manual of Outpatient Cardiology*, 407
DOI 10.1007/978-0-85729-944-4_16,
© Springer-Verlag London Limited 2012

murmur. Our aim is to generate a reference for the provider to formulate a differential diagnosis of findings and to identify pathology from physiology. These skills are introduced very early in training, but often require the length of a career to master.

What Is a Murmur?

A murmur results from audible vibrations caused by increased turbulence over a region of variable flow. This sound is created from high blood flow rate through normal or abnormal orifices, forward flow through a narrowed or irregular orifice into a dilated vessel or chamber, or backward (regurgitant) flow through an incompetent valve. The onset and cessation of the sound represent initiation and termination of physiologic pressure differences across the vascular beds.

M Leannec was credited with the invention of the primitive stethoscope near the beginning of the nineteenth century. Its birth came out of necessity as a young woman in with "diseased heart" was "laboring under general symptoms". Her large habitus limited the yield of manual palpation and percussion, which were the main instruments for examination at the time. And, with direct auscultation of a young woman being inadmissible at that time, he was forced to apply a rolled up pile of papers to her chest. With his ear applied to the other end, he was able to hear "more clear and distinct" than ever before [1]. Nine years later, a 21 year old physician named William Stokes (of the Cheyne-Stokes emponym), wrote the first textbook in auscultation, *An Introduction to the Use of the Stethoscope* [2]. From then on, the use of auscultation has continued to develop into one of the most important tools doctors have today.

Most patients with valvular heart disease were diagnosed through the auscultation of a murmur. While there is obviously variations in technical skill between providers, evidence suggests that auscultation yields an approximately 70% sensitivity and 98% specificity for the detection of significant valvular disease [3]. Both positive and negative predictive values ranged as high as 92% when compared to the gold-standard, transesophageal echocardiography.

Describing a Murmur

The more detail that goes into describing a murmur the more narrow a differential diagnosis will be. Paying particular attention to the salient features that accompany these sounds will be the key to correct identification. Historically, each murmur's description is accompanied with its characteristic timing, shape, grade, pitch, quality, location, and associated features. Routine inclusion of these findings is also useful in the surveillance of known valvular disease.

Timing

The timing of a murmur with systole and diastole is one of the main keys to identifying its origin. The onset of S1 (closing of the atrioventricular valves) classically signifies the onset of systole, while S2 (closing of the semilunar valves) marks the beginning of diastole. We have all been trained to use the radial pulse when auscultating in an attempt to decipher S1 from S2. Using the onset of the carotid upstroke is another way to make this distinction. S1, the onset of systole, will produce an ejection jet out of the ventricle and into the aorta. This movement of blood obviously precedes the transfer of forces to the more distal carotid arteries. Therefore S1 will occur just before the carotid upstroke, which is then followed by S2. Also, typically S2 is louder than S1 when auscultation points are more superior. This coincides with more direct contact with the closure of aortic and pulmonic valves [4]. Similarly, S1 is louder than S2 more apically as the mitral and tricuspid closures are anatomically closer.

The identification of these two sounds can be difficult in patients that are tachycardic, have electrical abnormalities, additional heart sounds, or other pathology altering their genesis.

Further classification into its relation to the timing of systole or diastole (early, mid, late, throughout) is also helpful in the diagnosis. We will review common findings of each time-frame later in the chapter.

Shape

Shape refers to the configuration of a murmur as its amplitude is expressed over time. The classical descriptors are crescendo, decrescendo, crescendo-decrescendo, and plateau.

Crescendo: a murmur that grows louder

Decrescendo: a murmur that becomes softer

Crescendo-decrescendo: a murmur that becomes louder, then softer

Plateau: a murmur with a fixed intensity throughout

Grade

The accepted grading of murmurs was initially described in 1933 by Samuel A. Levine [5]. Simply put, a grade I murmur is only heard after several seconds of auscultation. A grade II murmur is faint, but heard immediately. A grade III murmur is moderately loud. A grade IV murmur is loud with a palpable thrill. A grade V murmur can be heard with only the edge of the stethoscope on the chest. And, a grade VI murmur is heard without contact between the stethoscope and the skin. While grade is an important descriptor of a murmur, it does not necessarily correlate with severity.

Pitch and Quality

Pitch and quality are subjective interpretations of the murmur's character. Pitch is typically described as high, medium, or low. It is a marker of the frequencies of sound waves created by the flow. The higher the frequency, the higher the pitch will be. Quality refers to the idiosyncratic sounds generated such as blowing, harsh, rumbling, or musical sounds.

Location

While "normal" locations can vary from patient to patient, we recommend paying particular attention to the cardiac geography when listening to the chest. Placing the stethoscope directly over the desired structure is often not optimal due to overlying cardiac and chest walls. Often, just distal to flow pattern will yield the best results. This means at the second right sternal intercostal space for the aortic valve, second left sternal intercostal space for pulmonic valve, fifth right or left sternal intercostal space for the tricuspid valve, and fifth intercostal space at the mid-clavicular line for the mitral valve. Other places of interest for diagnosis ventricular septal defects, myxomas, or hypertrophic cardiomyopathy will be discussed later.

Associated Features

Radiation: Since blood vessel or chamber has a fixed volume and is organized in a series of circuits, the transmission of turbulent flow will move distally. In other words, the turbulence of flow will also move with blood flow. Therefore murmurs can be followed from their origin towards the pathway of flow. The orientation and angulation of structures where the murmur begins will also contribute to the pattern of distribution. This can be of help in describing and distinguishing murmurs.

Dynamic maneuvers designed to augment certain features of murmurs can be quickly performed when abnormalities are found. Several maneuvers and pharmacologic agents have been given to exploit pressure changes, which can narrow the diagnosis. Practically however, these maneuvers ultimately do one of two things: change right-sided volume or change left-sided volume. An increase in chamber volume will typically amplify the sound of pathology present, while decrease in volume should do the opposite. Historically, pharmacologic agents such as amyl nitrate and norepinephrine have been administered, but this is now impractical. More simply, right and left sided volumes can be manipulated through deep inspiration, position change, Valsalva maneuvers, and hand-gripping. A more complete physiologic review will be provided later in the chapter.

General Characteristics of Murmurs – Benign Versus Significant?

There is a high prevalence of functional flow. Studies estimate that murmurs can be detected in 60% of the general population. Of these patients, over 90% had a subsequently normal echocardiogram [6]. These "innocent" murmurs can be readily identified by location, grading, onset, and use of dynamic maneuvers.

Features of Innocent Murmurs [7]

- Location typically near left sternal border
- Grade <3
- Systolic ejection pattern
- Absence of other abnormal sounds
- Absence of hypertrophy
- Absence of increase with Valsava or position change

These murmurs are common in younger patients, pregnancy, anemia, and other high-output states.

The timing of the murmur with respect to the cardiac cycle is often a clue as to whether or not it represents a pathologic condition. For example, many systolic murmurs represent normal physiology, while diastolic continuous murmurs virtually always signify an underlying pathological condition. These require further cardiac evaluation. Other associated findings and symptoms would also suggest additional work-up as needed. The presence of angina, syncope, or heart failure should prompt further testing regardless of character or onset.

Imaging

ACC/AHA Recommendations for Echocardiography with Murmurs

Class I All evidence level C (should be done)	Diastolic murmurs
	Continuous murmurs
	Holosystolic murmurs
	Mild peaking systolic murmurs
	> or = Grade 3
	Presence of an ejection click
	Radiation into neck or back
	Any murmur with symptoms of ischemia, heart failure, syncope, systemic embolism, or suspected endocarditis
Class IIa All evidence level C (consider doing)	Murmur with abnormal ECG findings
	Murmur with abnormal chest x-ray finding
	Presence of other cardiac findings on physical examination (RV heave, displaced or sustained impulse, additional heart sounds, altered S1/S2 character
	Potential of cardiac cause not excluded
Class III All evidence level C (should not be done)	Grade 2 or less
	Diagnosis of innocent or functional murmur made at bedside

Some common questions we are asked pertain to the usage of transesophageal echocardiography, or TEE. This modality requires intubation of the esophagus and stomach, providing a detailed view of posterior cardiac anatomy and the aorta. The lack of interfering bone, cartilage, skeletal muscle, and subcutaneous tissue allows the sound waves to come in more direct contact with the heart. This yields a very clear view of semilunar and atrioventricular valves, the left atrium, and the aorta from root to descending. It is a much better test at defining pathology in these structures and is a test of choice if a diagnosis is not made with transthoracic echocardiography. It is helpful for diagnsosing valvular disease, endocarditis, aortic dissection, septal defects, or intracardiac thrombus. As a general rule, new, concerning murmurs should be assessed with transthoracic imaging first. Further discussion regarding TEE will be addressed in chapter 3 Echocardiography.

General Discussion About Possible Pathologies

Forming a Differential

Integrating the characteristics of a murmur is the key to defining its origin and ultimately its significance. One of the most recognizable ways to generate a differential diagnosis is to begin with the timing of the murmur within the cardiac cycle. When thinking about the timing we can identify a murmur and being present during systole, diastole, or both (continuous).

Murmurs in either systole and diastole can represent pathology over either the atrioventricular or semilunar valves. Regurgitant flow is produced as soon as valve closure occurs due to the increased pressure in the distal chamber. Therefore, semilunar regurgitation is heard at the onset diastole and atrioventricular regurgitation is heard at the onset of systole. One exception to this is mitral valve prolapse, which is a regurgitant murmur occurring in mid to late systole that develops after systolic pressure rises to drive a myxomatous leaflet into the left atrium. Once this occurs, backflow can then be heard.

Murmurs occurring in the mid to late cycle are produced when the pressure generated by the proximal chamber is high enough to generate turbulence over the affected valve. Therefore, murmurs of stenosis typically take some time after systolic or diastolic onset to be heard, occurring in the mid to late cycle.

The next section will provide a review of murmurs and their characteristics. Most of this pathology can be diagnosed at the bedside with a trained ear. To best organize them and to entrain a systematic way of identifying them, we elected to organize based on timing with the cardiac cycle.

Systolic Murmurs

Systolic murmurs are classified according to time of onset (early, mid, late, throughout) and component of termination (A2 or P2 due to whether on right or left side of heart). To further narrow the differential diagnosis, we elect to first identify the murmur in this way. This usually represents movement of blood across the semilunar valves and terminates with cessation of that flow.

Mid-systolic murmurs: Begins after S1 and terminates after S2.

Aortic stenosis: This is one of the simplest and most important diagnoses to make on the auscultory exam. Aortic stenosis is classically described as a systolic, crescendo-decrescendo murmur heard best at the right upper sternal borders (second intercostal space). A thrill can sometimes be palpated over this area. It typically radiates with the aorta into the carotid arteries. Much has been described about the characterization of the severity of disease based on its features and other associated findings.

- Parvus et tardus: The "slow and late" pulse is best appreciated with manual palpation of the carotid pulse and is a marker of more severe disease.
- S2 intensity: As the aortic valve leaflets become more diseased, they open less during systole. The softer A2 component of S2 reflects less velocity or impact of their closure. In some severe cases A2 can be entirely absent.
- Timing of peak: A larger gradient between the aorta and left ventricle will require more time and pressure to achieve forward flow through a stenotic valve. Therefore, the later in systole the peak murmur is appreciated, the more severe it typically is.

- Heart failure findings: Examples such as rales, S3, reduced PMI, or a sustained apical impulse can represent stigmata of severe aortic valve disease.

Aortic sclerosis is caused by the fibrocalcific confinement to the base with no restriction of the cusps. Therefore, they move freely without obstruction. This is the most common of mid-systolic murmurs and typically requires echocardiography to visualize absence of restricted movement. With severely calcified valves, the murmur can be transmitted towards the apex of the heart, possibly mistaking a murmur of aortic stenosis with one of mitral regurgitation. This is referred to as the Gallavardian phenomenon.

Pulmonic stenosis: This is typically a "harsh" murmur heard best over the second intercostal space left of the sternum with radiation into the left neck. A palpable thrill, split second heart sound, and diminished P2 component are often present. Severity correlates well with the duration of the murmur [2]. This can be best identified with its relation to A2. If the murmur persists past A2, it is typically in the mild to moderate range. Murmurs that extend after A2 are often more severe.

Outflow obstruction: This phenomenon is typically left-sided resulting from fixed stenosis over the valvular, subvalvular, or supravlalvular apparatus. Often the site of stenosis is difficult to differentiate on exam, however, subtle clues can be present. Valvular obstruction is most common with aortic stenosis (as described above). With supravalvular stenosis, the maximal intensity may be slightly higher than the right second interspace with greater radiation into the right carotid artery. Subaortic obstruction, typically from hypertrophic cardiomyopathy can be difficult to localize due to the lack of radiation and variable location within the ventricular cavity.

Murmurs of increased flow: Short soft mid-systolic murmurs can be "normal" due to transfer of rapid ejection of blood with pregnancy, fever, thyrotoxicosis, or anemia. They can also be due to neighboring pathology such as severe aortic insufficiency or atrial septal defects.

Still's murmur: A soft murmur heard over the precordium in children, thought to be due to the vibration of leaflets in the pulmonary trunk. It is also characterized as a benign or innocent murmur.

Holosystolic murmurs: Starts with S1 and terminates into S2. There are three significant settings where this occurs, mitral regurgitation, tricuspid regurgitation, and ventricular septal defects. The sounds occur from blood leaving a higher pressure chamber, entering into a lower system.

Mitral regurgitation: This is typically high pitched, of variable intensity, and best in the mid-clavicular space with the patient in the left lateral decubitus position. The radiation can also be variable with the jet projection dependent upon the affected leaflet and segments. With anterior leaflet incompetence, a posterolateral jet will often be heard in the axilla or inferior angle of the left scapula. If the posterior leaflet is insufficient, the murmur will typically radiate anteromedially along the aorta. This can often make the distinction of mitral regurgitation and aortic disease difficult. Decreases in the carotid pulse or S2, along with increased intensity after a pause (premature ventricular contraction or atrial fibrillation) support aortic stenosis. Along with intensity, secondary findings such as the presence of an S3, displaced apical impulse, or clinical heart failure correlate with severity.

Tricuspid regurgitation: Tricuspid murmurs are typically best appreciated over the lower left sternal border, are typically high pitched, and radiate inferiorly towards the cardiac apex and even epigastrium. This pattern and respiratory variability are its hallmark. Carvallo's sign refers to the increase in intensity with inspiration. This is due to the increased volume from more venous return as intrathoracic pressure declines. The change does not temporally correlate with inspiration, but in the subsequent 1–2 cardiac cycles. With severe right ventricular failure, the intensity of the murmur can be very soft. In this instance, other examination findings such as a prominent internal jugular v wave, pulsatile liver, or volume overload may be the only clues.

Ventricular septal defect: When VSD murmurs are isolated to systole, it represents shunting from left to right only. This usually is due to high velocity through a smaller communication and preservation of normal right-sided pressures and function. Depending on the location of the defect, the murmur can be heard from the second to fourth intercostal space along the left sternum. As VSD size increases, additional findings such as right ventricular heaves and increasing P2 components can be identified. If Eisenmeinger's phenomenon is present, then the murmur will be absent due to equalization in right and left sided pressures throughout the cardiac cycle.

Early systolic murmurs: Onset is with S1, but termination occurs before S2. These pathologies within this class include mitral and tricuspid regurgitation and ventricular septal defects where pressure between chambers is equalized (LV to LA, RV to RA, or LV to RV) prior to the termination of systole. This signifies a much more severe disease state and usually the need for emergent treatment. Since most of the flow occurs in early systole, the murmur shape is decrescendo.

Late systolic murmurs: Onset is after S1, but termination is into S2.

Mitral valve prolapse: This is by far the most common late systolic murmur. It is high pitched, begins with a click, and is typically crescendo in shape. It is best heard near the cardiac apex. Often difficult to distinguish from mid systolic murmurs, one can exploit its sensitivity to volume change to unmask the diagnosis. The intensity of the prolapse murmur is inversely proportional to left ventricular volume. With Valsalva or standing abruptly from the squatting position, preload sudden drops (and left ventricular diastolic volume), and the murmur lengthens and amplifies. Mitral valve prolapse flow can also be affected by isometric hand gripping. The sudden increase in afterload with cause more increase in left ventricular pressure, which generates a greater force against the incompetent valve. The murmur is accentuated and delayed, but the "click" remains present. The "click" and augmentation with hand-grip are important characteristics that distinguish mitral valve prolapse from the murmur of hypertrophic cardiomyopathy.

Other late systolic murmurs include tricuspid valve prolapse or papillary muscle displacement/dysfunction.

Diastolic Murmurs

Early diastolic murmurs: These begin with the second heart sound (either A2 or P2) and continue through diastole.

Aortic regurgitation: Beginning with A2 it is typically a low intensity, high-pitched, decrescendo murmur that occurs when left ventricular pressure drops below aortic. It can be difficult to elicit and is best appreciated while the patient is sitting forward during end exhalation over the right or left sternal border. It can be described as "blowing" and can radiate across the precordium or into the apex. The duration of the murmur is variable and typically proportional to severity. The exception would be acute or severe insufficiency where aortic and left ventricular pressures equalize early in diastole.

Additional features of severe and chronic aortic regurgitation have been described [8].

- Austin-Flint murmur: First described in 1862, it is a mid to late diastolic "rumble" over the mitral area reflective of turbulent antegrade flow through a prematurely closed anterior mitral leaflet secondary to high left ventricular diastolic pressures caused by severe aortic insufficiency [9]. This can also be confused with mitral stenosis, but lacks the opening "snap".
- Widening of the pulse pressure due to elevated systolic and diminished diastolic pressures (due to regurgitant volume loss)
- Water Hammer Pulse (Corrigan's Pulse): Bounding forceful and collapsing pulse due to increased pulse pressure
- Quincke's Pulse: Capillary pulsations seen with gentile distal pressure on the fingernail beds
- De Musset's Sign: Head-bobbing with each heartbeat
- Duroziez Sign: Presence of systolic murmur over the femoral artery when compressed proximally and a diastolic murmur when compressed distally.
- Müller's Sign: Visible pulsations in the uvula
- Reversed splitting of S2

Pulmonic regurgitation: Beginning with P2, it is typically from pulmonary hypertension (Graham-Steell murmur) or

Tetralogy of Fallot repair and is a high pitched, "blowing", decrescendo murmur of variable length, best appreciated at the left upper sternal border. With the Graham-Steel murmur P2 is often accentuated and can be more pronounced with inspiration. This is a contrast to a repaired tetralogy patient because pulmonary pressures should remain low.

Dock's murmur: This is a focal murmur of variable length that can rarely be appreciated over the second or third intercostal space, just lateral to the sternum. It is reflective of left anterior descending stenosis and is reversible with revascularization [10].

Mid and late diastolic murmurs: Occur after S2 and extend up to A2 or P2.

Mitral stenosis: A low-pitched, "rumbling", mid-diastolic murmur that is best heard at the left ventricular maximal impulse that represents turbulence across a narrowed mitral valve. Listening to the patient in the lateral decubitus position can increase sensitivity. It begins with an "opening snap" and its duration is typically directly proportional to severity.

Tricuspid stenosis: This is described also as a "rumbling", crescendo-decrescendo, mid-diastolic murmur, but is best appreciated along the left sternal border. Similar to tricuspid regurgitation, Carvallo's sign (increase in intensity with inspiration) can be present. It is almost universally associated with mitral stenosis, and if found independently, should concern for infection or malignancy should arise. Other associated findings on exam are enhanced internal jugular "a" wave and presystolic hepatic pulsation

Atrial myxoma: Myxomas are an uncommon finding on exam and would mimic the characteristics of either mitral or tricuspid stenosis, depending upon the affected chamber. Also called a "tumor plop", this murmur is typically diastolic, low pitched, and heard over the atrioventricular territories [11].

Continuous Murmurs

Continuous murmurs begin during systole and extend into diastole. They do not need to encompass the entire duration of either cycle to be included in this category. They represent turbulent flow from a higher pressure bed to a lower pressure, in which the gradient exists into diastole. These commonly include arteriovenous or arteropulmonary communications.

Patent ductus arteriosus: A persistent embryological communication between the aorta and the pulmonary artery. Because, aortic pressure is greater than pulmonary arterial pressure in both systole and diastole, a continuous "machine-like" murmur is heard. Auscultation is best appreciated at the upper sternal borders with a maximal intensity near S2.

Shunts, coarctation of the aorta, arteriovenous communications (ex: dialysis fistulas), coronary to pulmonary artery connections are other types of continuous murmur. A more benign continuous murmur called a "mammary soufflé" is a benign example notable during pregnancy that is a sign of increased flow to the superficial vasculature.

Physical Maneuvers and Pharmacologic Interventions [12]

Deep inspiration: Increase in right-sided volume, augmenting tricuspid and pulmonic murmurs.

Valsalva strain: Sudden decrease in preload that decreases the intensity of almost all murmurs. The exceptions are mitral valve prolapse (becomes longer and louder) and hypertrophic obstructive cardiomyopathy (becomes louder).

Standing: Also a sudden drop in preload that produces similar effects as the Valsalva strain.

Squatting: The abrupt increase and preload and afterload will typically augment most murmurs. This is the opposite of what happens with Valsalva strain and standing, producing the opposite effects (all murmur intensify, but HCM and MVP will shorten and soften). Passive leg raises can produce a similar effect.

Exercise: The increase in blood flow creates greater turbulence over normal or stenotic valves. This means accentuated stenosis murmurs.

Hand-grip: Increase in afterload, increases LV volumes, augments left-sided volume-dependent murmurs such as aortic regurgitation, mitral regurgitation, or ventricular septal defects.

Post-premature beats or atrial fibrillation: Electrical delay after premature beat or pause with atrial fibrillation will provide more time for the ventricles to fill and will likely cause greater ejection. This will augment systolic stenotic murmurs and the murmur of hypertrophic cardiomyopathy. The time delay will have no effect on the length or intensity of mitral valve prolapse.

Pharmacologic interventions: Traditionally, this has been done with inhaled amyl nitrate, which is a potent vasodilator. Vasodilatory effects are initially hypotension, then a reflex tachycardia. The decline in afterload will decrease the volume dependent murmurs murmurs such as aortic regurgitation, mitral regurgitation, or ventricular septal defects. However, the augmented stroke volume and cardiac output that follows will increase the flow over a stenotic aortic valve, increasing its intensity. The tachycardia phase will also augment mitral stenosis and right-sided murmurs.

Transient arterial occlusion: It can be achieved with external compression of both brachial arteries by increasing blood pressure cuff to 20 mmHg above systolic pressures. The increase in afterload will increase left sided volumes, thus enhancing volume dependent murmurs such as aortic regurgitation, mitral regurgitation, or ventricular septal defects.

New Murmurs in Acute Coronary Syndrome

An ischemic event can cause dysfunction of the vascular territory it supplies. When infarction of papillary muscles, the ventricular free wall, or in the interventricular septum occurs, this can be a medical emergency. Detection of this pathology can be difficult, but identifying these can expedite potential surgical intervention. All patients with suspicion of these events should receive an emergent echocardiogram.

The murmur of acute mitral regurgitation from a sudden rupture of papillary muscle or chordae tendinae can be lethal. Because the left atrium and left ventricle have free communication during diastole and systole (no valve closure), a murmur may be soft or absent. Identifying other features such as clinical heart failure, hypotension, large v waves, or the presence of an S4 can be valuable subtle clues.

Ventricular septal defects with infarction are also commonly lethal complications. As inflammation of the myocardium quells and tissue begins to necrose and thin, the incidence rises. This is why patients are at greatest risk of development 48–72 h from the event. Frequency is greatest with infarction of the left anterior descending artery territories, but posterior necrosis (whether supplied by the right coronary or left circumflex arteries) is not uncommon. The murmur is typically harsh, continuous, and radiates over a large area of the sternum and apex. If the posterior wall is affected, it can also produce mitral valve leaflet dysfunction and significant regurgitation. The dual presence may augment the systolic component of the murmur and should prompt urgent echocardiography.

Honing Skills

One of the most remarkable facts concerning murmurs is that the majority of them were first described decades and even centuries ago. It is a testament to those physicians that their findings have withstood the ever-changing field of medicine. However, we realize their shortcomings. Today's patients are larger, environments are typically with more background noise, pathology is often defined in a milder severity, and many patients have already have had echocardiography define their anatomy. However, the data gained from a thorough and integrated examination can produce as accurate a diagnosis in a much faster and cost efficient manner. It allows more regular surveillance and comparison of disease. The stethoscope can also identify pathology that may be frequently missed with echocardiography, such as pulmonic stenosis or ventricular septal defects. This skill set is learned with early training, but really does take a career to master. While practice is the key, we also recommend several websites for further training.

- http://www.merckmanuals.com/professional/resources/multimedia/name/audio.html
- http://www.med.ucla.edu/wilkes/inex.htm

References

1. Laennec RTH. De l'auscultation médiate ou traité du diagnostic des maladies des poumons et du coeur. Paris: Brosson & Chaudé; 1819 (The complete title of this book, often referred to as the 'Treatise' is *De l'Auscultation Médiate ou Traité du Diagnostic des Maladies des Poumons et du Coeur* (On Mediate Auscultation or Treatise on the Diagnosis of the Diseases of the Lungs and Heart)).
2. Perloff JK. The clinical recognition of congenital heart disease. Philadelphia: W. B. Saunders; 1994. p. 157–214.
3. Roldan CA, Bruce KS, Crawford H. Value of the cardiovascular physical examination for detecting valvular heart disease in asymptomatic subjects. Am J Cardiol. 1996;77:1327–31.
4. Bickley LS. Bates' guide to physical examination and history taking. 10th ed. Philadelphia: Lippincott Williams & Williams; 2009. p. 362–6.
5. Siverman ME, Wooley CF. Samuel A. Levine and the history of grading systolic murmurs. Am J Cardiol. 2008;102:1187.
6. Etchells E, Bell C, Robb K. Does this patient have systolic murmur ? Abnormal. JAMA. 1997;277(7):564–71.
7. Grewe K, Crawford MH, O'Rourke RA. Differentiation of cardiac murmurs by dynamic auscultation. Curr Probl Cardiol. 1988;13:669–721.
8. Libby P, Bonow RO, Mann DL, Zipes DL. Heart disease: A textbook of cardiovascular medicine. 8th ed. Philadelphia: Saunders; 2007. p. 1638–39.
9. Perloff JK. Physical examination of the heart and circulation. Shelton: People's Medical Publishing House; 2009, Chapter 6, p. 210.
10. Dock W, Zoneraich S. A diastolic murmur arising in a stenosed coronary artery. Am J Med. 1967;42(4):617–9.

11. Libby P, Bonow RO, Mann DL, Zipes DL. Braundwald's Heart disease: A textbook of cardiovascular medicine. 8th ed. Philadelphia: Saunders; 2007. p. 136.
12. ACC/AHA Guidelines for the management of patients with valvular heart disease. Am J Cardiol. 2006; 28(3):e9–11.

Chapter 17
Approach to the Patient with Dyspnea

Christopher D. Lang and Imran N. Chaudhary

Dyspnea is a common presenting symptom of cardiovascular disease in both the outpatient and inpatient setting. Despite its prevalence, the lack of specificity and variation in language used to describe sensation of shortness of breath, it poses unique diagnostic and management challenges. Often times, understanding of the underlying mechanisms of dyspnea in parallel with a focused history and exam can lead to an initial workup and differential. It is difficult to have one all-encompassing framework for evaluation of dyspnea; however, it is useful to have a general framework from which to proceed. This chapter will cover the general mechanisms of dyspnea as well as the basic workup for possible pulmonary disease causes. The focus will be specifically on dyspnea as it directly relates to diseases of the cardiovascular system.

C.D. Lang (✉)
Department of Internal Medicine,
University of Rochester Medical Center, Rochester, NY, USA
e-mail: christopher_lang@urmc.rochester.edu

I.N. Chaudhary
Department of Cardiology,
University of Rochester Medical Center, Rochester, NY, USA

J.D. Bisognano et al. (eds.), *Manual of Outpatient Cardiology*,   427
DOI 10.1007/978-0-85729-944-4_17,
© Springer-Verlag London Limited 2012

Characteristics and Mechanisms of Dyspnea

Regulation of the respiratory system comprises of a complex interaction between physiology, environmental factors, and behavioral control. Sensations from multiple areas of the cardio-pulmonary system, and the chest wall, receive information regarding respiratory status. This sensation is integrated in the brain, though different receptors and appears to cause different symptoms. These mechanisms will be explored further, along with a discussion of how alternate stimuli produce different sensation and descriptions of dyspnea.

According to the American Thoracic Society's consensus statement on dyspnea [1], the respiratory control center in the brainstem is responsible for organizing sensory information in order to maintain homeostasis. The sensation of dyspnea is associated with output from respiratory control centers which appears to provide a 'corollary' signal to the sensory cortex to stimulate a change in respiratory pattern. Dyspnea is considered to be "a mismatch between central respiratory motor activity and incoming afferent information from receptors in the airways, lungs, and chest wall structures" [1–3]. In other words, if the peripheral receptors send a signal to increase respiration, this sensation is likely to lead to dyspnea. Perception of dyspnea combined with social, behavioral and emotional factors ultimately result in the complaint of shortness of breath. This theory is often described as "neuro-mechanical" [4] dissociation.

While this theory plausibly explains the sensation of dyspnea, the mechanical and chemical triggers are extensive and varied, and often will lead to differing subjective interpretations of dyspnea. The recognized receptors implicated in maintaining regulation of the respiratory system are chemoreceptors (peripherally and centrally located), and mechanoreceptors (located in the airways, lungs and chest wall) [1].

Chemoreceptors are receptors that are stimulated by changes in PCO_2 and PO_2 levels. The centrally located chemorecepters are found in the medulla. Peripherally located chemoreceptors are found in the aortic arch and carotid bodies. There is direct evidence that increase of PCO_2 as sensed by the chemoreceptors can lead to subjective perception of dyspnea [5]. Similarly, research suggests hypoxia can stimulate dyspnea, presumably by chemoreceptor stimulation [6].

Mechanoreceptors are more diverse than chemoreceptors in their ability to sense various stimuli. These receptors are located in the airways, lungs and the chest wall. Upper airway temperature receptors respond by altering the subjective sensation of dyspnea. When air is cold, dyspnea is reduced [7]. In the lungs, the multiple pulmonary mechanoreceptors exist. The three main types are: pulmonary stretch receptors, Irritant receptors, and C-fibers. Pulmonary stretch receptors are stimulated by increased airway tension, acting as a surrogate for lung volume. The sensation that arise from these receptors is suspected to be the driving force between asthma related dyspnea.

Irritant receptors are located in the bronchial walls, and respond to irritation of the bronchial mucosa by touch, air, or smooth muscle constriction. C-fibers are located in near alveoli in the pulmonary parenchyma, and are stimulated by increases in pressure. Chest wall receptors, comprised of spindle and tendon organs, respond to restricted chest wall movements, and work in combination with pulmonary and chemoreceptors in sensing dyspnea in restrictive lung diseases [8].

Impaired oxygen delivery plays a significant role in perception of dyspnea, despite not being necessarily cardiac or pulmonary related. Anemia is a case where normal oxygen exchange takes place, but dyspnea is experienced. Hypotheses exist to describe why this occurs, including development of interstitial edema with sensation by J-fibers, along with reduced metabolic activity of key respiratory muscles, leading to development of acidosis. However, the exact mechanism remains unclear. Deconditioning can also lead to dyspnea. General deconditioning leads to exercise intolerance and quicker incidence of progressing to anaerobic metabolism during low levels of exercise. This often occurs in patients with significant COPD and those with a sedentary lifestyle. These patients are often symptomatically improved after undergoing outpatient exercise programs. Further areas with difficult physiologic interaction include the toxic ingestion, chronic dyspnea, anxiety, depression, which appear to have a significant behavioral component in addition to mechanisms noted above [9].

In summary, dyspnea is due to a dissociation between physiologic stimuli and the brain's sensation to increase respiration. The main receptors involved sensation are chemoreceptors, that sense oxygenation and carbon dioxide, and mechanical receptors that can sense stretch or the lung, inflammation and chest wall movement.

Initial Approach to the Dyspneic Patient

This section will provide a general framework for approaching dyspnea with focus on determination of the cardiac causes of dyspnea.

History

The multiple underlying mechanisms of dyspnea illustrate the varied patient presentation that is seen in the clinical setting. Further the "language of dyspnea," or the subjective experience of dyspnea, lends towards even greater variation in descriptions of shortness of breath [10]. It is critical to begin by obtaining a complete history with focus on several key factors important in the evaluation of dyspnea. Initially, a patient presenting with a chief complaint of dyspnea must be evaluated for life threatening causes. These are generally acute in onset, from minutes to hours. Basic screening for life threatening causes such as acute coronary syndromes, pneumothorax, tamponade are requisite, but generally can be disclosed with basic vital signs, and focused history and exam. After these causes are ruled out, further evaluation can proceed. There is an extensive amount of research regarding the language of dyspnea. Born from this, several categories of terminology have been defined to highlight the variable reports of subjective dyspnea [1].

There are several different categories of subjective language gleaned from research questionnaires regarding patient reports of dyspnea. The term "air hunger" refers to patients who subjectively feel the need to inspire. In normal subjects, this sensation arose both from hypercapnea and restricted thoracic motion, and is often found in patients who have CHF and bronchoconstriction. "Chest tightness" is also found often in cases of bronchoconstriction. CHF is also associated with a description of "suffocation." Increased work of breathing has been linked to ILD, COPD, and neurologic diseases. Cardiovascular deconditioning and anemia often produce deep heavy breathing [10–13].

In addition to identifying key subjective terms, it is necessary to define the further aspects of the history of dyspnea. In particular, duration, severity, associating and relieving factors are all important aspects of the initial evaluation. Past medical history does help to identity future clues. For example, the positive likelihood ratio for a CHF exacerbation in a patient with a history of COPD is 0.81, whereas a previous history of CHF has a positive likelihood ratio of 5.8 [14]. Further exploration of social history is important in eliciting potential causes for a patients dyspnea. Deconditioning can be present in the patient who is sedentary, smoking is a clear predictor of underlying pulmonary disease. Drug use, such as cocaine, can be related to dyspnea through several different mechanisms. Medication effect can directly cause a sensation of dyspnea (such as opioids) and can indirectly cause dyspnea if patients are not compliant or recently stopped taking requisite medications (such as lasix for fluid overload, or brochodilators for COPD) [15].

Physical Examination and Testing

The physical exam plays an important role in evaluating the dyspneic patient. With many diagnostic possibilities, careful consideration during the exam can help narrow the differential. Key elements to evaluate include inspection of the upper airways. JVD should always be assessed, as this can point to elevated pressure in the venous system, which is important in multiple cardiac causes of dyspnea. Full cardiac and pulmonary exams are also components of the workup.

After basic evaluation, formulating a hypothesis of whether there is primary cardiac, pulmonary, or neurologic pathology is useful. However, it is often difficult to pinpoint one organ system or one leading hypothesis. Additionally multiple systems may be impacted simultaneously.

Initially, laboratory testing may be of benefit. Basic labs can indicate the elevated CO_2 levels, acidosis and electrolyte abnormalities. Identification of anemia is useful and can be done by checking a complete blood panel. Patients who are dyspneic because of anemia will generally improve when the anemia is corrected. An EKG can give insight into underlying heart rhythms, as well as pericardial disease and occasionally PE. Troponin testing to evaluate for myocardial ischemia is important, especially in atypical presentations of MI such as dyspnea.

Recently, the use of BNP and nt-pro-BNP has been purported as test to rapidly separate dyspnea due to CHF versus other, predominately pulmonary, causes. The studies evaluating BNP were completed in the context of evaluating patients with dyspnea, and posted a *sensitivity* of 90% and a *specificity* of 76% for patients eventually found to be in heart failure [16]. Several drawbacks exist to using this modality in the evaluation of dyspnea. Of patients who do have CHF, heart failure may not be the primary or only cause. Since CHF remains a clinical diagnosis, it is unlikely that a patient would not be treated for CHF if symptomatically considered to be in heart failure. BNP, especially nt-pro-BNP, is significantly impacted by renal failure and age. In patients who have low BNPs, CHF still may be an active issue, as BNP may not reflect acute pulmonary edema [17]. This topic is controversial, and remains at the discretion of individual providers to decide whether BNP would be a useful adjunct in the context of a patient's presenting symptoms [18].

A standard chest X-ray has several roles in identifying causes of dyspnea. A CXR has ability to identify pulmonary disease, pneumonia, pulmonary edema, and a variety of other diseases that may contribute to dyspnea. Chest X-ray should be obtained in most cases of dyspnea. CT scan of the chest can be utilized during evaluation for pulmonary embolism, and a multitude of pulmonary and vascular diseases.

Echocardiography can be used in patients who have dyspnea, suspected of being cardiac in origin. Echocardiogram has the ability to analyze valvular and wall motion abnormalities (especially under stress), pulmonary pressures, in addition to assessing systolic function. Depending on accessibility, echo can be a useful tool in assessing dyspnea [19].

Cardiopulmonary exercise testing is a modality used in situations where difficulty exists identifying the primary cause of dyspnea. This is often best applied in cases of exertional dyspnea, generally when cardiac or pulmonary disease is at early stages. In this form of testing, patients are monitored and breathing and ventilatory patterns are studied during incremental exercise. The difference in adaptation to exercise can determine whether dyspnea is caused by primary cardiac or pulmonary process [20].

Specific Cardiac Causes of Dyspnea

A majority of diseases in the cardiac system can have a component of dyspnea. This section will focus on multiple common cardiac conditions, how they cause dyspnea, and basic evaluation and management.

Congestive Heart Failure

Mechanisms of Dyspnea

There are multiple hypothesized mechanisms by which congestive heart failure can lead to dyspnea [21]. Given the wide range of physiologic and emotional factors related to this disease process, nearly all the modalities of dyspnea discussed above can be involved. Increased respiratory drive, which in turn leads to increased demand can occur from two sources in CHF. Increased LVEDP in CHF can lead to pulmonary venous congestion, which stimulates the pulmonary mechanoreceptors. This impulse is transmitted by vagal afferents to respiratory control centers, thereby sensing dyspnea. Alternatively, pulmonary venous congestion can lead to ventilation-perfusion mismatch, leading further to impaired oxygen delivery and hypoxemia. Hypoxemia can stimulate peripheral and central chemoreceptors, which is then transmitted to the respiratory center [1].

Increased work of breathing and a sense of "air hunger" likely originates from an alternate mechanism. The pathophysiology underlying this arises from increased pulmonary venous congestion, leading to reduced compliance, increased airway resistance and ultimately increased work of breathing.

Other factors that may contribute to sensation of dyspnea in CHF are weakness of respiratory muscles and psychological factors. Respiratory muscles can break down catabolically in CHF, leading to a mismatch between diminished respiratory muscle function and mechanoreceptor sensation [1, 22].

Initial Evaluation, Workup and Management

Key features of evaluating a patient with suspected CHF include clarifying the quality of dyspnea, as well the presence of orthopnea, and paroxysmal nocturnal dyspnea. Physical exam maneuvers which should be assessed include determination of JVD and evaluation of lower extremity edema. A thorough cardiopulmonary exam with careful auscultation for rales, S3 and potentially mitral regurgitation murmur depending on LV enlargement have high predictive value for CHF [21].

Major causes of CHF fall into several broad categories. Dilated cardiomyopathy leads to a primarily systolic functional impairment, and often is idiopathic, though viral causes have been well established. Ischemic cardiomyopathy is the most common cause in the US, and arises from dysfunctional myocardium after coronary ischemia. Cardiotoxic agents, including alcohol, are a potentially reversible cause of non-ischemic cardiomyopathies. Valvular diseases such as MR and AR are potential causes of underlying systolic heart failure [19].

Further workup can include EKG, Troponins, BNP, and echocardiography. This will be discussed extensively elsewhere the book.

Initial treatment depends on the severity of presentation. Initial supplemental oxygen can help overcome hypoxemia [19]. Often, judicious use of diuretic therapy can be used to promote rapid relief. Vasodilators such as nitroglycerin can be useful as well. If the patient has hemodynamic instability, inpatient admission and ionotropic support should be considered. Further treatment will be discussed in Chap. 11.

Pulmonary Hypertension

Mechanism of Dyspnea

Up to 60% of patients with pulmonary hypertension present with dyspnea, making dyspnea by far the leading symptom of this rare disease [23]. There are at least three primary mechanisms which contribute to dyspnea in this patient population. First, ventilation-perfusion mismatch stimulates pulmonary receptors which sense lack of perfusion to oxygenated alveoli. Second, acidosis frequently occurs during exertion, changing the pH, sensed by peripheral chemoreceptors. The third mechanism is hypoxemia, which occurs in some patients, either due to left to right shunt from a PFO, or reduced time for oxygen transport due to elevated pulmonary capillary pressures. This decreases pO_2 and pH, which again is sensed by chemoreceptors [24].

Overview, Initial Evaluation, Workup and Management

The gold-standard definition of pulmonary hypertension is a right heart catheterization measurement of mean pulmonary artery pressure greater than 25 mgHg. The natural history of idiopathic pulmonary hypertension caries a life expectancy of 3 years. There are five WHO classifications of Pulmonary hypertension. Class I is known as Pulmonary arterial hypertension, and includes sporadic idiopathic pulmonary hypertension, PAH due to diseases affecting the pulmonary muscular arterioles, which include connective tissue diseases and HIV. Classes II-V refer to pulmonary hypertension resulting from left heart disease, hypoxemia, thromboembolic disease, and that caused by unclear multifactorial mechanisms [25].

Initial history will generally illicit exertional dyspnea, and early fatigue, as the patient cannot increase cardiac output with exercise. The patient may describe exertional chest pain, and syncope. Edema and hepatic congestion can arise, causing lower extremity swelling and abdominal pain, which the patient may be endorse [26].

Physical exam in patients with pulmonary hypertension has several striking features. Right ventricular heave may be noted along the left sternal border. Jugular venous distension is common, notable for large positive waveforms. The second heart sound generally has an intense P2 component. Auscultation may also reveal a S4, and tricuspid regurgitation. RV failure can lead to typical exam findings of JVD, S3, as well as peripheral edema and crackles [26].

Initial workup of patients with suspected of pulmonary hypertension begins with screening at risk individuals. Connective tissue disorders, such as scleroderma, have a strong association with pulmonary hypertension. According the ACCF/AHA guidelines, the most appropriate initial test after CXR and EKG is echocardiography. Confirmation of pulmonary hypertension with a right heart catheterization is essential, and acute vasodilator testing provides useful therapeutic information. Others studies to evaluate the etiology of pulmonary hypertension are crucial to help determine additional underlying or contributing causes. PFTs can give information regarding ventilatory function and gas exchange. A sleep study may also be an important step in the workup, giving insight into sleep disorders. PH has been associated with HIV, ANA, and LFT abnormalities (point to hepatopulmonary syndrome). Functional tests, such as the

6 min walk test, can give information about functional status and prognosis [25].

Treatment of pulmonary hypertension is complex, and many new therapies are being studied. Calcium channel blockers have often been used as a modality to improve hemodynamic and clinical endpoints. However, only a subset of patients with pulmonary hypertension benefit from calcium channel blockers (based on IV vasodilator challenge). Further specialized therapies are prostacyclin anaglouge, including Epoprostinil (Flolan), Treprostinil (Remodulin), endotheline antagonists, such as Bosenten (Tracleer), and PDE-5 inhibitors like Sildenefil (Revatio), or Tadalafil (Adcirca). They have been studied and provide some experimental benefit. These therapies should be directed by experienced providers who are knowledgeable regarding side effects and titration parameters of these medications [27].

Myocardial Infarction

Mechanisms of Dyspnea

Dyspnea is not the most common presenting symptom of myocardial ischemia; however, it is associated with increased mortality when it is the chief complaint [22]. Myocardial infarction has been documented to cause diastolic dysfunction [28]. This high pressure system reflects back to the pulmonary capillaries, leading to pulmonary edema. This then can activate pulmonary "stretch" receptors to signal increased drive to breath and dyspnea. Additionally, MI can result in the rupture of chordae tendinae, and severe mitral regurgitation can led to pulmonary edema and thereby dyspnea. Further, anxiety regarding chest pain may add a behavioral component of shortness of breath in some patients.

Evaluation, Workup and Management

Dyspnea is often present in the presenting symptoms of MI, but is rarely the only symptom. If an acute coronary syndrome is suspected an EKG should be obtained as soon as possible, while a focused history is acquired. Common complaints are crushing substernal chest pain, radiation to the arm, and impending sense of doom. Associated problems include diaphoresis, nausea/vomiting, lightheadedness, palpatations, and fatigue.

The physical exam does not often assist in the diagnosis of MI, but can be usefully in ruling out other diagnoses. There are associated physical exam findings which may portend worse outcome, such as blowing systolic murmur of MR with chordae tendinae rupture, or cardiomyopathy after event [19].

Work up begins with obtaining an EKG. Evaluation for ST segment elevations, new LBBB, or other changes are important in the initial workup. Laboratory work-up is important in the setting of less than concrete EKG changes, with testing for markers of myocardial injury (such as CK-MB and troponins). Echocardiography can be a useful test in this setting, which can indicate wall motion abnormalities or valvular changes, potentially giving insight to underlying locations of coronary artery plaque rupture.

Immediate stabilization is needed in patients with myocardial infarction. Aspirin has demonstrated early mortality benefits [29]. Supplemental oxygen and nitroglycerin should be given as well. Treatment of acute MI is reperfusion as it has the greatest mortality benefit. Discussion about further diagnosis, therapy and management of acute MI will occur elsewhere in this book (see Chap. 8?) [19].

Pulmonary Embolism

Mechanisms of Dyspnea

One of the leading clinical symptoms associated with pulmonary embolism is dyspnea. Essentially, thrombi traveling from most commonly the lower extremities will proceed through the right heart to the pulmonary vasculature. Depending on the size, the clot can deposit in the periphery of the lung whereas a large clot may get stuck at the major bifurcation of the pulmonary artery. The major mechanism of dyspnea is suspected to be ventilation perfusion mismatch. This occurs in part due to vascular blockage, as well as stimulation of the irritant receptors in the pulmonary stroma, sensing inflammation from coagulation [30].

Initial Findings, Exam and Workup

Historical symptoms of PE include acute onset of dyspnea, chest pain, syncope and hemoptysis. Classically, in these patients pleuritic chest pain dyspnea and hemoptysis suggest pulmonary infarction [31]. Those who present with symptoms of sudden dyspnea, cyanosis, shock or syncope central PE should be suspected with potential of cardiovascular collapse. Initial physical exam findings are often non-specific, but are most likely to find a patient with tachypnea and/or tachycardia. Patients may have a friction rub on auscultation, though this is a rare finding [32].

Workup of pulmonary embolism is multifaceted. Wells criteria can be used for risk stratification prior to testing. Laboratory tests can be obtained, none of which are specific. Troponins can be elevated, are generally associated with right heart strain, and are associated with greater mortality and in-hospital complications. BNP may be obtained and high levels indicate RV dysfunction. ABG may be normal, but often will indicate low PaO_2 and elevated a-a gradient. CXR can demonstrate classic signs such as Westermark Sign or Hamptons hump, but these are rarely observed and non-diagnostic. EKG should be obtained in ruling out MI, but may indicate a S1Q3T3 pattern, which is the most specific finding for PE. Most commonly, ST and T wave changes that are non-specific are seen [19].

Imaging tests can give important diagnostic and prognostic information. The standard imaging technique to evaluate the presence of PE is CT imaging with contrast. The gold standard remains pulmonary angiography, but this is an invasive test with potential for complications compared with CT, for little added benefit. VQ scans remain an option in patients in whom contrast dye is contraindicated. Echocardiography has a important role in PE. In patients with suspected right ventricular dysfunction, TTE can provide a rapid assessment of RV function in these patients. Typical findings on echocardiogram include RV dilation, hypokinesis, TR, septal flattening, paradoxical septal motion, D-sign, and diastolic left ventricular displacement secondary to abnormal septal motion. Pulmonary hypertension and lack of inspiratory collapse can occur, along with potential direct visualization of the thrombus. Large PEs often have sparring of the RV apex, and free wall hypokinesis, known as McConnell's sign, and has a 71% PPV for PE [19].

Treatment of PE is highly individualized. In patients who are hemodynamically stable, the cornerstone of treatment is anticoagulation with heparin or low-molecular weight heparin. Generally heparin needs to be continued for 4–5 days at a minimum, and coumadin can be started for maintenance of long term anticoagulation. Coumadin is to be titrated to achieve an INR of 2.0–3.0, and a patient should be anticoagulated for a minimum of 3 months, though depending on the inciting cause, this could be longer, and potentially indefinitely. If a patient is hemodynamically unstable, thrombolysis and embolectomy are also potential options, both which carry risks. Thrombolysis with TPA has a benefit in patients who are hemodynamically stable, but it is unclear if patients with RV strain without hemodynamic instability are likely to benefit. Thrombolysis has an increased risk of severe bleeding associated with it and should be used with extreme caution, especially in those that are bleeding risks. Embolectomy can be sought if hemodynamic stability exists and there is a disadvantage or contraindication to thrombolysis. Further work up for causes of PE, such as hypercoagulable state can be explored as an outpatient if the patient has recurrent PE/DVT or unprovoked clot. Common hypercoagulable states include Factor V leiden mutation, Protein C, Protein S and antithrombin deficiency, antiphospholipid antibody, malignancy, and Heparin induced thrombocytopenia [19].

Valvular Disease

In general, stenosis or regurgitation of any valve, if significant enough, can produce dyspnea. The mechanisms of dyspnea vary between valves, and sometimes imply ventricular dysfunction prior to the onset of dyspnea. Mitral regurgitation, especially in the acute presentation, is the most likely to cause rapid dyspnea due to regurgitation in the pulmonary venous system. This type of dyspnea is generally present at rest, and orthopnea is likely also present. Chronic MR can lead to LV dysfunction, and be associated with exertional dyspnea, PND and orthopnea. Further, longstanding MR can lead to pulmonary hypertension. Dyspnea is also common in mitral stenosis, generally exertional and also PND, reflecting elevated pulmonary pressures. Tricuspid stenosis can produce early fatigue and potentially exertional dyspnea due to fixed cardiac output. Similarly, TR will be associated with reduced cardiac output and RV failure and sometimes be associated with dyspnea. PS will be evident over time with right sided heart failure and DOE. PR also presents like PS with DOE and RV failure. AS typically presents with angina or syncope, but LV dysfunction leads to exertional dyspnea and HF symptoms. AR will also present with symptoms of LV dysfunction and DOE if chronic, while acute AR will rapidly progress with severe SOB and cardiovascular collapse [19].

Exam, Workup and Treatment

In depth exploration of valvular disease will be presented in other chapters. Typically, these patients will present either with symptoms, a murmur or have a echocardiogram obtained for an alternate reason showing evidence of valvular disease. If valvular disease is suspected, and echocardiogram should be obtained. Treatment is specific to the valve involved and ranges from medication optimization to valve replacement.

Other Cardiovascular Causes of Dyspnea

Many other cardiac conditions exist that elicit dyspnea. Many congenital heart diseases can produce dyspnea especially at severe forms of the disease. Classically, if there is a left to right shunt, hypoxemia will occur and produce dyspnea, though development ventricular dysfunction can occur, producing dyspnea from alternative mechanisms.

Pericardial disease can also cause dyspnea. Typically constrictive pericarditis can initially progress from exercise intolerance to dyspnea on minimal exertion. Pericardial effusions can lead to lung compression and atelectasis, and thereby a mechanical form of dyspnea. Cardiac tamponade often presents with dyspnea with low cardiac output.

Aortic aneurysm can produce dyspnea depending on its location, if it is compressing on the trachea or major airways.

References

1. Dyspnea. Mechanisms, assessment, and management: a consensus statement. American Thoracic Society. Am J Respir Crit Care Med. 1999;159:321.
2. Schwartzstein RM, Simon PM, Weiss JW, Fencl V, Weinberger SE. Breathlessness induced by dissociation between ventilation and chemical drive. Am Rev Respir Dis. 1989;139:1231–7.
3. Schwartzstein RM, Manning HL, Weiss JW, Weinberger SE. Dyspnea: a sensory experience. Lung. 1990;168:185–99.
4. O'Donnell DE, Webb KA. Exertional breathlessness in patients with chronic airflow limitation. Am Rev Respir Dis. 1993;148:1351–7.
5. Banzett RB, Lansing RW, Reid MB, Adams L, Brown R. 'Air hunger' arising from increased PCO_2 in mechanically ventilated quadriplegics. Respir Physiol. 1989;76:53–67.
6. Lane R, Cockcroft A, Adams L, Guz A. Arterial saturation and breathlessness in patients with chronic obstructive airways disease. Clin Sci. 1987;72:693–8.

7. Schwartzstein RM, Lahive K, Pope A, et al. Cold facial stimulation reduces breathlessness induced in normal subjects. Am Rev Respir Dis. 1987;136:58.
8. Burki NK, Lee L. Mechanisms of dyspnea. Chest. 2010;138: 1196–201.
9. Schwartzstein R. Approach to the patient with dyspnea. In UptoDate, Basow, DS (Ed), UpToDate, Waltham, MA 2011.
10. Scano G, Stendardi L, Grazzini M. Understanding dyspnoea by its language. Eur Respir J. 2005;25:380.
11. Mahler DA, Harver A, Lentine T, et al. Descriptors of breathlessness in cardiorespiratory diseases. Am J Respir Crit Care Med. 1996;154: 1357.
12. O'Donnell DE, Bertley JC, Chau LK, Webb KA. Qualitative aspects of exertional breathlessness in chronic airflow limitation: pathophysiologic mechanisms. Am J Respir Crit Care Med. 1997;155:109.
13. Simon PM, Schwartzstein RM, Weiss JW, et al. Distinguishable types of dyspnea in patients with shortness of breath. Am Rev Respir Dis. 1990;142:1009.
14. Wang CS, FitzGerald JM, Schulzer M, Mak E, Ayas NT. Does this dyspneic patient in the emergency department have congestive heart failure? JAMA. 2005;294(15):1944–56.
15. Eurman DW, Potash HI, Eyler WR, Paganussi PJ, Beute GH. Chest pain and dyspnea related to "crack" cocaine smoking: value of chest radiography. Radiology. 1989;172(2):459–62.
16. Hosenpud JD, Greenberg BH. Congestive heart failure. 3rd ed. Philadelphia: LWW; 2006.
17. Schneider HG, Lam L, Lokuge A, et al. B-type natriuretic peptide testing, clinical outcomes, and health services use in emergency department patients with dyspnea: a randomized trial. Ann Intern Med. 2009;150:365.
18. Maisel AS, Krishnaswamy P, Nowak RM, et al. Rapid measurement of B-type natriuretic peptide in the emergency diagnosis of heart failure. N Engl J Med. 2002;347:161.
19. Griffin B, Topol E. Manual of cardiovascular medicine. 3rd ed. Philadelphia: LWW; 2009.
20. Messner-Pellenc P, Ximenes C, Brasileiro CF, Mercier J, Grolleau R, Préfaut CG. Cardiopulmonary exercise testing: determinants of dyspnea due to cardiac or pulmonary limitation. Chest. 1994;106: 354–60.
21. Braunwald E. Heart failure. In: Braunwald E, Fauci AS, Kasper DL, et al., editors. Harrison's principles of internal medicine. 15th ed. New York: McGraw-Hill; 2001. p. 1318–29.
22. Canto JG, Shlipak MG, Rogers WJ, Malmgren JA, Frederick PD, Lambrew CT, et al. Prevalence, clinical characteristics, and mortality among patients with myocardial infarction presenting without chest pain. JAMA. 2000;283(24):3223–9.

23. George RB. Chest medicine: essentials of pulmonary and critical care medicine. Philadelphia: LWW; 2005. p. 224.
24. Sun XG, Hansen JE, Oudiz RJ, Wasserman K. Exercise pathophysiology in patients with primary pulmonary hypertension. Circulation. 2001;104(4):429–35.
25. Simonneau G, Robbins IM, Beghetti M, Channick RN, Delcroix M, Denton CP, et al. Updated clinical classification of pulmonary hypertension. J Am Coll Cardiol. 2009;54(1 Suppl):S43–54.
26. Runo JR, Loyd JE. Primary pulmonary hypertension. Lancet. 2003;361(9368):1533–44.
27. McLaughlin VV, McGoon MD. Pulmonary arterial hypertension. Circulation. 2006;114:1417–31.
28. Persson H, Linder-Klingsell E, Eriksson SV, Erhardt L. Heart failure after myocardial infarction: the importance of diastolic dysfunction. A prospective clinical and echocardiographic study. Eur Heart J. 1995;16(4):496–505.
29. Randomised trial of intravenous streptokinase, oral aspirin, both, or neither among 17,187 cases of suspected acute myocardial infarction: ISIS-2. ISIS-2 (Second International Study of Infarct Survival) Collaborative Group. Lancet. 1988;2(8607):349–60.
30. Nakos G, Kitsiouli EI, Lekka ME. Bronchoalveolar lavage alterations in pulmonary embolism. Am J Respir Crit Care Med. 1998;158 (5 Pt 1):1504–10.
31. Walker HK, Hall WD, Hurst JW, editors. Clinical methods: the history, physical, and laboratory examinations. 3rd ed. Boston: Butterworths; 1990.
32. Simel DL, Rennie D. The rational clinical exam. Evidence based clinical diagnosis. 1st ed. New York: McGraw-Hill; 2009.

Chapter 18
Preoperative Cardiovascular Risk Assessment for Non-cardiac Surgery

John E. Reuter and John C. Teeters

Introduction

The purpose of preoperative evaluation is to optimize the patient's status before surgery and thereby minimize risk. Generally the most feared post-operative cardiac complications are myocardial infarction, heart failure, malignant arrhythmias, and death. Factors to consider during the preoperative evaluation are patient risk factors, patient functional capacity, and the type of surgery the patient will undergo. Patients with comorbidities such as peripheral arterial disease have higher incidences of underlying coronary artery disease and left ventricular dysfunction. Deconditioned patients also have a higher incidence of cardiac complications. Finally, certain procedures, such as vascular surgery or major thoracic and abdominal procedures, predispose to myocardial ischemia due to greater blood loss, fluid shifts, increased myocardial oxygen demand (due to increased heart

J.E. Reuter (✉)
Department of Cardiology, University of Rochester Medical Center, Rochester, NY, USA
e-mail: john_reuter@urmc.rochester.edu

J.C. Teeters
Division of Cardiology, Highland Hospital,
University of Rochester Medical Center,
Rochester, NY, USA

J.D. Bisognano et al. (eds.), *Manual of Outpatient Cardiology*,   445
DOI 10.1007/978-0-85729-944-4_18,
© Springer-Verlag London Limited 2012

rate and blood pressure), and increased post-operative plate-let reactivity.

History, Physical Exam, and EKG

The interview should determine whether the patient has any history of coronary artery disease, myocardial infarction, angina, peripheral arterial disease, congestive heart failure, valvular disease, and/or arrhythmias. Whether the patient has a pacemaker or implantable cardioverter defibrillator (ICD) is also important for intra-operative management (i.e., disabling tachytherapies prior to surgery so that the electrocautery does not interfere with proper device function). The patient's functional capacity should also be assessed (Table 18.1) as this plays an important role in the ACCF/AHA algorithm that will be discussed later in this chapter. In addition to the routine cardiovascular and pulmonary exam, the physical examination should include assessment for the presence of aortic stenosis and congestive heart failure. Table 18.2 summarizes the recommendations for obtaining a preoperative electrocardiogram. In general, a preoperative EKG is not indicated for asymptomatic patients scheduled for low risk procedures.

Estimation of Cardiac Risk

The most commonly used and best validated clinical prediction model for the estimation of surgical cardiac risk is the Revised Cardiac Risk Index (RCRI) [1]. This model incorporates six independent variables to predict cardiac death, myocardial infarction, cardiac arrest, complete heart block, and pulmonary edema. These predictors are high risk surgery, ischemic heart disease (defined as history of myocardial infarction, positive exercise stress test, current angina, use of nitrates, or Q waves on EKG), history of heart failure, cerebrovascular disease, diabetes mellitus being treated with

TABLE 18.1 Functional capacity

1 MET	Can you …	4 METs	Can you …
→	Take care of yourself?	→	Climb a flight of stairs or walk up a hill?
	Eat, dress, or use the toilet?		Walk on level ground at 4 mph (6.4 kph)?
	Walk indoors around the house?		Run a short distance?
	Walk a block or 2 on level ground at 2–3 mph (3.2–4.8 kph)?		Do heavy work around the house like scrubbing floors or lifting or moving heavy furniture?
4 METs	Do light work around the house like dusting or washing dishes?		Participate in moderate recreational activities like golf, bowling, dancing, doubles tennis, or throwing a baseball or football?
		Greater than 10 METs	Can you ….
			Participate in strenuous sports like swimming, singles tennis, football, basketball, or skiing?

Obtained from Fleisher et al. [2] and used with permission from Elsevier.
kph indicates kilometers per hour, *MET* metabolic equivalent, *mph* miles per hour

TABLE 18.2 ACCF/AHA recommendations regarding preoperative EKGs[a]

Class I – A preoperative resting 12-lead EKG is recommended for:	• Patients with ≥1 clinical risk factor[b] who are undergoing vascular surgery. • Patients with known coronary artery disease, peripheral artery disease, or cerebrovascular disease who are undergoing intermediate risk surgery.
Class IIa – A preoperative resting 12-lead EKG is reasonable for:	• Patients without clinical risk factors[b] who are undergoing vascular surgery.
Class IIb – A preoperative resting 12-lead EKG may be considered for:	• Patients with ≥1 clinical risk factor[b] who are undergoing intermediate risk surgery.
Class III – A preoperative resting 12-lead EKG is not recommended for:	• Asymptomatic patients undergoing low risk surgery.

[a]For stable patients in whom a resting 12-lead EKG is recommended, the consensus suggests that an ECG within 30 days of surgery is adequate.
[b]See the "ACCF/AHA Guidelines" section below for the definition of clinical risk factors.

insulin, and preoperative serum creatinine >2 mg/dL. Subjects with none of the above variables had a 0.5% rate of the outcomes listed above, and those with three or more risk factors (the highest risk patients based on the RCRI) had a 9.1% incidence of the primary outcome (Table 18.3).

One caveat is that this model does not predict all-cause mortality. Only one third of perioperative deaths are due to cardiac causes. Another caveat is that subsequent validation studies have shown higher event rates. This is likely due to the fact these studies had patients that were older with more comorbidities than the original derivation and validation populations. In addition, the RCRI used CK-MB for the detection of post-operative myocardial infarction, which is less sensitive than the troponin assays used in later studies. Nonetheless, the RCRI provides a simple model to estimate risk for non-emergent cases.

ACCF/AHA Guidelines

The American College of Cardiology Foundation (ACCF) and American Heart Association (AHA) have published thorough guidelines on preoperative evaluation. These guidelines were revised and simplified in 2007 with a focused update in 2009 [2]. Figure 18.1 shows the algorithm.

The first step is to determine whether the patient requires emergent surgery. In this case, further testing and interventions that would delay the procedure are unlikely to be beneficial, and despite the elevated risk, patients should proceed directly to the operating room. Perioperative beta blockers may be helpful in certain patient populations, and this will be discussed later in the chapter. Such patients should be followed closely post-operatively.

TABLE 18.3 Revised cardiac risk index

Variables	• High risk surgery • Ischemic heart disease[a] • History of heart failure • Cerebrovascular disease • Diabetes mellitus being treated with insulin • Preoperative serum creatinine >2 mg/dL.
Risk of cardiac death, myocardial infarction, cardiac arrest, complete heart block, and pulmonary edema	Score 0: 0.5% Score 1: 1.3% Score 2: 3.6% Score ≥3: 9.1%

[a]Ischemic heart disease is defined as history of myocardial infarction, positive exercise stress test, current angina, use of nitrates, or Q waves on EKG.

The second step is to assess for what the guidelines term "Active Cardiac Conditions" (Table 18.4) such as severe or unstable angina, myocardial infarction within the last 7–30 days, decompensated congestive heart failure, certain arrhythmias such as high-grade AV block or uncontrolled tachycardias, or severe aortic stenosis. These conditions generally require further intensive management preoperatively and could require delay or cancellation of elective or urgent surgeries. For example, most experts advise waiting at least 6 weeks after myocardial infarction to perform elective surgery.

If there are none of the above conditions, then advance to the next step. Step 3 states that patients undergoing low risk surgery can proceed to the operating room without further testing.

Step 4 entails an assessment of the patient's exercise capacity/functional ability, which is expressed in metabolic equivalents (METs). One MET is equivalent to basal resting energy expenditure. Table 18.1 lists the METs for other common activities. However, it is important to recognize confounders such as claudication, arthritis, and pulmonary disease that may caused reduced exercise capacity. The assessment of functional capacity is important because patients with poor functional status are at higher risk of complications. Conversely, asymptomatic patients with good functional capacity (≥ 4 METs) may proceed with the planned surgery, regardless of the type/risk of surgery.

In patients with poor (<4 METs) or unknown functional capacity, then the next step (Step 5) is to assess for what the guidelines term "Clinical Risk Factors." These are ischemic heart disease (includes stable angina, history of prior MI, or Q waves on the EKG compatible with prior MI), compensated or prior CHF, history of stroke or transient ischemic attack, diabetes mellitus, and renal insufficiency (serum creatinine >2 mg/dL). You'll notice that these five risk factors are also components of the Revised Cardiac Risk Index discussed earlier in this chapter. Patients with no clinical risk factors may proceed with the planned surgery. Other patients

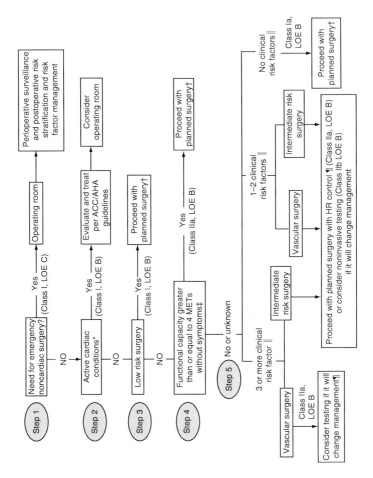

FIGURE 18.1 ACCF/AHA algorithm Obtained from Fleisher et al. [2] and used with permission from Elsevier.

*See Table 18.4 for cardiac conditions. See Table 18.1 for estimated MET level equivalent. §Noninvasive testing may be considered before surgery in specific patents with risk factors if it will change management. ||Clinical risk factors include ischemic heart disease, compensated or prior heart failure, diabetes mellitus, renal insufficiency, and cerebrovascular disease. ¶Consider preoperative beta blockade for populations in which this has been shown to reduce cardiac morbidity/mortality. ACC/AHA indicates American College of Cardiology/American Heart Association; HR, heart rate; LOE, level of evidence; and MET, metabolic equivalent

TABLE 18.4 Active cardiac conditions

Conditions	Examples
Unstable coronary syndromes	• Severe or unstable angina
	• Myocardial infarction within the last 7–30 days
Decompensated congestive heart failure	• New onset or worsening CHF
	• NYHA functional class IV CHF
Significant arrhythmias	• High grade AV block
	• Mobitz II AV block
	• Complete heart block
	• Newly recognized ventricular tachycardia
	• Symptomatic ventricular arrhythmias
	• Supraventricular arrhythmias (including atrial fibrillation) with uncontrolled ventricular rates (HR > 100 bpm at rest)
	• Symptomatic bradycardia
Severe valvular disease	• Severe aortic stenosis (aortic valve area <1 cm^2 or mean pressure gradient >40 mmHg)
	• Symptomatic mitral stenosis (progressive dyspnea on exertion, exertional presyncope, or heart failure)

Adapted from Fleisher et al. [2]

are to be further stratified by the estimate of the surgery-specific cardiac risk (Table 18.5).

Note that vascular surgeries are generally high risk, with the exception of carotid endarterectomies which are

Table 18.5 Surgery-specific risk

Risk stratification	Procedure examples
Vascular (report cardiac risk often more than 5%)	Aortic and other major vascular surgery
	Peripheral vascular surgery
Intermediate (reported cardiac risk generally 1–5%)	Intraperitoneal and intrathoracic surgery
	Carotid endarterectomy
	Head and neck surgery
	Orthopedic surgery
	Prostate surgery
Low[b] (reported cardiac risk generally less than 1%)	Endoscopic procedures
	Superficial procedure
	Cataract surgery
	Breast surgery
	Ambulatory surgery

[a]Combined incidence of cardiac death and nonfatal myocardial infarction
[b]These procedures do not generally require further preoperative cardiac testing

intermediate risk. Orthopedic surgeries are generally of intermediate risk. Low risk surgeries include cataract surgery, breast surgeries, endoscopies, and superficial surgical procedures. Follow the ACCF/AHA algorithm for further recommendations based on the number of Clinical Risk Factors and the risk of surgery. In some scenarios, it is appropriate to obtain noninvasive testing and/or treat with perioperative beta blockers.

Finally, there are certain minor risk factors that are not included in the ACCF/AHA guidelines. These include advanced age, hypertension, left bundle branch block, and atrial fibrillation with controlled ventricular rate.

Preoperative Testing

The first general principle behind preoperative cardiac testing such as echocardiography, noninvasive stress testing, or cardiac catheterization is that these additional studies should only be performed if the results will change the management of the patient. Second, the negative predictive value of a preoperative stress test (i.e., the likelihood that a patient with a negative stress test does not have obstructive CAD) is high, >95% in many studies. In contrast to the above, the positive predictive value of a preoperative stress test (i.e., the likelihood that a patient with a positive stress test has obstructive CAD) is quite low, only 18% in one review [3]. Exercise should be used over pharmacologic stress whenever possible, as the patient's exercise ability carries independent predictive value. Please also see Chapter 4 in this text for further discussion of stress tests.

Regarding echocardiograms, the ACCF/AHA guidelines state that it is reasonable to assess ventricular function in patients with dyspnea of unknown origin or those with prior/current heart failure with worsening symptoms. Echocardiography can also be used to assess for significant valvular disease in a patient with a cardiac murmur. The ACCF/AHA advises against routine perioperative echocardiograms in all patients.

Preoperative Revascularization: The CARP Trial

One of the questions that cardiologists are often asked is whether patients with known obstructive coronary artery disease should undergo revascularization prior to elective surgery. Older and/or retrospective data provided conflicting recommendations about whether such revascularization was beneficial. The best evidence to date for answering this question comes from the Coronary Artery Revascularization Prophylaxis (CARP) trial [4].

This trial enrolled patients at 18 Veterans Affairs medical centers who were scheduled for elective major vascular surgery – 67% for lower extremity peripheral arterial disease and 33% for repair of expanding abdominal aortic aneurysm. Patients felt to be at increased risk for perioperative cardiovascular complications underwent coronary angiography and were eligible for the study if they had a stenosis of at least 70% in at least one of the major coronary arteries and said stenosis was amenable to revascularization. Patients were excluded if they had at least 50% stenosis of the left main coronary artery, if the left ventricular ejection fraction was <20%, or if there was severe aortic stenosis. Patients were also excluded if they required urgent or emergent surgery, had a severe coexisting illness, or had undergone prior revascularization without evidence of recurrent ischemia.

The 510 patients (98% male) who met all of the eligibility requirements were randomly assigned to preoperative revascularization or no revascularization. Of the patients who were revascularized, 59% underwent percutaneous coronary intervention (PCI) and 41% underwent coronary artery bypass grafting (CABG). The fraction of included patients with a Revised Cardiac Risk Index score ≥ 2 was 49%, while 13% had a score ≥ 3.

The CARP trial's primary end point was long-term mortality. At an average follow-up of 2.7 years, mortality was 22% in the revascularization group and 23% in the non-revascularization group (p-value 0.92). There was no significant difference in the long-term use of beta blockers, aspirin, ACE inhibitors, and statins between the two groups either. Further statistical analysis demonstrated no survival benefit to revascularization in any high risk subgroup, such as positive nuclear stress test, high risk category on the Revised Cardiac Risk Index, or three vessel CAD with LV dysfunction.

Examination of the trial's secondary end points revealed no difference in post-operative myocardial infarction (11.6% of the revascularization group and 14.3% of the non-revascularization group, p-value 0.37) or rate of death within 30 days after vascular surgery (3.1% vs. 3.4%, p-value 0.87). Furthermore, there was no difference in the rates of postoperative stroke, limb loss, hemodialysis, reoperation, days spent in the ICU, and total length of hospital stay.

However, revascularization significantly delayed the elective vascular surgery, with a median time to surgery of 54 days after randomization in the revascularization group, and 18 days in the non-revascularization group (p-value < 0.001). Otherwise, there were no significant differences in perioperative management. The use of perioperative beta blockers, aspirin, statins, and heparin was similar between the two groups.

Based on this evidence, it is reasonable to conclude that in patients with stable CAD and none of the above exclusion criteria, routine coronary revascularization prior to elective major vascular surgery is not recommended. That said, revascularization should be performed under the usual standard of care for patients with unstable angina/acute coronary syndromes/myocardial infarction, severe left main CAD, and depressed left ventricular ejection fraction.

Preoperative Revascularization: Patients Who Require PCI and Need Subsequent Surgery

This is a complex situation where multiple factors including the need/urgency/timing of surgery, the risk of surgical bleeding, the risk of coronary lesion restenosis, and the risk of stent thrombosis should be considered. In general, if the risk of surgical bleeding is low, then stenting could be performed and dual antiplatelet continued perioperatively. If the risk of surgical bleeding is intermediate-to-high, then balloon angioplasty without stenting could be considered for surgeries needed within the next 2–4 weeks. Drug eluting stents should not be used if surgery is necessary within the next year. For these decisions, a cardiologist should be consulted.

Perioperative Medications: Antiplatelet Agents

Multiple studies have demonstrated an increased risk of death and myocardial infarction in patients who underwent noncardiac surgery within 6 weeks of PCI with bare metal stent (BMS). This is often due to stent thrombosis, caused by increased post-operative platelet reactivity and/or early discontinuation of dual antiplatelet therapy. For instance, if a patient has received a BMS and clopidogrel is discontinued within the first month, then the risk of stent thrombosis is 3% [5]. Conversely, studies have shown that the risk is much lower 6 weeks after BMS. Therefore, in patients who are status post PCI, it should be considered whether the proposed surgery can be delayed (Fig. 18.2). If this is not possible, then consideration should be given to operating on dual antiplatelet therapy. At least aspirin should be continued throughout the perioperative period unless a severe contraindication exists.

Perioperative Medications: Beta Blockers

Prior guidelines recommended more widespread use of beta blockers than the current version. Some of the evidence behind perioperative beta blockade comes from an extremely large retrospective cohort study of 663,635 patients who received noncardiac surgery in 2000–2001 [6]. Analysis revealed an increase in the in-hospital death rate in the lowest risk groups who received beta blockers, with odds ratios of 1.36 for RCRI score 0 and 1.09 for RCRI score 1. However, beta blockers were beneficial for the higher risk groups, with odds ratios of 0.88, 0.71, and 0.58 for RCRI scores 2, 3, and 4, respectively. It should be noted that the study was retrospective and that only 10% of the study population had RCRI score 2 and only 2% had RCRI score 3–4.

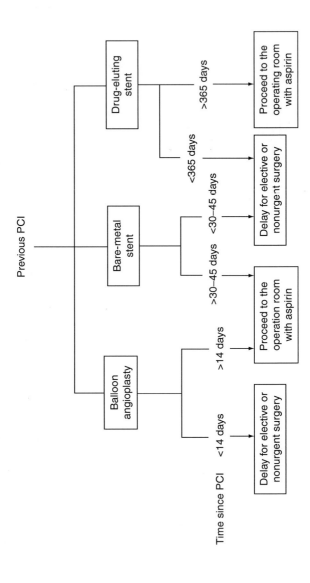

FIGURE 18.2 Management of patients with recent PCI who require noncardiac surgery. PCI indicates percutaneous coronary intervention. Obtained from Fleisher et al. [2] and used with permission from Elsevier

To date, the largest prospective randomized study of beta blockers is the POISE trial, which enrolled 8,351 patients undergoing noncardiac surgery (42% vascular surgery [9]). Most patients were intermediate risk, with RCRI scores of 1–2. They were randomized to a high fixed dose of extended release beta blocker (metoprolol succinate 100 mg given 2–4 h before surgery) or placebo. The beta blocker group received an additional 100 mg dose 0–6 h after surgery, and on subsequent days received 200 mg daily so long as the heart rate was ≥ 50 bpm and the systolic blood pressure was ≥ 100 mmHg. This regimen was continued for 30 days post-surgery. The primary end point at 30 days was a composite of cardiovascular death, nonfatal MI, and nonfatal cardiac arrest, the incidence of which was 5.8% in the beta blocker group and 6.9% in the placebo group (p-value 0.04). This reduction in the primary end point seemed to derive entirely from the reduction in MI (4.2% vs. 5.7%, p-value 0.002). However, all cause mortality was increased in the beta blocker group (3.1% vs. 2.3%, p-value 0.03), as was the rate of stroke (1.0% vs. 0.5%, p-value 0.005), which seemed to stem from increased hypotension in the beta blocker group (15.0% vs. 9.7%, p-value < 0.0001). Criticisms of the POISE study are that the dose of beta blocker was too high, the dose was fixed and not adjusted for heart rate, and that beta blocker therapy was initiated too shortly before surgery.

In contrast, the DECREASE-IV trial [7] was a randomized open-label 2 × 2 factorial design trial of 1,066 intermediate risk (estimated risk of perioperative event 1–6%) patients undergoing non-cardiovascular surgery (general surgery 39%, urologic surgery 19%, orthopedic surgery 16%, ENT surgery 12%) who were randomized to bisoprolol, fluvastatin, combination therapy, or placebo. Medications were started a median of 34 days prior to surgery and continued for 30 days after surgery. Bisoprolol was started at the modest dose of 2.5 mg daily and titrated to a resting heart rate of 50–70 bpm. Bisoprolol was temporarily withheld for HR < 50 bpm, systolic blood pressure <100 mmHg, heart failure, bronchospasm, first degree AV block >300 ms, and second or third degree AV block. The primary end point was the composite of cardiac death and myocardial infarction at 30 days. Those patients randomized to bisoprolol had a 2.1% rate of the primary outcome versus 6.0% in the bisoprolol-control group (*p*-value 0.002, hazard ratio 0.34, 95% CI 0.17–0.67). Ischemic stroke occurred at a rate of 0.8% in the bisoprolol group and 0.6% in the bisoprolol-control group (*p*-value 0.68). There was also no significant difference in the number of patients who developed heart failure, hypotension, or clinically significant bradycardia (0.6% vs. 0.4%, *p*-value 0.65). The results from the fluvastatin arms of this trial will be discussed in the next section below.

In summary, current data is mixed regarding the use of beta blockers for reducing perioperative cardiovascular events in patients undergoing noncardiac surgery. The ACCF/AHA guidelines were updated in 2009 to reflect this new data. Briefly, it is strongly recommended to continue beta blockers if the patient is already taking one prior to surgery (e.g., for CAD, compensated heart failure, or hypertension). There is a weak recommendation to initiate beta blockers in patients with >1 clinical risk factor scheduled for vascular or intermediate risk surgery. It is reasonable to use beta-1 selective agents such as metoprolol. The ACCF/AHA recommend starting the beta blocker days-to-weeks before surgery and carefully titrating the dose to a resting heart rate in the 60s, but hypotension and symptomatic bradycardia must be avoided. Intravenous metropolol can be used if oral intake is transiently infeasible. If the beta blocker is not going to be continued long-term post-surgery, then it should be tapered carefully (Table 18.6).

Perioperative Medications: Statins

HMG-CoA reductase inhibitors (statins) are well-known to have beneficial effects in post-MI patients. There is mounting evidence that statins have pleiotropic effects including plaque modification and stabilization, improved endothelial function,

TABLE 18.6 ACCF/AHA recommendations regarding preoperative beta blockers[a]

Class I – Preoperative beta blockers are recommended:	• Patients who are already taking beta blockers should be continued on them.
Class IIa – Preoperative beta blockers may be beneficial for:	• Patients undergoing vascular surgery who are at high risk due to known CAD or cardiac ischemia on preoperative stress testing.
	• Patients undergoing vascular or intermediate risk surgery with ≥2 clinical risk factors.[b]
	• Patients undergoing intermediate risk surgery in whom preoperative assessment identifies CAD.
Class IIb – The utility of preoperative beta blockers is uncertain for:	• Patients undergoing vascular or intermediate risk surgery without known CAD but with 1 clinical risk factor.[b]
	• Patients undergoing vascular surgery without any clinical risk factors[b] who are not currently taking beta blockers.
Class III – Preoperative beta blockers are not recommended:	• Beta blockers should not be given to patients undergoing surgery who have absolute contraindications to beta blockade.
	• Routine administration of high dose beta blockers in the absence of dose titration is not useful and may be harmful to patients not currently taking beta blockers who are undergoing non-cardiac surgery.

[a]Beta blockers should be titrated to heart rate and blood pressure as detailed in the text
[b]See the "ACCF/AHA Guidelines" section above for the definition of clinical risk factors

and anti-inflammatory properties. A recent meta-analysis [8] included 4,805 patients in 21 trials and determined that the use of pre-procedural statins significantly reduced post-procedural (PCI, coronary artery bypass grafting, and non-cardiac surgery) myocardial infarction (risk ratio 0.57, 95 % CI 0.46–0.70, p-value < 0.0001). Subgroup analysis showed this benefit in post-PCI and post-non-cardiac surgery patients, but not post-CABG patients. All-cause mortality was non-significantly reduced. The three non-cardiac surgery trials that were included were DECREASE-III and DECREASE-IV which compared fluvastatin 80 mg versus control, and a small 100 patient study of elective vascular surgery patients by Durazzo et al in 2004 that compared atorvastatin 20 mg versus control. In all three studies the statin was started approximately 1 month prior to surgery and continued for 30 days post-surgery. All three individual studies showed a non-statistically significant trend towards reduction in post-procedure MI and this benefit became statistically significant when the studies were pooled (RR 0.47, 95 % CI 0.28–0.78).

The ACCF/AHA guidelines recommend the following with regard to statin therapy in the peri-operative period:

- Statins should be continued for patients already taking them (class I recommendation).
- Statin use is reasonable for patients undergoing vascular surgery, with or without clinical risk factors (class IIa recommendation).
- Statin use may be considered in patients with ≥1 clinical risk factor who are undergoing intermediate risk surgery (class IIb recommendation).

References

1. Lee TH et al. Derivation and prospective validation of a simple index for prediction of cardiac risk of major noncardiac surgery. Circulation. 1999;100:1043.

2. Fleisher LA et al. 2009 ACCF/AHA Focused Update on Perioperative Beta Blockade Incorporated into the ACC/AHA 2007 Guidelines on Perioperative Cardiovascular Evaluation and Care for Noncardiac Surgery: a Report of the American College of Cardiology Foundation/American Heart Association Task Force on Practice Guidelines. J Am Coll Cardiol. 2009;54:e13.
3. Mangano DT, Goldman L. Preoperative assessment of patients with known or suspected coronary disease. N Engl J Med. 1995;333:1750.
4. McFalls EO et al. Coronary-artery revascularization before elective major vascular surgery. N Engl J Med. 2004;351:2795.
5. Leon MB et al. A clinical trial comparing three antithrombotic-drug regimens after coronary-artery stenting Stent Anticoagulation Restenosis Study Investigators. N Engl J Med. 1998;339:1665.
6. Lindenauer PK et al. Perioperative beta-blocker therapy and mortality after major noncardiac surgery. N Engl J Med. 2005;353:349.
7. Dunkelgrun M et al. Bisoprolol and fluvastatin for the reduction of perioperative cardiac mortality and myocardial infarction in intermediate-risk patients undergoing noncardiovascular surgery: a randomized controlled trial (DECREASE-IV). Ann Surg. 2009;249:921–6.
8. Winchester DE et al. Evidence of pre-procedural statin therapy: a meta-analysis of randomized trials. J Am Coll Cardiol. 2010;56:1099–109.
9. POISE Study Group, Devereaux PJ, et al. Effects of extended-release metoprolol succinate in patients undergoing non-cardiac surgery (POISE trial): a randomized controlled trial. Lancet. 2008;371:1839.

Chapter 19
Approach to the Patient with Cardiovascular Disease and Activity Limitations

Ryan W. Connell and Duncan D. Wormer

Introduction

Patients with cardiovascular disease often have functional limitations and an increased risk of activity-related cardiac events. The impact of cardiovascular disease on the daily lives of some patients is quite apparent, while others may be asymptomatic and unknowingly at high risk for adverse events. Cardiologists and primary care physicians frequently encounter questions about activity limitations in patients with, or at risk for, cardiac disease. This can be a challenging question to address as there are many variables involved. It is important to consider each patient individually when making such decisions.

This chapter will address a general approach to this issue as well as some of the common diseases and activities that are encountered. This chapter should be used as a general guide only when evaluating individual patients. The unique characteristics of each patient must be considered when making these decisions.

R.W. Connell (✉) • D.D. Wormer
Division of Cardiology, Department of Internal Medicine,
University of Rochester Medical Center, Rochester, NY, USA
e-mail: ryan_connell@urmc.rohester.edu

J.D. Bisognano et al. (eds.), *Manual of Outpatient Cardiology*,   465
DOI 10.1007/978-0-85729-944-4_19,
© Springer-Verlag London Limited 2012

Physiologic Response to Exercise

It is important to understand the basic physiologic response to exercise when assessing activity tolerance and safety. The normal cardiac and hemodynamic changes that occur with exercise may be altered in patients with cardiac disease. Additionally, some cardiac medications may diminish typical hemodynamic responses of heart rate and blood pressure. Subjective exercise tolerance from noncardiac factors may also lead to limitations in activity.

The normal cardiac response to exercise has been well established with predictable hemodynamic changes occurring within a few minutes of exercise initiation [1, 2]. Exercise results in increased muscle oxygen consumption and carbon dioxide production. Therefore, there is a need for increased cardiac output and ventilation to accommodate sustained exercise. Increased cardiac output is accomplished in multiple ways that are reflected in the following basic calculation:

$$\text{Cardiac output} = \text{Heart rate} \times \text{Stroke volume}$$

Heart rate increases primarily from increased sympathetic activity with exercise. Increases in stroke volume are a result of multiple factors. Decreased systemic vascular resistance at the muscular level leads to afterload reduction and increased stroke volume. Additionally, contractility increases with sympathetic stimulation and beta-receptor activation. An increase in venous return from skeletal muscle contractility also modestly increases preload. The resulting endpoint is an increase of cardiac output 4–6 times normal. There is an increase in systolic blood pressure and mean arterial blood pressure with this process. Diastolic blood pressure does not change significantly with exercise.

The overall pulmonary response to exercise is an increase in ventilation. This allows for both increased oxygenation and release of carbon dioxide. Increased levels of carbon dioxide are normally the trigger for increased respirations. Pulmonary blood flow can increase substantially in healthy patients without significant increases in pulmonary pressures. Ventilation is typically limited by maximal sustained ventilation and respiratory muscle fatigue.

The type of exercise performed has an impact on the hemodynamic changes. Aerobic activity generally has a more substantial increase in cardiac output, predominantly as a result of increased HR, decreased SVR and increased SV. Isometric exercise (i.e., weight training) has only a moderate increase in cardiac output, but has a significant increase in mean arterial pressure.

The change from aerobic metabolism to anaerobic metabolism has a significant effect on activity tolerance. As oxygen demand increases in muscles, there is increased blood supply to meet this demand for aerobic metabolism. Anaerobic metabolism occurs to provide additional energy when oxygen supply is limited. Anaerobic metabolism is not as efficient and produces lactic acid. Lactic acid buildup causes muscle fatigue and pain and is an activity limiting factor. Lactic acid also results in increased ventilation and can lead to respiratory fatigue.

The point at which anaerobic metabolism exceeds aerobic metabolism is referred to as the anaerobic threshold. The anaerobic threshold is a function of cardiac output, pulmonary function, maximal oxygen consumption (VO_2 max) and muscle composition. This is different for each patient and can be measured with formal cardiopulmonary testing. An indirect measure of this can be determined by maximum heart rate. In normal individuals, the activity level at which maximum heart rate occurs is presumed to be the point of VO_2 max and anaerobic threshold. Maximum heart rate is estimated as follows:

$$\text{Maximum heart rate} = 220 - age$$

Maximum exercise can only be maintained for a brief period of time because of the anaerobic threshold and lactic acid accumulation. Submaximal exercise can be maintained much longer if oxygen supply and CO_2 removal are adequate. Exercise-related hemodynamic changes tend to remain steady with submaximal exercise.

Response to Exercise with Cardiovascular Disease

Patients with cardiovascular disease often have an inadequate or altered response to exercise compared to normal subjects. Cardiovascular-related exercise limitations are primarily the result of decreased cardiac output or angina. Additionally, typical exercise-induced changes may be blunted in the setting of cardiac disease [1, 2].

Heart failure, or cardiomyopathy, results in decreased cardiac output. This may not always be significant at rest, but often becomes apparent during exercise. This is irrelevant of the cause of cardiomyopathy (ischemic, nonischemic, valvular, etc.). High levels of activity can result in the need for cardiac output 4–6 times normal, beyond what may be possible in the setting of heart failure. Additionally, chronic hypoperfusion results in changes at the muscular level that lead to decreased strength and efficiency.

The typical hemodynamic changes that occur with exercise do not always occur appropriately in the setting of cardiac disease. Increased sympathetic activity with exercise causes increases in heart rate and contractility in normal patients. There is decreased beta-receptor activity in patients with heart failure and this response can be quite diminished. Underlying conduction can also limit heart rate augmentation.

Coronary artery disease can impact the ability to increase cardiac output with activity. As cardiac contractility and heart rate increase, there is increased oxygen demand in the cardiac muscle. Coronary artery disease can limit the increased blood flow that is required to accomplish this. The result is myocardial ischemia which can cause angina and ventricular dysfunction. Additionally, myocardial ischemia with exercise can result in cardiac arrhythmias including ventricular tachycardia or ventricular fibrillation. This concept is the basis of exercise testing.

Some commonly used cardiac treatments can also cause an indirect limitation on activity. Beta-blockers reduce heart rate and cardiac contractility and thus limit cardiac output. This may affect maximal exercise performance for competitive athletes. Anti-platelet medication can increase bleeding and should be a consideration with contact sports or activities with a high risk of trauma. Pacemakers-dependent patients may have limitation related to the need for increased heart rate with exercise. This is less of an issue with newer rate responsive pacemakers. Patients with pacemakers or defibrillators should also avoid activities that could result in direct trauma to the device itself.

General Approach

Assessing a cardiac patient for appropriate levels of activity is an individualized process. There are certain factors to consider in specific diseases and activities. However, from a practical standpoint, the decision involves an evaluation of three general clinical assessments: functional capacity, ischemic risk and arrhythmias.

The role of the physician is to help navigate the acceptable level of risk for each individual. Ultimately, it is impossible to completely eliminate the risk of adverse events. Along with the medical background, this decision should take into consideration the patient's comfort level of risk, the physician's professional opinion and any outside regulations.

Evaluating Functional Capacity

The functional assessment is the evaluation of a patient's physical ability to perform a specific task. The impact of cardiac disease on activity or exercise tolerance is discussed above, but there are many other factors that contribute to functional tolerance beyond cardiac function. Pulmonary disease, musculoskeletal limitations, neurological disease, and general conditioning are just a few of the contributing issues. These should be considered along with any cardiac limitations.

Subjective evaluation of functional abilities is often the most helpful and practical approach. A detailed and accurate history of baseline activity tolerance offers immense insight into a patient's abilities and is the most important and useful piece of information available. Baseline activities and associated symptoms should be clearly established. Additionally, it is helpful to understand at what level of activity a person typically becomes symptomatic (i.e., 3 flights of stairs, 10 min of walking, etc.).

If the planned activity is consistent with what a patient tolerates at baseline, then no further testing is necessary. If the planned activity is at or above a level that has previously brought on unacceptable symptoms, then the activity should generally be avoided. Some patients who live sedentary lives have not established a baseline upper limit of activity tolerance. It may be unclear what level of activity causes symptoms if they do not achieve that level at baseline. If the anticipated new activity is in this unclear range, then further testing could be considered.

The exercise portion of any exercise stress test (i.e., Bruce protocol) can be useful to demonstrate the level of tolerable activity. This is in addition to the ischemic evaluation which is often the primary purpose of the test. Stress testing and protocols are discussed in full detail in Chap. 4.

The exercise stress protocols can be roughly converted to other activities using a metabolic equivalent of task (MET) measurement. One MET is defined as the amount of energy used at rest. Increased levels of activity result in increased energy exertion. Examples of activities and corresponding METs are listed in Table 19.1. This can be useful when comparing actual activities to the standard stress protocols that are discussed in Chap. 4.

Formal cardiopulmonary testing offers a detailed evaluation of cardiopulmonary function. This includes assessment of anaerobic thresholds and calculation of VO_2 max. This test has important prognostic value and is often a part of a work up for cardiac transplantation. However, it is less clear how this translates to specific activities and it is rarely necessary to pursue this for activity clearance.

Cardiac rehabilitation offers a valuable way to assess and increase functional capacity in patients with CHF or CAD [3].

TABLE 19.1 MET levels and activities

1	1-2	3-4	5-6	7-8	9-10	11+
Resting	• Talking	• Walking at a brisk pace	• Stairs while carrying objects	• Stairs while carrying objects >25 lbs	• Slow jogging	• Running >6 mph
	• Walking at a slow pace	• Playing with children	• Using heavy power tools	• Dancing (fast)	• Moving heavy furniture	• Cycling at a brisk pace
	• Light gardening	• Washing car	• Heavy yard work	• Canoeing/ kayaking	• Heavy manual labor	• Competitive sports
	• Light house work	• Working with hand tools	• Chopping wood	• Swimming laps		
	• Playing a musical instrument	• Vacuuming	• Carrying heavy objects	• Shoveling heavy snow		
	• Playing cards	• Mopping				
		• Painting				

It can be particularly useful in patients with recent cardiac events who have not clearly established a peak activity threshold. Cardiac rehabilitation programs have a set protocol that gradually increases the level and duration of exercise while patients are being monitored. This is most appropriate for patients who have had a recent cardiac event (MI) or who have chronic symptomatic heart failure. Participation in cardiac rehabilitation is an ideal way for patients with CAD or CHF to transition to a regular exercise program.

The 6-min walk test is a useful way to monitor changes in activity tolerance in patients with chronic cardiac issues. This simply consists of measuring the distance a person can walk over a 6-min period. It can easily be done in the office setting, often by counting the number of times someone can comfortably walk the length of a premeasured hallway in 6 min. This test is most useful for trending changes over time rather than as a single assessment.

Evaluating Ischemic Risk

Assessment of ischemic risk relates directly to the safety of participating in various activities. This can be a more difficult question to answer than functional tolerance alone.

As with the functional assessment, a good history from the patient is often the most useful piece of information. It is important to find out what types of activities a patient typically can tolerate. General descriptions are helpful, but specific quantifications (such as distance walking/running, number of stairs, minutes of exercise) are more useful. It is also important to know what the "limit" is with these activities. Stopping because of fatigue is nonspecific. It could possibly represent ischemia, but also may be a function of pulmonary disease, muscle issues or general conditioning. Alternatively, activity limitations because of classic angina symptoms are more specific for coronary artery disease. It is also worth noting that stress-induced ischemia does not always produce symptoms, especially in diabetic patients. For higher risk patients, it may be necessary to proceed with other testing to better assess a safe level of activity tolerance.

Testing options are available to further assess ischemic risk. A resting EKG is reasonable to assess for evidence of underlying cardiac disease (Q waves, loss of R waves, inverted T waves, nonspecific ST changes). These finding have been associated with an increased risk of future cardiac events. However, the sensitivity and specificity are low which limits the utility [4–6]. Exercise or stress testing may offer more information than a resting EKG alone.

Exercise ECG testing is generally the most cost-effective and accessible initial evaluation and has been widely studied as a screening tool to diagnose CAD [7]. An exercise ECG may be combined with imaging (echocardiography or nuclear imaging) to confirm and better define the extent of CAD. Exercise echocardiography and nuclear studies are more useful in patients with established CAD or a high pretest probability. Pharmacologic stress testing is of limited utility as part of an evaluation for activity tolerance. Compared to exercise stress testing, there is no way to correlate symptoms or ischemic changes with activity levels when pharmacologic stress testing is done. The indications and limitations of various stress tests are discussed in detail in Chap. 4.

Angiography plays a limited role in the evaluation of ischemic risk. Angiography does not assess function or activity. Its utility in this setting is mainly as an additional test following abnormal exercise or stress testing with associated angina. It should not be the sole assessment when determining activity tolerance.

The appropriateness of work up and testing to assess activity tolerance in specific patient groups is discussed further below. This is divided into sections based on the presence of underlying CAD and risk factors.

No History of CAD, No Risk Factors

Asymptomatic patients without a history of coronary artery disease and without risk factors have a low pretest probability of having significant coronary artery disease. In this setting, there is little role for stress testing to further risk stratify.

A low pretest probability dramatically decreases the positive predictive value of a positive stress test.

The presence of typical angina symptoms raises the pretest probability significantly despite having no prior CAD or risk factors. In this setting, stress testing could be considered to better assess ischemic burden in a controlled setting. However, it should be noted that in extremely low-risk patient groups (i.e., young healthy patients) even typical angina only results in an intermediate risk of true coronary disease. In the setting of a low pretest probability, stress testing can result in more frequent false positives, thus decreasing its utility.

The 2004 USPTF task force and the updated 2002 ACC/AHA guidelines recommend against routine screening for low-risk patients [8, 9].

No History of CAD, CAD Risk Factors

Multiple risk factors have been identified to independently increase the risk of coronary artery disease. These are discussed in detail in Chap. 8. When assessing pre-activity risk stratification, the goal is to determine if someone actually has undiagnosed CAD that could limit safe participation. Risk calculators can be used to better assess the pretest probability. In higher risk patients, noninvasive testing may be useful if the anticipated activity level is beyond what a patient has demonstrated can be tolerated.

In the setting of cardiac risk factors, a positive exercise ECG test has been shown to predict future cardiac mortality and events [7, 10–13]. The predictive power of an exercise ECG is significantly higher in the setting of cardiac risk factors when compared to no risk factors [11]. However, specific interventions (beyond medical management) have never been shown to change this prognosis. Risk factor reduction should be pursued from a general cardiac standpoint, but does not necessarily affect activity limitations [3]. The identification of a significant coronary artery obstruction may require interventions such as PCI or CABG. This is discussed in more detail in Chap. 5.

The presence of diabetes is not only a risk factor, but considered to be a CAD equivalent [14]. The presence of DM is also of particular concern because it can be associated with silent ischemia, presumably as a result of neuropathy and decreased sensation. Given this, the updated 2002 ACC/AHA guidelines do recommend evaluation of asymptomatic diabetic patients prior to the initiation of a vigorous exercise program [9].

2004 USPS Task force and the ACC/AHA have not made recommendations for or against screening nondiabetic patients at higher risk [8, 9]. Some organizations have recommended routine screening for high-risk patients in certain situations that affect public safety; however, there is no consensus at this time. It would be reasonable to pursue stress testing in patients who are felt to be at higher risk for underlying CAD.

Stable CAD

Patients with stable coronary disease often have slow changes in the degree of coronary artery stenosis. However, they are generally still at increased risk for acute plaque rupture given the higher baseline disease burden. By definition, patients with stable coronary artery disease do not have ischemia at rest and any angina is predictable and reproducible based on the level of activity. As activity increases, the myocardial demand proportionally increases as well. Angina occurs when the demand exceeds the supply of oxygen the blood flow can provide. Establishing a baseline level of tolerable activity is essential to identify general levels of safe activity tolerance.

The extent of coronary disease is correlated with the risk of cardiac events. Multivessel disease and large territories of ischemia increase the risk of future events. This should be considered when assessing a patient's risk.

The presence of stable CAD does not mean that all aerobic activity should be avoided. In fact, symptom limited exercise regimens for patients with CAD are generally recommended. This has been shown to decrease the risk of future MI and mortality [15].

High intensity, strenuous activity is associated with a transient increase in the risk of an acute MI [16]. However, CAD patients who participate in regular exercise are generally at a lower overall risk of MI [15]. The highest risk tends to be in patients who do not engage in regular physical activity and then suddenly undergo significant exertion [16, 17]. This should be interpreted carefully as it should not lead to recommendations of avoiding all exercise. Rather, a framework should be created for how to participate in it. Periodic episodes of extreme activity should be avoided in the setting of CAD. Regular activity can be increased slowly to a level of tolerance and is beneficial in the long term. Maximal exercise capacity should be avoided and symptom should generally limit peak activity (SOB, chest pain, extreme fatigue, and extreme diaphoresis).

There are no specific recommendations or guidelines regarding activity limitations in patients with established coronary artery disease. Reasonable individualized guidelines can be established for each patient using the above information. Generally, a safe level of activity should be established based on baseline history/activity. In diabetic patients, it may be reasonable to pursue exercise echo or nuclear perfusion studies given the distinct possibility of silent ischemia. Periodic episodes of transient strenuous activity should be avoided given the increased risk of MI during that time. Regular, symptom limited exercise can and should be recommended for long-term risk reduction.

Stress testing is a reasonable option to evaluate activity tolerance in the setting of CAD. No specific society guidelines exist to recommend the most appropriate test. Generally, just as in choosing any stress test, the pretest probability of a clinically significant blockage should guide the choice of tests. Exercise testing or cardiac rehabilitation is reasonable for a patient with stable CAD who is planning to start an exercise program or participate in a higher level of activity. Exercise echocardiography or nuclear stress testing provides a higher sensitivity and specificity. This may be more useful to evaluate activity-related symptoms or lower levels of ischemia.

Unstable CAD

Patients with unstable coronary artery disease are a very high risk group. This includes patients who have angina that has become more intense, occurs with less activity or even at rest. Patients with unstable angina are at high risk for MI and should be evaluated immediately and treated as acute coronary syndrome. This needs to be evaluated acutely before considering any type of activity recommendations.

Arrhythmia Risk

Cardiac arrhythmias may lead to increased risk with certain activities. Generally, most of these risks are present regardless of activity. The evaluation and work up of various arrhythmias is discussed extensively in Chap. 10. The two main concerns with arrhythmias impacting activity tolerance are syncope- and exercise-induced arrhythmias.

Syncope related to arrhythmias is typically the result of sudden tachycardia, bradycardia or heart block. Exertional syncope is also encountered with aortic stenosis or outflow tract obstructions. Syncope is discussed in detail in Chap. 14.

Exercise-induced arrhythmias are rare events, but potentially devastating. Exercise-induced ventricular arrhythmias are most commonly the result of hypertrophic cardiomyopathy, ischemia-induced VT or catecholamine-induced ventricular arrhythmias. Certain subtypes of long QT syndrome also result in ventricular arrhythmias with exercise.

Hypertrophic cardiomyopathy is the most common cause of sudden cardiac death in young athletes. It is generally screened for during pre-sports physicals and sometimes with echocardiography. It should be considered in patients with exercise-induced syncope.

Ischemia-induced VT with exercise is typically the result of coronary disease with increased mycocardial demand. History may include exertional angina associated with palpitations, pre-syncope or syncope. However, the ischemia may not always be associated with angina and the only clinical presentation may only be related to the arrhythmia. Prior to any activity clearance, patients with this type of presentation should be worked up for ischemia urgently.

Catecholamine-induced arrhythmias are a rare group of diseases that can result in ventricular tachycardia or ventricular fibrillation with exercise. These patients typically present with exertional palpitations or syncope in adolescents or as young adults. Standard exercise ECG testing often reveals frequent PVCs and ventricular tachycardia. These patients may require antiarrhythmic medications and implantable defibrillators.

Activity-Specific Approach

Driving

The presence of underlying medical conditions impacts a patient's ability to safely drive. This is certainly true of many cardiac issues as well. The concern with driving and medical issues involve to danger to the driver, passengers in the car, passengers in other cars and bystanders. This is clearly a sensitive issue that can have significant social impacts. Overly conservative driving restrictions may unnecessarily limit the daily activities of low-risk drivers. Alternatively, a driver who is at high risk for driving impairments may pose a significant public health risk. Physicians are often put in the difficult position of making these decisions. Regulations and restrictions do exist, but are different for each state. The local regulations in place should be consulted before making any final decisions about a patient's ability to drive.

Driving limitations from cardiac disease are primarily because of risks of syncope or loss of consciousness. Cardiac disease that results in a generalized functional inability to drive (i.e., NYHA class IV CHF) is also a clear contraindication. The majority of the time, however, the concern is centered on arrhythmias and the potential for syncope.

Any patient with uncontrolled arrhythmias that result in hemodynamic instability should not operate a motor vehicle.

This may be the result of an underlying primary arrhythmia or ischemia-induced arrhythmias related to CAD. Driving abilities can be reassessed once the arrhythmia is under control.

It is generally recommended that driving should be restricted for at least 6 months after a documented VT or VF arrest. This is more of a concern with primary arrhythmias than with an arrest secondary to a specific cause (i.e., MI) that has resolved. A defibrillator should be implanted before the 6-month waiting period begins.

There is no clear evidence or guidelines regarding driving restrictions after implantation of an ICD for primary prevention. It is reasonable to have someone withhold from driving for 1–2 weeks after implantation. This could theoretically be an increased risk of arrhythmia after implantation due to inflammation/irritation at the lead site or device malfunction. This is an individualized decision at the discretion of the electrophysiologist.

Driving should be avoided for at least 6 months after an appropriate ICD shock for VT/VF. The arrhythmia should be well controlled prior to resuming driving. Inappropriate ICD shocks could result in transient loss of control while driving. The reason for the inappropriate shock should be addressed and corrected prior to driving.

It is worth noting that some commercial drivers are not allowed to drive after an ICD has been implanted. This varies with each state and driving company. Pacemakers generally do not have this limitation.

Competitive Athletes

Competitive athletes are a unique population from a cardiac standpoint. They are frequently exposed to intense levels of activity that require increased cardiac output and place extraordinary demand on the heart. This is beyond the demands seen with recreational sports or standard exercise programs. Low level or recreational level athletics can be approached similar to general activity limitations as described above, but competitive athletes need special consideration.

Athletes with Known Cardiovascular Disease

Recommendations for competitive athletes with established cardiovascular disease have been clearly established by the Bethesda guidelines. The Bethesda Conference meets periodically and releases updated guidelines addressing these specifics in detail. These recommendations are designed to specifically address competitive sports and are not necessarily applicable to recreational athletes. The recommendations for each specific disease vary with the severity of disease and the level or activity. Reviewing all of these recommendations is beyond the scope of this chapter, but the major points will be highlighted below. Full details can easily be found in the published guidelines [2].

Competitive athletics can be classified into varying levels of intensity. This is obviously an imprecise process as individual athletes will have different levels of exertion. However, it is helpful to categorize these activities in order to make broad comparisons. Table 19.2 provides examples of low-, moderate- and high-intensity sports based on cardiovascular demands.

In adult cardiology, ischemic heart disease and valve diseases are frequently encountered. General recommendations from the Bethesda Guidelines for various levels of competitive sports are summarized in Tables 19.3 and 19.4. Readers

TABLE 19.2 Cardiovascular demands with competitive sports

Low intensity	Low-moderate	Moderate intensity	Moderate-high	High intensity
Bowling, golf, billiards	Archery, equestrian, baseball, softball, fencing, volleyball	Field events, martial arts, weight lifting, football, figure skating, long distance running, soccer	Body building, snowboarding, skiing, wrestling, basketball, hockey, swimming, middle distance running	Boxing, cycling, decathlon, rowing, speed skating, triathlon

Adapted from Maron and Zipes [2]

TABLE 19.3 Valve disease and participation in competitive sports

	Low intensity	Moderate intensity	High intensity
Mild MS	Yes	Yes	Yes
Moderate MS	Yes	Yes	No
Severe MS	No	No	No
Mild MR, normal LV	Yes	Yes	Yes
Mild MR, LV dilation	Yes	Yes	No
Moderate MR, normal LV	Yes	Yes	Yes
Moderate MR, LV dilation	Yes	Yes	No
Severe MR	No	No	No
Mild AS	Yes	Yes	Yes
Moderate AS	Yes	Yes[a]	No
Severe AS	No	No	No
Mild AI, normal LV	Yes	Yes	Yes
Mild AI, LV dilation	Yes[a]	Yes[a]	No
Moderate AI, normal LV	Yes	Yes	Yes
Moderate AI, LV dilation	Yes[a]	Yes[a]	No
Severe AI	No	No	No
Mild/Moderate AI and enlarged aorta (not including Marfans)	Yes	No	No
Bicuspid valve, no aortic dilation	Yes	Yes	Yes
Bicuspid valve, aortic root 40–45 mm	Yes	Yes	No

(continued)

TABLE 19.3 (continued)

	Low intensity	Moderate intensity	High intensity
Bicuspid valve, aortic root >45 mm	Yes	No	No
TR, normal RV	Yes	Yes	Yes
TS	Yes[a]	Yes[a]	Yes[a]
Significant multivalve disease	No	No	No
Prosthetic mitral, no anticoagulation	Yes	Yes	No
Prosthetic aortic, no anticoagulation	Yes	Yes	No
Any prosthetic with anticoagulation	No	No	No

Adapted from Maron and Zipes [2]
MS mitral stenosis, *MR* mitral regurgitation, *LV* left ventricle, *AS* aortic stenosis, *AI* aortic insufficiency, *TR* tricuspid regurgitation
[a]Exercise testing should be done to confirm

TABLE 19.4 CAD and competitive sports

	Clinical features	Low intensity	Moderate intensity	High intensity
Lower risk CAD	• Normal EF • Normal stress test • <50% CAD stenosis	Yes	Yes	No
Higher risk CAD	• Abnormal EF • Abnormal stress test • >50% CAD stenosis	Yes[a]	No	No

Adapted from Maron and Zipes [2]
[a]Exercise testing should be done to confirm

are encouraged to review the guidelines directly for specific patient questions.

Screenings for Young Competitive Athletes

Sudden cardiac death in young competitive athletes is a rare but devastating event. The majority of cases are found to be the result of undiagnosed hypertrophic cardiomyopathy or congenital heart disease. This leads to the understandable question of whether widespread screening should be done to identify these patients.

It remains controversial whether intense screening of all competitive athletes is appropriate. The prevalence of underlying structural heart disease in this population is very low (0.3%) while the total number of estimated participants in the United States is enormous (estimated >10 million). Additionally, even when structural heart disease is identified, the incidence of sudden cardiac death is still thought to be relatively low [2]. The cost and time to intensely screen all competitive athletes can be prohibitive with a relatively low yield of preventing any events. It could also unnecessarily restrict many athletes from sports participation. That being said, sudden cardiac death in a young, healthy appearing athlete is a tragic and dramatic event. These cases, although rare, often gain substantial public and media attention.

At this time, pre-participation screening and physical exam is the only universal screening recommendation in the United States [2]. This screening should assess for high-risk features as described by AHA recommendations (Table 19.5). High-risk features identified can then be followed up with further testing such as ECG and echocardiogram as indicated.

Universal screening programs with modalities such as ECG or echocardiogram are not currently a standard recommendation in the United States. Other countries have initiated these types of programs with varying success in identifying high-risk patients. Local programs have been initiated in some schools and communities, but there are currently no specific recommendations for or against this.

Table 19.5 Pre-participation athletic screening

Family history	Personal history	Physical exam
• Sudden cardiac death	• Heart murmur	• Blood pressure
• Heart disease in family member <50 y/o	• Hypertension	• Heart murmur
	• Fatigue	• Femoral artery pulses
	• Syncope	• Marfan syndrome
	• Excessive exertional dyspnea	
	• Exertional chest pain	

Adapted from Maron and Zipes [2]

Airline Travel

The safety of airline travel by patients with cardiovascular disease has not been well studied. It should generally be safe for patients who can functionally manage the physical demands of traveling, but a few risks should be considered.

High-altitude flights, even with pressurization, result in a slightly lower oxygenation level. Patients with marginal arterial oxygenation saturations on room air may require supplemental oxygen when flying. Patients on chronic supplemental oxygen therapy may require higher levels of supplementation.

Airline travel does not appear to add specific increased risk of cardiovascular events [18, 19]. However, there is minimal medical care available while flying so access to treatment is limited for acute events. Patients with unstable cardiac disease of any etiology should generally avoid airline travel. Additionally, recommendations have been suggested to avoid flying for 2–6 weeks after an acute myocardial infarction by various medical societies. At this time, there are no ACC/AHA guidelines on this issue.

Airline travel itself does not interfere with the function of pacemakers and implantable defibrillators. Magnetic-based security screenings in airports can potentially interfere and should be avoided if possible. Magnetic security wands could also impact these devices if placed directly over them and should be avoided if possible.

Sexual Activity

Patients with cardiovascular disease, especially coronary artery disease, frequently inquire about cardiac risks with sexual activity. Studies have shown that sexual activity has similar hemodynamic effects on heart rate and blood pressure as moderate exercise (3–4 METS). This is generally lower than the peak activity levels encountered in day to day life [20].

A small increase in relative risk of MI has been shown during the 2 h after sexual activity [21]. This is similar to the small increase in cardiac events that has been shown following any intermittent period of increased activity. However, cardiac patients who exercise on a regular basis have a lower overall incidence of cardiac events.

Patients with cardiac disease may be more prone to problems with sexual dysfunction. This results from a combination of concomitant vascular disease risk factors, medication side effects and anxiety about potential cardiac events. Medical therapy for sexual dysfunction can be considered for cardiac patients, but vasodilators (i.e., Viagara) are contraindicated in patients using nitroglycerin.

Return to Work

Returning to work following a cardiac event can be a difficult decision for patients, employers and physicians. This is complicated by not only patient safety, but also financial pressure, disability coverage and liability. Unfortunately, no standard set of guidelines exist to address this specific issue. As described extensively above, the decision should be made while considering the individual's specific medical condition and the anticipated level of activity that is likely to be encountered. The goal is to find an acceptable level of risk and make reasonable activity recommendations. Approaching this difficult task can be done similar to approaching any type of activity limitation. This chapter can be used to help guide that process.

References

1. Fletcher GF, Balady GJ, Amsterdam EA, Chaitman B, Eckel R, Fleg J, et al. Exercise standards for testing and training: a statement for healthcare professionals from the American Heart Association. Circulation. 2001;104(14):1694–740.
2. Maron B, Zipes D. 36th Bethesda Conference: Eligibility Recommendations for Competitive Athletes With Cardiovascular Abnormalities JACC. 2005; Vol. 45, No. 8:1312–1375.
3. Clark AM, Hartling L, Vandermeer B, McAlister FA. Meta-analysis: secondary prevention programs for patients with coronary artery disease. Ann Intern Med. 2005;143(9):659–72.
4. Knutsen R, Knutsen SF, Curb JD, Reed DM, Kautz JA, Yano K. The predictive value of resting electrocardiograms for 12-year incidence of coronary heart disease in the Honolulu Heart Program. J Clin Epidemiol. 1988;41(3):293–302.
5. Daviglus ML, Liao Y, Greenland P, Dyer AR, Liu K, Xie X, et al. Association of nonspecific minor ST-T abnormalities with cardiovascular mortality: the Chicago Western Electric Study. JAMA. 1999;281(6):530–6.
6. De Bacquer D, De Backer G, Kornitzer M, Myny K, Doyen Z, Blackburn H. Prognostic value of ischemic electrocardiographic findings for cardiovascular mortality in men and women. J Am Coll Cardiol. 1998;32(3):680–5.
7. Rautaharju PM, Prineas RJ, Eifler WJ, Furberg CD, Neaton JD, Crow RS, et al. Prognostic value of exercise electrocardiogram in men at high risk of future coronary heart disease: Multiple Risk Factor Intervention Trial experience. J Am Coll Cardiol. 1986; 8(1):1–10.
8. U.S. Preventive Services Task Force. Screening for coronary heart disease: recommendation statement. Ann Intern Med. 2004; 140(7):569–72.
9. Fraker Jr TD, Fihn SD, 2002 Chronic Stable Angina Writing Committee, American College of Cardiology, American Heart Association, Gibbons RJ, Abrams J, Chatterjee K, et al. 2007 Focused updated of the ACC/AHA 2002 guidelines for the management of patients with chronic stable angina: a report of the American

College of Cardiology/American Heart Association Task Force on Practice Guidelines Writing Group to develop the focused update of the 2002 guidelines for the management of patients with chronic stable angina. J Am Coll Cardiol. 2007;50(23):2264–74.

10. Ekelund LG, Suchindran CM, McMahon RP, Heiss G, Leon AS, Romhilt DW, et al. Coronary heart disease morbidity and mortality in hypercholesterolemic men predicted from an exercise test: the Lipid Research Clinics Coronary Primary Prevention Trial. J Am Coll Cardiol. 1989;14(3):556–63.

11. Gibbons LW, Mitchell TL, Wei M, Blair SN, Cooper KH. Maximal exercise test as a predictor of risk for mortality from coronary heart disease in asymptomatic men. Am J Cardiol. 2000;86(1):53–8.

12. Laukkanen JA, Kurl S, Lakka TA, Tuomainen TP, Rauramaa R, Salonen R, et al. Exercise-induced silent myocardial ischemia and coronary morbidity and mortality in middle-aged men. J Am Coll Cardiol. 2001;38(1):72–9.

13. Myers J, Prakash M, Froelicher V, Do D, Partington S, Atwood JE. Exercise capacity and mortality among men referred for exercise testing. N Engl J Med. 2002;346(11):793–801.

14. Haffner SM et al. Mortality from coronary heart disease in subjects with type 2 diabetes and in nondiabetic subjects with and without prior myocardial infarction. N Engl J Med. 1998;339(4):229–34.

15. Thompson PD, Franklin BA, Balady GJ, Blair SN, Corrado D, Estes 3rd NA, et al. Exercise and acute cardiovascular events placing the risks into perspective: a scientific statement from the American Heart Association Council on Nutrition, Physical Activity, and Metabolism and the Council on Clinical Cardiology. Circulation. 2007;115(17):2358–68.

16. Willich SN et al. Physical exertion as a trigger of acute myocardial infarction. Triggers and Mechanisms of Myocardial Infarction Study Group. N Engl J Med. 1993;329(23):1684–90.

17. Giri S, Thompson PD, Kiernan FJ, Clive J, Fram DB, Mitchel JF, et al. Clinical and angiographic characteristics of exertion-related acute myocardial infarction. JAMA. 1999;282(18):1731–6.

18. Gong Jr H-SO. Exposure to moderate altitude and cardiorespiratory diseases. Cardiologia. 1995;40(7):477.

19. Beighton PH, Richards PR-SO. Cardiovascular disease in air travellers. Br Heart J. 1968;30(3):367.

20. Nemec ED, Mansfield L, Kennedy JW. Heart rate and blood pressure responses during sexual activity in normal males. Am Heart J. 1976;92(3):274.

21. Hellerstein HK, Friedman EH. Sexual activity and the postcoronary patient. Arch Intern Med. 1970;125(6):987.

Index

J.D. Bisognano et al. (eds.), *Manual of Outpatient Cardiology*,   489
DOI 10.1007/978-0-85729-944-4,
© Springer-Verlag London Limited 2012